Occupational Therapy in Orthopaedics and Trauma

Edited by

Madeleine Mooney, Dip COT
Senior Occupational Therapist, Royal Liverpool and Broadgreen
University Hospitals NHS Trust, Liverpool, UK
Chair of the College of Occupational Therapists Specialist Section:
Trauma and Orthopaedics 1999–2004

and

Claire Ireson, Dip COT, Diploma in Management
Learning Environment Lead, Oxfordshire and Buckinghamshire Mental
Health NHS Foundation Trust, UK
(Formerly Head of Occupational Therapy Services – Nuffield Orthopaedic
Centre NHS Trust, Oxford, UK)
Chair of the College of Occupational Therapists Specialist Section:
Trauma and Orthopaedics 2004–2008

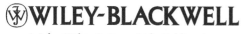

A John Wiley & Sons, Ltd., Publication

Library of Congress Cataloging-in-Publication Data

Occupational therapy in orthopaedics and trauma / edited by Madeleine Mooney, Claire Ireson.
p. ; cm.
Includes bibliographical references and index.
ISBN 978-0-470-01949-8
1. Occupational therapy. 2. Orthopedics. I. Mooney, Madeleine. II. Ireson, Claire.
[DNLM: 1. Occupational Therapy–methods. 2. Orthopedic Procedures–methods.
3. Wounds and Injuries. WB 555 O1446 2009]
RM735.O343 2009
615.8′20727–dc22
2009008872

A catalogue record for this book is available from the British Library.

Set in 10 on 12.5 pt Sabon by SNP Best-set Typesetter Ltd., Hong Kong

1   2009

Contents

Contributors

Daniel Brown, MB ChB, FRCS (Trauma and Orthopaedics)
Consultant Orthopaedic Surgeon
Royal Liverpool and Broadgreen
  University Hospitals NHS Trust
Liverpool
UK

Fiona Carnegie, Dip COT
Senior Occupational Therapist
Amputee Therapy Team
Queen Mary's Hospital
Roehampton
London
UK

Neil Davidson, MB ChB MRCS
Specialist Registrar
Orthopaedics and Trauma Mersey
  Rotation
Royal Liverpool and Broadgreen
  University Hospitals NHS Trust
Liverpool
UK

Natalie Evans (nee Schroder), BOccThy
  (Hons)
University of Queensland
Head Occupational Therapist –
  Rehabilitation
Royal Brisbane and Women's Hospital
Australia
Formerly, Paediatric Occupational
  Therapist
Nuffield Orthopaedic Centre NHS Trust
Oxford
UK

Chris Harris, MB ChB, FRCS (Trauma
  and Orthopaedics)
Orthopaedic Surgeon
Royal Children's Hospital
Melbourne
Australia

Heather McDowell, BSc (Hons) OccThy,
  Certificate in Management (Open)
Head of Therapies
Royal National Orthopaedic Hospital
  NHS Trust
Stanmore
Middlesex
UK
and
Chair of the College of Occupational
  Therapists:
Specialist Section in Trauma and
  Orthopaedics
(2008 – present)

Dawn Miller, Dip COT
Occupational Therapy Professional
  Lead
Worthing Wheelchair Service
West Sussex Primary Care Trust
Worthing
West Sussex
UK
Formerly, Head Occupational Therapist
Orthopaedics and Trauma
St George's Hospital NHS Trust
Tooting
London
UK

Alis Moores, MSc Advanced Health Care
Practice, BHSc (Hons) OccThy, Post
Graduate Certificate in Academic
Practice
Senior Lecturer and Teaching Fellow
York St John University
York
UK

Neil M. Orpen, MB ChB, FRCS Ed
(Trauma and Orthopaedics)
University of Stellenbosch
South Africa
and
Spinal Fellow
Frenchay Hospital
Bristol
UK

Oliver Pearce, MB BS, MRCS Engl.
Specialist Registrar Trauma and
Orthopaedics
Oxford Rotation
Nuffield Orthopaedic Centre NHS Trust
Oxford
UK

Kerry Sorby, MSc, Dip COT
Senior Lecturer
York St John University
York
UK

Julie Upton, Dip COT
Head Occupational Therapist
Nottingham University Hospitals NHS
Trust
City Campus
Nottingham
UK
Formerly, Senior Occupational Therapist
Nottingham Shoulder and Elbow Unit
Nottingham City Hospital
Nottingham
UK

Andrew M. Wainwright, MB ChB, BSc
(Hons) FRCS (Trauma and
Orthopaedics)
Consultant Children's Orthopaedic
Surgeon
Nuffield Orthopaedic Centre NHS Trust
and
Honorary Senior Lecturer
University of Oxford
Oxford
UK

Foreword

Occupational therapy has played a key and well-established role in the lives of people with disabling or potentially disabling conditions for a number of years. Currently health care practices are being revolutionised with, for example, the use of keyhole and robotic surgery and the reduction in lengths of hospital stay, so occupational therapy, like all other health care professions, is rapidly changing too.

The pressures of working in today's demanding health care environment mean that occupational therapists new to the field of orthopaedics and trauma need quick access to up-to-date and trusted information. This includes the aetiology and current treatment techniques of the most common musculoskeletal conditions matched with evidence based occupational therapy. The aims are as always, to ensure that patients achieve the maximum benefits from surgery and have safe and effective hospital discharges as well as to enable them to maintain independence and quality of life in their own terms.

This book has been compiled with the needs of a busy practitioner in mind. The editors, Madeleine Mooney and Claire Ireson, are both highly respected and experienced specialists in the field of orthopaedics and trauma. They have drawn on their years of experience and the knowledge and best practice of eminent surgical colleagues and other specialist occupational therapists to create a book that can be studied in depth or dipped into for reference.

Spanning assessment, short-term and long-term rehabilitation, together with inpatient and outpatient care, this book has something to offer everyone. Students and occupational therapists returning to work, junior occupational therapists new to orthopaedics and trauma who need to 'hit the ground running', rehabilitation assistants and other members of the rehabilitation team working in hospital or in the community, will all find this text an invaluable resource. Although written in the UK, its application is international.

I congratulate Madeleine and Claire for their excellent editing skills and all the authors for their expert and highly readable contributions and I heartily recommend this much needed addition to the occupational therapy literature.

Ann E Stead OBE, MA, DipCOT, SROT
Consultant in Health, Social Care and Inclusion
Formerly, Director of Disability Services at the Nuffield Orthopaedic Centre NHS Trust, Oxford, UK (1992–2002)
and
Chairman of the Boards of RADAR – the UK Disability Network (2001–2005) and the DARE Foundation (2001–2004)

Preface

In our respective roles as a senior occupational therapist working in a trauma unit within an acute general hospital, and head of occupational therapy services within a specialist orthopaedic centre, colleagues, staff and students regularly questioned us regarding occupational therapy practice within these musculoskeletal settings.

These clinical enquiries were usually received from newly qualified occupational therapists embarking on their first post. This was often within a mixed speciality rotation and these practitioners wished to develop their orthopaedic and trauma skills and knowledge. It was evident that many had not had the opportunity to obtain clinical experience in these areas during their clinical placements when training. Pre-registration occupational therapy students undertaking their practice placement education within a trauma or orthopaedic service were also seeking practical and evidence based knowledge to support their learning in the clinical environment.

Also, as leading committee officers (chair and secretary) of the College of Occupational Therapists Specialist Section: Trauma and Orthopaedics (UK), we received many national and international musculoskeletal occupational therapy practice enquiries. These not only included students and junior occupational therapists, but also practitioners who had recently changed their field of practice, commenced working in new and emerging services providing continuity of care for people with musculoskeletal conditions with which they had limited or out-of-date experience and knowledge or for those who rarely encountered an individual with a musculoskeletal condition in their caseload.

Throughout our collaborative working, while providing support, information and guidance to these practitioners, we became very aware that a well-recognised, practical and evidenced based text, specifically written for occupational therapists working in the field of trauma and orthopaedics was not available to support learning. There are a number of excellent well known orthopaedic textbooks and separate occupational therapy practice texts, but none of these are combined to give easy and quick access to information for busy practitioners.

We were approached to consider producing such a text by Colin Whurr, (then Whurr Publications), who wished to add to the range of occupational therapy publications. Following discussion, we were encouraged and persuaded to embark upon the task. Writing for publication was a new venture for both of us, but proved to be an irresistible challenge. Our agreed scope for the book was to cover the conditions, treatment and management of people with trauma and orthopaedic conditions most commonly encountered by occupational therapy practitioners. We acknowledged that we were by no means experts in all these fields and therefore we agreed we would approach specialist and expert contributors from both occupational therapy and surgical practice to help develop the content of the book.

For ease of reference, the book is divided into two parts: orthopaedics and trauma, with chapters linking the anatomy, aetiology and medical and surgical management of the condition, followed by the application of occupational therapy theory and practice. The chapters describe the most common musculoskeletal conditions and trauma that occupational therapists encounter in their daily practice. With over 200 musculoskeletal conditions affecting millions of people worldwide, there are many more conditions, syndromes and injuries that occur that we are not able to cover here. More information regarding these can be located in the classic orthopaedic texts, via specialist websites and interactive media (some of which are listed at the end of the book).

We have described the theory of occupational therapy intervention and processes, and have presented practical treatment media that is evidence based, and those that are considered best practice by our expert occupational therapy colleagues. We have suggested frames of reference or models of practice and treatment approaches and interventions that are appropriate in this area of practice.

The text has been written to ensure it is appropriate for a wide international readership. Therefore reference to country specific guidelines and legislation has been avoided in most cases. We therefore encourage readers to review their own government, health and professional bodies' guidelines, legislation and policies and adopt these within their service development and clinical practice. We also acknowledge that access to resources and services will also range tremendously from region to region and from country to country, therefore we have tried to avoid being prescriptive or too specific in terms of recommending equipment or services. We believe our book is unique, and that it demonstrates collaboration and an inter-professional approach to sharing expert knowledge regarding the management of people with musculoskeletal conditions.

The fields of orthopaedics and trauma are constantly developing and evolving as advances in medicine, surgery and technology are made. Occupational therapy practitioners will need to ensure that they remain up to date and that their practice continues to develop and adapt so they remain flexible and innovative in the skills and approaches to the problems people referred to them may face resulting from trauma or musculoskeletal disease. It is certain that the population will continue to be affected by musculoskeletal conditions that limit functional ability and capacity, and that those with functional impairment will continue to need and benefit from the skills and interventions of occupational therapists in the future.

Occupational therapists must ensure that they continue to meet the challenge of being an inter-disciplinary team member who remains focused on the individual's psycho-social needs, and impact of disease or trauma on their occupations, rather than narrowing their interventions solely on the management of a specific joint or injury. We will see throughout the text that occupational therapists offer a unique and holistic approach to the management of people, ranging from those with acute trauma to those living with a long-term musculoskeletal condition.

We have both learnt many new skills and acquired new knowledge during our editing and publishing journey. We are delighted that *Occupational Therapy in Orthopaedics and Trauma* has brought together contemporary talents in this field and hope that our book will become the definitive and indispensable text that enhances and develops the reader's knowledge. Our aspiration is that the reader will be inspired to continue and learn more about this challenging but satisfying area of clinical practice. Ultimately, we anticipate that this will lead to additional reading, study and investigation, thus contributing and expanding the body of research and knowledge base to inform future occupational therapy practice. This will ensure that best practice that is reliable and valid is disseminated. In turn, this will assist in providing the best quality of occupational therapy intervention for people in our care.

Madeleine Mooney and Claire Ireson

Acknowledgements

The editors would like to extend their appreciation to the many friends and colleagues who have helped and supported them in putting this book together.

In particular we are extremely grateful to all our contributors, we appreciate the time and effort you have put into your chapters, while working in demanding jobs, studying for examinations and striving to achieve a healthy work–life balance.

We are also indebted to those of you who read and provided constructive comments on individual chapters, in particular, Dr Chris Mayers for her helpful comments which guided revision of Chapter 3, Badri Narayan for his advice and guidance on Chapter 9 and Fiona Cashin for her thoughts and comments on Chapter 13.

We would also like to thank those of you who have supplied our contributors with photographs and X-rays, including Harry Brownlow, Peter Burge, Sulfi Rahimtula, and Nicola Orpen.

Our gratitude also goes to Philip Hall for his illustrations in Chapters 4 and 11 and Figures 5.1 and 5.2, from originals by T. J. C. Upton. We would also like to thank him for his computer 'know how' and invaluable assistance with the photographs throughout the book.

We also acknowledge the kind permission of Emis and Pip 2005 and Elsevier Publications for their kind permission to reproduce photographs, figures and tables, respectively.

Finally, to the publishing staff who have helped and supported us along the way, in particular, Colin Whurr for his enthusiasm in getting us started and to the many staff at Wiley Blackwell, in particular to Emma Hatfield and Catriona Dixon, who have helped us complete the journey.

Part I
Orthopaedics

Chapter 1

Principles of orthopaedic surgery

Neil M. Orpen

Introduction

In this chapter we will explore some of the more recent developments in orthopaedic surgery, in particular, those aspects that form the basis of everyday practice. In recent years there has been a rapid expansion in the treatment options available to people with musculoskeletal disease. This has resulted from the development of safe anaesthesia, improved engineering of implant materials and refinement of surgical techniques. With this improvement, a greater emphasis has been placed on the person's recovery from surgery which, in turn, has led to the development and importance of rehabilitation and the multi-disciplinary approach to people's care.

History and early development

Orthopaedics derives from the Greek words 'straight' and 'child' and was a term described by Nicholas Andry (1658–1759) in his book *Orthopaedia: or the Art of Correcting and Preventing Deformity*. Much of the early practice of orthopaedics was concerned with the correction of deformity. More recently, as our population age has changed, the conditions that form part of our everyday practice have changed too. To mention all the important developments in the process of orthopaedic history would be exhausting, but some names of interest follow.

Ambroise Pare (1510–1590) was a prominent surgeon in France in the sixteenth century and published on anatomy and physiology and later on surgery. He described a number of surgical techniques relating to amputation such as the use of ligatures for large vessels, and tourniquets. He also designed a number of surgical instruments and artificial limbs. At times of conflict, limb amputations were common and often the only treatment for limb injury and deformity. Limb amputation skills were displayed with amazing speed and precision in experienced hands.

Antonius Mathysen (1805–1878) invented the plaster of Paris (POP) bandage which remains part of everyday orthopaedic and trauma practice. Little has changed in the principle of this form of splintage since its creation and only some of the indications have been altered to keep up with alternatives offered by surgery. Joseph Lister (1827–1912) became James Syme's (of Syme amputation fame 1942) house surgeon and later married his daughter. While working as assistant surgeon to the Royal Infirmary in England he introduced antisepsis, which had a dramatic effect in reducing infection, and infection related mortality. This paved the way for further developments in surgical techniques and is a crucial part of successful surgery and specifically to orthopaedic surgery today. Wilhelm Conrad Rontgen (1845–1923) was a professor of Physics at Wurzburg and discovered roentgen rays (X-rays). The first radiograph taken was of his wife's hand and this was allegedly offered to her as a Christmas present. Something he may not get away with today! In 1901 he received the Nobel prize for his work in this area.

Gathorne Robert Girdlestone (1881–1923) was the first professor of orthopaedics in Britain and has a long association with a number of prominent centres, including the Nuffield Orthopaedic Centre in Oxford. His technique of excision arthroplasty of the femoral head is a procedure now used mainly as a salvage procedure after failed hip replacement and carries his name. Originally it was commonly used to treat hip tuberculosis prior to the advent of antibiotic therapy and joint replacement surgery. In 1942, an American, Austin Moore (1899–1963), performed and reported the first metallic hip replacement. Although it involved replacing the entire upper portion of the femur with a vitallium prosthesis, this was the start of a rapid development in better designs and techniques. Sir John Charnley (1911–1982) improved the design of the total hip replacement and was also involved with the development of self-curing acrylic cement. Many of the hip joint arthroplasties performed in the 1960s by him are still surviving well. It is open to debate as to whether his excellent design was luck or brilliance, but it was to form the benchmark for total hip replacements for the next 40 years.

Other centres such as Exeter have now proven results of joint replacement while those such as Birmingham are in the early stages of producing promising long-term results with newer designs. The Birmingham hip resurfacing arthroplasty, designed by Derek McMinn and colleagues at the Royal Orthopaedic Hospital in Birmingham in the early 1990s has had widespread interest due to a successful return to early design principles but now with better manufacturing techniques and better results. Other designs of this metal on metal resurfacing arthroplasty have followed and these types of replacement are now widely used throughout Europe, the USA and Canada.

Although huge strides have been made in the past century in the field of orthopaedics, it is expected that similar ongoing advances will continue to be made. Developments in cartilage replacement options hold promise as alternatives to joint replacement and there is continued development in the field of stem cell research. These and many others offer tremendous therapeutic options for an ever-increasing population of people with orthopaedic problems.

Prevention of infection

Prevention and management of infection in orthopaedic surgery has been one of the most important advances over the past century, which has allowed rapid development in our practice. Over 70% of hospital-acquired infections occur in people who have undergone surgery and these lead to considerable morbidity and rise in surgical costs.

Treatment of infection in bone can be very difficult, and following implant surgery even more of a challenge, and so the prevention of infection is where we place a great deal of our efforts.

Definitions

- **Decontamination** – a process of removing microbial contaminants which can be carried out by cleaning, disinfection or sterilisation.
- **Cleaning** – a process that removes visible contaminants but does not necessarily destroy microorganisms.
- **Disinfection** – reduces the number of viable organisms to an acceptable level but may not inactivate some viruses, hardy organisms such as mycobacteria, or spores. A topical disinfectant that can be safely applied to epithelial tissue (like skin) is called an *antiseptic*.
- **Sterilisation** – this involves complete destruction of all viable microorganisms, including spores, viruses and mycobacteria. This may be accomplished by heat, radiation or chemical means and often the choice depends on the nature of the material being sterilised.

Prevention strategies

Handwashing has been shown to be the single most important method of controlling the transmission of hospital-acquired infection, as organisms are passed from one person to the next via staff caring for them. Washing the hands before and after physical contact with people and after activities where they are likely to become contaminated cannot be overemphasised.

Soaps, detergents or alcohol-based agents are now commonly provided in areas such as wards, clinics and outpatient departments where staff come into direct contact with people. A set of 'universal precautions' are typically taught and are available as a way of reminding staff of ways to prevent the transmission of infection. These include instructions on wearing gloves, dealing with wounds, sharp instruments and contaminated products. All staff should make themselves familiar with local policies and guidelines relating to these.

Screening of at-risk patient groups is important especially in the more controlled environment of planned or elective surgery. Organisms that can be detected and controlled, such as methicillin-resistant *Staphylococcus aureus* (MRSA), are important to detect prior to high-risk surgery and particularly in implant surgery. It is advisable to isolate a person found to be carrying these organisms so as to prevent the transmission to other people in the ward.

Antibiotics are used routinely in implant surgery and have been shown to reduce the risk of postoperative wound and deep infection. Broad-spectrum prophylactic antibiotics given prior to starting the surgical procedure are required for implant surgery and the choice of antibiotics is often dependent on local microbiological guidelines. The widespread use of antibiotics in all clinical settings, however, has led to certain organisms becoming resistant to various agents, for example:

- MRSA
- Vancomycin-intermediate *S. aureus* (VISA)
- Vancomycin-resistant *Staphylococcus epidermidis* (VRSE).

The appropriate use of antibiotics, however, is an essential part of prevention of infection in orthopaedic surgery.

Theatre strategies include sterile gowns, drapes, double gloves, and the use of masks and caps. Air-borne bacteria are a source of postoperative sepsis and now laminar-flow ventilation systems in theatres are becoming the norm to supply ultra-filtered air to the operative field and thereby reduce infection. Evidence exists to show that the use of ultra-clean air conditions will reduce the incidence of deep periarticular infections by half (from 3.4% to 1.6%). The addition of antibiotics will further reduce this to 0.19%. This is of particular benefit in prosthetic implant surgery (Lidwell et al. 1987).

All staff in contact with the operative field or instruments involved in surgery are required to disinfect their hands prior to placing sterile gloves on for surgery. This is aimed at reducing the volume of viable organisms, which may otherwise contribute to postoperative infection. A number of preparations are available, and many are alcohol or iodine based.

The surgical area is prepared with an **antiseptic solution** and care is taken that nothing contaminates this during surgery. Sterile drapes are used and all instruments used are sterilised to ensure no viable organisms are likely to contaminate the operative field.

Main conditions, diagnosis and treatment principles

Osteoarthritis

Osteoarthritis is a non-inflammatory degenerative joint disease. It is characterised by loss of articular cartilage and associated with new bone formation and capsular fibrosis that results when chondrocytes fail to repair damaged cartilage. The causes fit into two broad groups:

- **Primary/idiopathic** – no obvious cause
- **Secondary** – identifiable cause:
  - Previous trauma
  - Congenital deformity
  - Infection
  - Metabolic disorders.

Typically this condition is progressive and results in pain and stiffness in the joint involved. This may lead to:

- Alteration of limb length
- Fixed deformity in the joint limiting movement
- Progressive wasting of muscles as the limb is used less.

People who experience symptoms and signs of non-inflammatory arthritis have the clinical diagnosis confirmed with X-rays. Radiological signs include (Figure 1.1):

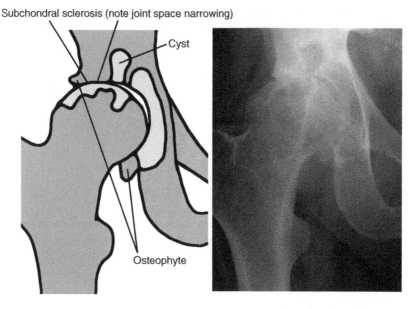

Subchondral sclerosis (note joint space narrowing)

Cyst

Osteophyte

Figure 1.1 Radiological signs of osteoarthritis.

- Joint space narrowing – initially at maximal load area before progressing to the entire joint
- Development of osteophytes as the joint endeavours to repair itself
- Subcortical/ subchondral sclerosis indicated by thickening of the bone below the joint surface
- Subchondral pseudo-cyst formation.

Initially treatment should always involve conservative/non-operative options. Once non-operative measures have been exhausted, surgery may be considered. The non-operative/ conservative measures recommended are:

- Protection of joint overload by achieving weight loss and using walking aids
- Exercise of supporting muscles to avoid wasting and prevent stiffness
- Pain relief in the form of analgesics and anti-inflammatory drugs
- Intra-articular corticosteroid injections
- Intra-articular hyaluronic acid injections (Snibbe and Gambardella 2005)
- Glucosamine and chondroitin (Richy et al. 2003).

Operative measures (for people with persistent pain and symptoms despite conservative measures) include:

- Arthroplasty – unicompartmental or total joint arthroplasty
- Realignment osteotomies in younger persons.

Some treatments are being used but do not yet have convincing evidence to prove their benefit and at this stage should be considered experimental. For example, soft tissue grafts, such as:

- Chondrocyte transplants (Bentley et al. 2003)
- Mosaicplasty (Bentley et al. 2003)
- Fresh osteochondral grafts (Ma et al. 2004)

As this condition is such a large part of everyday practice in orthopaedics, it is also part of massive financial investment into newer forms of treatment, many of which do not have good evidence to prove their benefit. These do form an essential part of the on-going development of our practice but must be used in controlled environments and with caution.

Rheumatoid arthritis

Rheumatoid arthritis (RA) is a chronic systemic autoimmune disease with an unclear aetiology and a number of joint sequelae. The symptoms are that of an inflammatory arthritis and typically the person experiences acute or chronic episodes throughout their life. Much of the treatment is aimed at controlling the condition and preventing the chronic changes usually associated with RA. Early aggressive medical treatment can control the condition and limit joint damage and thus prevent or limit the chronic disability typically associated with rheumatoid arthritis in the past.

Usually RA progresses through three stages:

(1) Swelling of the synovial lining of the joint causing warmth, redness, joint swelling and pain
(2) Rapid division and growth of cells resulting in pannus formation/thickened synovium
(3) Damage to the cartilage and bone by the inflammation, throughout the joint causing stiffness, pain and deformity typical of the end stage.

Rheumatoid joint disease

Symptoms should be considered as either systemic or local to the joint. They are typically symmetrical and can affect any joint, although most commonly begin in the smaller joints of the fingers, hands, and wrists. People with RA are more susceptible to infection. Systemic symptoms include:

- Fatigue
- Early morning stiffness or stiffness after rest
- Flu-like symptoms
- Rest pain
- Flares in symptoms followed by disease inactivity
- Rheumatoid nodules (occur in one-fifth of patients)
- Loss of appetite, anaemia, weight loss
- Sjögren's syndrome – involvement of the glands around the eyes and mouth causes decreased production of tears and saliva.

Diagnosis of RA is based on a collection of information rather that one specific test. This includes the person's history, clinical examination, laboratory tests and radiological investigations; specific criteria must be met before a diagnosis is made.

Current treatment methods focus on relieving pain, reducing inflammation, slowing or preventing joint damage, and improving function. Medication/therapeutic categories are based on those that are aimed at controlling the progression of disease and those aimed at symptomatic relief.

- **Non-steroidal anti-inflammatory drugs (NSAIDs)** – reduce inflammation, pain and fever. A side effect is an increase in bruising and bleeding and care should be taken when handling patients with RA.
- **Analgesic drugs** – relieve pain.
- **Corticosteroids** – low doses to reduce inflammation and to prevent joint damage. These may be administered systemically or as local intra-articular injections. Oral steroids should never be stopped abruptly.
- **Disease-modifying anti-rheumatic drugs (DMARD's)** – used in combination with other drugs to slow joint destruction over time, e.g. methotrexate, penicillamine, azathioprine. Care needs to be taken due to known side effects and drug interactions.
- **Immunotherapies** – such as anti-tumour necrosis factor (TNF) drugs. These are biological agents and immunoactive drugs, which principally inhibit cytokines in the immune system to control inflammation. There are no long-term studies that have looked at the effects of these on disease outcome.
- **Alternative therapies** – many people may have been given advice, or may have done their own research, on alternative therapy strategies. Although there may not be good evidence to support many of these, an open mind should be kept regarding those which people choose to take. Medical practitioners should be careful not to advise on therapies unless they are knowledgeable or trained in this field.

We now know that combination therapy is usually most effective in controlling the disease and therefore a person will usually be on more than one form of medication. However, despite medication and orthoses, many people will eventually require some form of surgery and techniques often used are:

- **Synovectomy** – to reduce the amount of inflammatory synovium in the joint. This can usually be performed arthroscopically or as keyhole surgery in the knee, but as an open procedure in other joints. Imminent tendon rupture in the hands is best treated with early synovectomy rather than later reconstruction (Gibbons et al. 2002; Ryu et al. 1998).
- **Joint replacement/arthroplasty** is used when pain is not controlled by medication alone and a person is limited in their movement. Typically partial replacement of joint (e.g. unicompartmental knee replacement or hemiarthroplasty of the hip) is not suitable as the whole joint is involved in rheumatoid arthritis.
- **Arthrodesis/fusion** can be used to control pain although it does prevent movement in the joint. This is more commonly employed in the foot and ankle.

Osteomyelitis

Osteomyelitis is an acute or chronic infection of the bone, which is usually caused by bacteria. In children the source of infection is typically via the blood (haematogenous) from another site in the body in the form of a bacteraemia or septicaemia whereas in adults the source is usually exogenous (e.g. after trauma or surgical intervention). Risk factors for development of osteomyelitis include:

- Local trauma, such as open fractures
- Previous orthopaedic surgery
- Diabetes mellitus
- Immunosuppression, such as in RA, chronic steroid therapy, human immuno-deficiency virus (HIV)/acquired immune deficiency syndrome (AIDS) or chronic illness
- Drug misuse
- Malnutrition.

In children, the presentation is early and symptoms typically occur before radiological signs. Haematogenous spread may occur to any bone but the vertebral bodies are the most commonly affected. Symptoms and signs of acute osteomyelitis include:

- Systemic
  - Fever
  - Malaise
  - Weight loss
  - Sweating
- Local
  - Swelling
  - Redness
  - Heat
  - Drainage of pus through the skin
  - Pain and local tenderness with muscle spasm.

History taking and examination should elicit the symptoms and signs and the diagnosis can be confirmed by further special laboratory and radiological investigations.

Laboratory investigations are aimed at evaluating the systemic response to infection and include full blood counts, C-reactive protein levels (CRP), and erythrocyte sedimentation rate (ESR). Blood cultures may offer a microbiological diagnosis prior to commencing antibiotic treatment and are positive in up to 50% of people tested. These may also be used to monitor the response to treatment.

Radiological investigations include radiographs of the affected bone although in acute infection there may be a delay in radiographic appearances of up to ten days. Ultrasound may be useful in the early stages in children with increased fluid in an affected joint and periosteal lift-off from an affected bone. Magnetic resonance imaging (MRI) (almost 100% sensitive) and computed tomography (CT) can be used to provide additional information regarding the diagnosis and extent of spread; these investigations can also aid in aspiration procedures to gain a microbiological diagnosis prior to commencing antibiotic therapy. Two conditions, which may often feature in the differential diagnosis are malignancy and tuberculosis (TB) and should always be considered, especially if the history is not typical. Although TB is uncommon in developed countries its incidence is increasing with increases in population migration and immunosuppressive illnesses such as HIV.

Treatment strategies are aimed at either suppression or eradication of the infection. One of the difficulties in dealing with bone infection is that penetration of antibiotics into bone is often limited and the environment of dead tissue further inhibits antibiotic penetration and activity. Bacteria can then live for prolonged periods causing recurrence of infection years after the initial infection is treated.

Eradication therapy may involve a combination of prolonged antibiotic therapy, together with surgical debridement. Debridement implies the removal of all dead material from the infection site as well as any foreign material (such as joint replacements). When involvement is extensive, surgery may result in large areas of bone loss, which will require further surgical correction when the infection is eradicated.

Septic arthritis

Joint infection is an important but less common cause of acute joint pain and is of vital importance to diagnose and treat early. A delay in the diagnosis can lead to rapid irreversible joint destruction and therefore treatment should be considered a surgical emergency. It is most common in the larger joints, and particularly in the adult it is often seen in the hand joints following hand trauma and in the foot in conditions such as diabetes mellitus. The clinical features in the infant are considerably different from those in adults, but here we will consider them together.

Symptoms and signs include:

- Children:
  - Septicaemia – which may be indicated by lack of progress, presence of septic focus such as umbilical stump infection, cyanosis with feeding, irritability or pyrexia
  - Failure to thrive
  - Local infection may be obscured by antibiotics given for another cause
  - Joint pain, swelling or lack of movement of the limb. The joint takes on the position of greatest capacity (hip: abduction, flexion, external rotation; knee: 20° flexion).
- Adults
  - Loss of joint motion due to pain
  - Swelling and joint tenderness
  - May have underlying rheumatoid or joint disease
  - Constitutional symptoms of fever, malaise, decrease in appetite
  - These may be absent in older patients or in patients taking steroids.
- Look for septic focus or history of recent illness.

In a child a high index of suspicion is required so as not to miss the diagnosis, whereas in the adult a clear history may steer one onto the correct path to a good clinical examination and then special investigations. Laboratory investigations are similar to those used to diagnose acute osteomyelitis but joint aspiration is essential to acquiring a microbiological diagnosis before starting antibiotic treatment. Aspiration of the knee is easy to perform in the clinic setting. As access to the hip is more difficult, the assistance of a radiologist may be required as an ultrasound-guided aspiration may be useful. This is particularly the case in a child, whereas in the adult this may simply be done under X-ray guidance.

Establishing the diagnosis early is crucial as the differential diagnosis may include much less serious conditions:

- Trauma
- Acute osteomyelitis
- Rheumatic fever
- Transient synovitis
- Gout
- Acute rheumatoid flare.

The treatment of this condition should always include a washout and antibiotics. The antibiotic course may be prolonged. When septic arthritis is complicating a joint replacement or other surgery involving a prosthesis or metal work, it may only be possible to clear the infection by removing the metal component.

Avascular necrosis

Avascular necrosis (AVN)/osteonecrosis/aseptic bone necrosis refers to a condition of bone cell death following loss of the blood supply. Although potential causes are multiple and in 25% not clearly defined, they more commonly include:

- Trauma
- Joint dislocation
- Steroid use
- Perthes' disease
- Fractures
- Heavy alcohol use
- Deep sea diving (Caison's disease) (Kenzora and Glimcher 1985).

Very often the true pathogenesis is unclear but the result is ischaemia at a cellular level followed by cell death and then a period of attempted repair, which may take place to varying degrees. Diagnosis can be difficult and early radiological features may be indistinguishable from other conditions. X-rays are therefore often of limited use. The advent of MRI has made the diagnosis much easier and features on MRI scan are typically present much earlier in the disease process.

Treatment is generally aimed at either helping the bone to repair itself or protecting the affected bone while the remodelling process occurs. When the diagnosis is made late or the remodelling process is inadequate, additional procedures may be required, aimed at reducing the pain in associated degenerated joints. This may take the form of fusion procedures, realignment operations or joint replacements and often depends on the joint affected and the age of the patient.

Bone grafting

Bone grafting involves the implantation of bone into an area of the skeleton for a specific surgical need. The sources of bone graft and surgical situations are mentioned in the list below but ultimately the aim is to encourage new bone formation.

Definitions

- **Autograft** – tissue grafted from one part of the body in the same individual to another part of the body in that individual (e.g. bone from the hip placed in the femur).
- **Isograft** – graft taken from a donor who is genetically identical to the recipient (tissue from one identical twin to another).
- **Allograft/homograft** – a graft of tissue from one individual to another of the same species with a different genotype (i.e. not from an identical twin).
- **Xenograft** – a graft of tissue taken from one species to a different species such as from a pig to a human.

There are a number of situations where bone grafting may be useful in orthopaedic and trauma surgery:

- Bone loss following trauma, infection, previous surgery where a space needs to be filled
- Delayed union/non-union of fractures, where bone with its various bone morphogenic proteins (BMPs) can be introduced into the site of poor healing to stimulate the formation of new bone
- Structural support in a bone defect such as revision joint replacement or a depressed articular surface in tibial plateau fractures
- Large bone defects where a large element of the bone is missing and another bone is harvested to bridge the defect/provide support and take over the function of the missing bone (bone tumours resulting in a large resection of bone such as vascularised fibular grafting following femoral resection for osteosarcoma)
- Encourage bone formation in arthrodesis/fusion surgery.

Most commonly autograft, and then specially prepared allograft, is used as this provides the least possible risk of tissue rejection. When only small amounts of bone are required, this can be harvested from the patients themselves with ease. This has the benefit of providing living tissue with all the bone stimulating factors that come with it. The iliac crest, distal femur, distal radius and fibula are commonly sources of donor bone tissue. Bone grafting is not without complications, however, and the risk of pain, nerve injury and infection are some of the things that must be taken into account when considering this procedure. This has led to research into newer bone substitutes being developed. Many of these are used purely for the structural element but some have the addition of bone stimulating proteins and other substances to encourage bone formation and therefore the additional benefits usually only provided with autograft.

Bone tumours

By far the most common tumour found in bone is that of a secondary deposit from a primary tumour elsewhere in the body. Typically malignant spread from lung, breast, kidney, prostate and thyroid occurs to bone but more uncommon metastatic tumours and haematological malignancies may also be found. We will mainly deal with primary bone tumours in the following text but for detail on specific tumours, the reader is referred to the recommended reading at the end of the chapter. Bone tumours are classified as follows:

- Benign:
  - Osteoid osteoma/osteoblastoma
  - Chondroblastoma
  - Enchondroma
  - Chondromyxoid fibroma
- Malignant – primary:
  - Osteosarcoma – 35%
  - Chondrosarcoma – 25%
  - Ewing's sarcoma – 20%
  - Spindle-cell sarcoma – 15%
- Malignant – secondary
  - Especially from bronchus, breast, prostate, kidney, thyroid
  - Haematopoietic tumours of the bone
  - Lymphoma
  - Plasmacytoma or myeloma.

People typically present with pain, which may occur with movement but also occurs with rest and at night. They may develop swelling and reduction of muscle bulk as the limb is used less. Systemic features of a tumour may exist, such as weight loss, anaemia, lymph node swelling, malaise, or those symptoms related to the primary elsewhere in the body. Temperature and sweating may suggest Ewing's sarcoma, but, of course, are also part of the clinical spectrum of infection and thus form part of the differential diagnosis. It is not unusual for the history to relate to a particular sporting or trivial injury and this risks a delay in diagnosis as health professionals, while treating it as a minor sporting or musculoskeletal injury, follow a conservative approach. (Musculo et al. 2003).

The first presentation may be of a pathological fracture or it may even be a coincidental finding. Following a good history and clinical examination some special investigations will offer further assistance in clarifying the diagnosis. Radiographs of the affected limb are mandatory and if concern is raised that a tumour is present then a chest radiograph should also routinely be requested. Tumours may be bone forming or bone destroying in nature. Further screening blood tests are aimed at diagnosis of the specific lesion and also to search for other causes, bearing in mind that bacterial osteomyelitis and TB infection should always form part of the differential diagnosis. Full blood counts, ESR, CRP and biochemical profiles are routine. If one is considering prostate carcinoma in men, then a prostate specific antigen (PSA) level is necessary and in older people being screened for myeloma, protein electrophoresis is requested. In searching for a primary tumour, a CT scan of the bone and other body regions can be useful and an MRI can determine the extent of the lesion within the bone. MRI is also the study of choice for soft tissue lesions and when the extent of soft tissue involvement is to be evaluated. Unless the diagnosis is certain, a biopsy is obtained for confirmation of the diagnosis and to assist in staging and planning surgery. When a specialist centre is available, this is best done under the supervision of an experienced surgeon or radiologist. Staging of tumours is necessary to determine the prognosis. The various prognostic factors used to define tumour stage include:

- Location and relative size
- The presence or absence of regional or distant metastases
- The histologic grade of the tumour.

Good histopathological and microbiological expertise is vital. In children cytogenetic samples can be useful and this requires the necessary backup to be available. Once staging is complete, a treatment plan can be devised and this is specific for the tumour type.

The three modalities available to treat bone tumours are chemotherapy, radiotherapy and surgery. The tumour variety will dictate the regimen and timing of surgery. Osteosarcoma for instance responds to chemotherapy which is offered prior to surgery and again following excision whereas chondrosarcomas do not respond to chemo- or radiotherapy and complete excision is the treatment offered. Ewing's on the other hand is treated by a combination of chemotherapy and surgical resection and if the response is incomplete it is treated with radiotherapy. Following surgical resection of a tumour, consideration must be given to reconstruction if necessary. Excision also often involves an envelope of soft tissue (muscles, tendons, etc.) which is important in ensuring a good prognosis and minimising recurrence; this will also be important in the reconstructive options available (Les et al. 2001). Endoprostheses, vascularised fibula grafts, bone grafts in combination with muscle flaps are options and good plastic surgical backup is often a prerequisite to satisfactory treatment. When the tumour is a secondary deposit, the aim of surgery in these circumstances is to improve the person's function to as near to normal as possible, to control pain and the treatment or prevention of pathological fractures. Plates and screws are seldom adequate as the bone is not expected to heal and therefore bridging of the diseased part of the bone with an intramedullary device is often required. A number of other devices are available and the best option depends on the specific site and tumour being treated. The life expectancy of a person presenting with a secondary metastatic lesion to the bone is 12 months in the UK but this is worse in people with lung metastasis and much better in carcinoma of the breast and kidney.

Nerve injury

Nerve injury is a common presentation of trauma but unfortunately is also a realistic risk following a number of therapeutic interventions and surgical procedures. In trauma the risk of an associated neurological injury increases in open injuries but even in closed injuries may occur at the time of injury or later from conditions such as compartment syndrome.

Aetiology of nerve injury may include:

- Trauma
- Metabolic
- Malignancy
- Toxins
- Thermal
- Infection
- Scarring
- Callus in fractures
- Ischaemia
- Arteriovenous malformations.

Some terms to be familiar with, which provide a useful classification, are as follows.

- **Neuropraxia** – this is a physiological interruption in function in a nerve that is anatomically intact. The axons remain intact but conduction stops because of segmental demyelination. The lesion is transient and full spontaneous recovery is expected within weeks to months.
- **Axonotmesis** – in this lesion the axons are separated and this results in the distal end of the axon degenerating by a process called Wallerian degeneration. Because the myelin sheath remains intact, the nerve regenerates along the previous path and recovery is likely, although slow. Sensory recovery is better than motor.
- **Neurotmesis** – this is complete transaction (by neurotmesis) of the nerve such as would occur in a surgical transection. There is a limited ability for nerve regeneration in peripheral nerves if the two cut ends are brought into apposition as would occur with surgical repair. Even after a good repair, only partial recovery can be expected.

Following an injury, the nerve goes through four pathological phases:

- Retraction
- Inflammation
- Degeneration – *retrograde* (primary) to the next proximal node of Ranvier but histologically the same as Wallerian; *Wallerian* (secondary) distal to point of injury
- Regeneration.

Diagnosis requires a good knowledge of the nerve anatomy and testing of the motor, sensory, and autonomic function of the nerve involved, bearing in mind that different signs are present during the various stages of the nerve injury process.

Although a good history and clinical examination may provide most of the information necessary to determine the type of injury present, when there is doubt, further information may be provided by neurophysiological studies. These are best performed two to three weeks after injury to distinguish a neuropraxia from an axonotmesis/neurotmesis. This therefore may provide useful information on the extent of the lesion and also the prognosis but prior to this has a limited role. Usually neurophysiological testing is reserved for those injuries which at six to eight weeks are not showing the recovery that was expected. MRI investigation of nerves is currently a research tool. Surgical exploration early in the course of a lesion may however be of more use, in that a conclusive diagnosis will be provided and repair may be undertaken at the same time. This is particularly true in trauma where neurotmesis is more likely and in this situation early repair is likely to be easiest and provide a better long-term result. When there is a delay to surgery, retraction often makes primary repair impossible and nerve autografts are considered. This of course means loss of a nerve elsewhere and also is not always as successful as could be expected if the repair was performed early.

Following repair it may be necessary to protect the soft tissues and the repair, and splinting may be required. This may also be necessary for the associated injuries and much of the treatment relies on good rehabilitation support while recovery occurs. When repair of the nerve is not achievable the emphasis may shift to tendon transfers to improve joint movement and prevent contractures or procedures directly aimed at the control of pain secondary to nerve injury.

Surgical approaches to symptomatic joint disease

Joint disease forms a prominent part of general orthopaedic practice and as the population ages this becomes even more the case. Conditions of the joints are not confined to older people, and this should become clear in the following chapters.

Surgery in the young is very often aimed at preventing the later development of joint degeneration such as in developmental dysplasia of the hips (DDH) and creating mobile painless joints. In older patients, however, surgery is usually reserved for failure of medical control of painful degenerative changes or inflammatory joint disease such as RA. Broadly, procedures are grouped into:

- **Joint debridement** – this may be aimed at removing inflamed synovium in inflammatory conditions to prevent destructive changes (RA) or removing bony osteophytes (OA), which through impingement may cause pain or impair movement. The true benefit of debridement and joint washout in OA is of some debate. This can usually be performed arthroscopically in larger joints.
- **Arthrodesis/fusion** – as pain in the joint can be caused by two degenerative surfaces rubbing against one another, fusing the joint prevents any movement and therefore stops pain, and is particularly useful in the small joints of the ankles, feet and hands and in the spine. It can also be used in specific situations in the hips and knees. One must bear in mind, however, that loss of movement in one joint may have an effect on adjacent joints, which may therefore later also require additional procedures.
- **Joint excision/excision arthroplasty** – This was practised historically in the treatment of infected and degenerate joints, and in the 1940s for the treatment of tuberculosis of the hip. The modern indications include failed infected joint replacement, recurrent dislocation of hip replacement and in specific cases of rheumatoid arthritis where a painful joint may be excised and the joint space filled with soft tissue which will eventually fibrose and thereby reduce and treat pain. The loss of stability and movement need to be considered and this is only suitable when a limited functional demand exists. In the large joints it is generally a salvage procedure and function is usually poor. Girdlestone described an excision arthroplasty of the hip, which bears his name (Horan 2005).
- **Osteotomy** – an osteotomy is a surgical technique involving a cut through the bone to realign or change the orientation of the axis of the bone. In joint disease this may be useful when trying to offload a particular articular surface such as to realign the joint. The chances of success are greater in younger patients; examples include high tibial osteotomies in unicompartmental arthritis of the knee where joint replacement may be less desirable. Osteotomies, however, can be used in a number of other circumstances and this will be highlighted in other chapters too.
- **Arthroplasty** – successful joint arthroplasty or replacement is one of the major advances in orthopaedic surgery and forms a prominent part of routine work performed in all units. The replacements are typically manufactured from a combination of metal alloys depending on the metal properties desired such as stainless steel and titanium. These are combined with an articulating component of polyethylene, metal or ceramic; the benefits and disadvantages of each are large discussions on their own. The prosthesis can be cemented or uncemented and design elements are

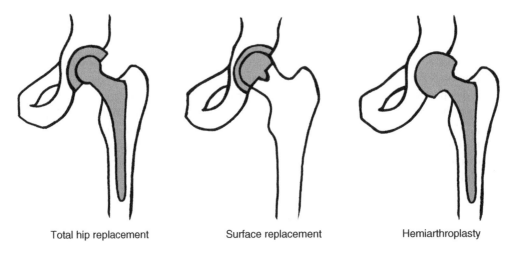

Total hip replacement   Surface replacement   Hemiarthroplasty

Figure 1.2 From left to right: examples of total hip replacement, surface replacement and hemiarthroplasty of the hip.

used to ensure a good, firm contact with the bone. A variety of terms are used to indicate which and how much of the joint is removed and replaced (Figure 1.2).

  – **Hemiarthroplasty** – only one articular surface is replaced and these are most commonly used in hip fractures and arthritis or fractures of the glenohumeral (shoulder) joint.

  – **Unicompartmental arthroplasty** – in the knee we often find that the degenerative changes are confined to either the medial or lateral half of the joint and in these cases good results can be achieved by only replacing the degenerative part.

  – **Total joint replacement/arthroplasty** – this is perhaps the gold standard for joint replacement and the form of arthroplasty that is most commonly performed. The whole (both sides) articular surface is removed and replaced with a prosthetic implant. Examples include replacements of the hips, knees, and ankles.

- **Surface replacement** – a modification of a total joint replacement involving only removing the articular cartilage and a minimal amount of subchondral bone. This provides the benefit of making further procedures and revision surgery easier as more bone is preserved. This is a refinement of an early technique made possible by better manufacturing methods in the production of prosthetic materials and articular surfaces. More detail will be provided in individual chapters.

Although joint replacement is a prominent part of orthopaedic practice, it is not without risk and these need to be considered carefully. The potential need for revision surgery in the future needs to be considered and in younger patients this may be required on more than one occasion. General risks of joint replacement include:

- Infection (1–5%)
- Dislocation
- Loosening (5%)
- Periprosthetic fracture
- Future revision

- Reduced movement
- Persistent pain
- Neurovascular injury.

Bearing in mind that none of the surgical options available are without risk, careful consideration should be given to the best option for each individual with the patient and multi-disciplinary team being actively involved in the decision-making process.

References

Bentley, G., Biant, L. C., Carrington, R. W., Akmal, M., Goldberg, A., Williams, A. M., Skinner, J. A., & Pringle, J. (2003). A prospective, randomised comparison of autologous chondrocyte implantation versus mosaicplasty for osteochondral defects in the knee. *Journal of Bone and Joint Surgery, British Volume, 85,* 223–230.

Gibbons, C. E., Gosal, H. S., & Bartlett, J. (2002). Long term results of arthroscopic synovectomy for seropositive rheumatoid arthritis: 6–16 year review. *International Orthopaedics, 26*(2), 98–100.

Horan, F. T. (2005). Robert Jones, Gathorne Girdlestone and excision arthroplasty of the hip. *Journal of Bone and Joint Surgery, British Volume, 7,* 104–106.

Kenzora, J. E., & Glimcher, M. J. (1985). Accumulative cell stress: the multifactoral etiology of idiopathic osteonecrosis. *Orthopedic Clinics of North America, 16,* 669–679.

Les, K. A., Nicholas, R. W., Rougraff, B., Wurtz, D., Vogelzang, N. J., Simon, M. A., & Peabody, T. D. (2001). Local progression after operative treatment of metastatic kidney cancer. *Clinical Orthopaedics and Related Research, 390,* 206–211.

Lidwell, O. M., Elson, R. A., Lowbury, E. J., Whyte, W., Blowers, R., Stanley, S. J., & Lowe, D. (1987). Ultraclean air and antibiotics for prevention of postoperative infection. A multicentre study of 8052 joint replacement operations. *Acta Orthopaedica Scandinavica, 58*(6), 4–13.

Ma, H. L., Hung, S. C., Wang, S. T., Chang, M. C., & Chen, T. H. (2004). Osteochondral autografts transfer for post- traumatic osteochondral defect of the knee-2 to 5 years follow-up. *Injury, 35,* 1286–1292.

Musculo, D. L., Ayerza, M. A., Makino, A., Costa-Paz, M., & Aponte-Tinao, L. A. (2003). Tumours about the knee misdiagnosed as athletic injuries. *Journal of Bone and Joint Surgery, American Volume, 85,* 1209–1214.

Richy, F., Bruyere, O., Ethgen, O., Cucherat, M., Henrotin, Y., & Reginster, J. Y. (2003). Structural and symptomatic efficacy of glucosamine and chondroitin in knee osteoarthritis: a comprehensive meta-analysis. *Archives of Internal Medicine, 163*(13), 1514–1522.

Ryu, J., Saito, S., Honda, T., & Yamamoto, K. (1998). Risk factors and prophylactic tenosynovectomy for extensor tendon ruptures in the rheumatoid hand. *Journal of Hand Surgery (Edinburgh, Scotland), 23*(5), 658–661.

Snibbe, J. C., & Gambardella, R. A. (2005). Treatment options for osteoarthritis. *Orthopaedics, 23*(2), S215–216.

Further reading

Kirk, R. M., & Ribbans, W. J. (2004). *Clinical Surgery in General* (4th edition). London: Churchill Livingstone.

Schajowicz, F. (1994). *Tumours and Tumour-like Lesions of Bone* (2nd edition). Berlin: Springer Verlag.

Vaccaro, A. R. (2005). *Orthopaedic Knowledge Update: Home Study Syllabus* (8th edition). USA, Illinois: American Academy of Orthopaedic Surgeons.

Walker, J. M., & Helewa, A. (2004). *Physical Rehabilitation in Arthritis* (2nd edition). St Louis: W.B. Saunders.

Chapter 2

Orthopaedic surgery for the lower limb

Neil M. Orpen

Total hip replacement

The aim of any joint replacement is to provide pain free, flexible, stable, sterile joints, which will last a long time. Although there have been many advances in the original designs first proposed, the greatest advance has been the reduction of infection rates which were a prominent cause of failure in early joint replacement surgery. Modern deep infection rates of 0.5% are achievable through the following measures:

- Surgery in ultra-clean theatre environments with sterile preparation
- Prophylactic antibiotics
- Disinfection of the surgical site
- Waterproof drapes and gowns
- Double gloving during surgery
- Correct patient preparation regarding microorganisms e.g. methicillin resistant *Staphylococcus aureus* (MRSA) eradication prior to surgery
- Good surgical technique with minimal soft tissue injury.

Indications and contraindications

For total joint replacement these are similar regardless of the joint being replaced, although some specific indications do exist for each joint. The absolute indication is for the management of pain when non-surgical measures have failed. Pain at night or at rest is a good indication for total hip replacement but a rapidly decreasing walking distance can assist in timing surgery.

Pain and disability can be assessed by using a number of **scoring systems**; most hospitals will follow a particular scoring system based on local policies. These scoring systems should assess pain, function and joint motion and can be useful to grade disability before and after surgery. Not only are these useful to assess outcome but they can also provide useful research data for long-term follow-up. Some of those in common use are the Medical Outcome Survey Short Form 36 (SF-36), Western Ontario and McMaster's Universities Osteoarthritis Index (WOMAC), Harris Hip Score, and Oxford Knee Score.

Age should not be considered a contraindication to surgery but patients should be warned of the potential for loosening and the possible need for further surgery. Heavy manual duties should be avoided following total hip replacement as well as impact exercise.

Other contraindications include:

- Uncontrolled medical problems
- Active infection
- Neuropathic joints (Charcot's joint)
- Muscle wasting around the joint
- Skeletally immature patients.

Preoperative assessment

This is routinely performed in most hospitals undertaking total hip replacements. It is aimed at assessing patients' suitability for surgery and early implementation of interventions that may aid or speed up recovery. A large joint replacement is to be considered major surgery and patients should be assessed as to their ability to withstand potential blood loss and adequate cardiac reserve. As patients are typically older, the preoperative assessment clinic also provides a good setting to discuss social care issues and tackle potential mobility issues that with the correct intervention prior to surgery may ensure a rapid recovery and early discharge from hospital following the surgical procedure. For this reason the preoperative assessment clinic should follow a multi-disciplinary approach with all members of the team represented.

Design considerations

Hip prosthesis design usually involves a metal femoral stem and an ultra-high molecular weight polyethylene (UHMWPE) acetabular component. These may either be cemented in place or be uncemented if the design allows this. Various surface finishes are applied to the prosthesis to avoid the need for cementing and encourage bone ingrowth to ensure prosthesis stability. These include beads, mesh, plasma sprayed titanium particles and hydroxyapatite. Uncemented acetabular components in conjunction with a cemented femoral component are in widespread use and constitute a 'hybrid'. The prosthesis is typically made of combinations of stainless steel, cobalt/chromium alloy and titanium, and prosthesis breakage is rare. To reduce the amount of wear-particles created by the articulating surfaces (felt to contribute to loosening), alternative designs have been created. These include metal-on-metal, ceramic-on-ceramic as variations from the typical metal on polyethylene. The efficacy of many of these remain unproven.

Potential complications

All patients should be given a careful explanation of the risks and potential complications of surgery. These include but are not confined to:

- Deep infection with a rate of 0.5–1.5%. After the second year <0.2% infections occur per year. Rates vary from unit to unit but when a deep infection does occur usually the only treatment available is revision surgery where the results are never as good as could be expected with primary surgery (Berbari et al. 1998).
- Deep vein thrombosis (DVT) occurs more often than is clinically evident and even with prophylaxis the clinical incidence is about 3%. The ideal prophylactic regimen is controversial but most would agree that some form of prophylaxis is required (British Orthopaedic Association 2006).
- Fatal pulmonary embolism (PE) occurs in 0.5% of patients.
- Dislocation occurs in 1–5% of patients and various hip precautions are often followed to prevent this. Surgeons differ in their opinions as to the need for these and local protocols should be implemented and followed (Berry et al. 2004).
- Loosening. This has decreased as techniques of cementing and designs have improved but still occurs in a significant number, with 5% of patients requiring revision surgery for aseptic loosening at 20 years (Klapach et al. 2001).
- Periprosthetic fractures.
- Limb length inequality – usually when the patients are counselled about this potential issue, they are tolerant of differences up to 1 cm (Edeen et al. 1995). It should be noted that idiopathic differences of up to 2 cm can occur in patient groups not undergoing hip replacement. When the difference is less than 2 cm following surgery, a heel wedge usually suffices in providing symptomatic relief (Cameron 1997).
- Limping – this is a greater problem in revision surgery where it can occur in up to 20% of patients.
- Depending on the surgical approach used certain nerves are at risk of being injured with the femoral and sciatic nerves of particular interest.

Rehabilitation

Patients are typically in hospital for less than seven days and rehabilitation is started as soon as possible following surgery. Again surgeons differ in what they recommend in the postoperative period and local protocols should be implemented. This avoids confusion for the rehabilitation team and patients who will often talk among one another to compare their care or progress. Limitations may be placed on the amount of flexion and rotation allowed of the hip and these fall into the broad category of hip precautions. There is a continued risk of dislocation and these are aimed at preventing this while the soft tissues and stabilising structures recover following surgery.

Revision surgery

About 10% of cases of arthroplasty are revision cases. Prior to undertaking surgery a clear indication should be sought as to the reason for failure. Typically this is either septic or aseptic loosening. If infection is the cause, this must be eradicated prior to the final implant being reinserted. Surgery is typically more difficult, the patients older and perioperative complications are more common.

Joint registries

A large numbers of patients have to be studied to be able to determine the effect of any one factor on the survival of the hip replacement. The most detailed information comes from the Swedish Hip Register onto which every total hip arthroplasty performed in Sweden since 1979 has been entered. Invaluable information has been made available and this has led to other countries adopting similar registries. The National Joint Register has been set up in England and Wales to collect similar data. From the Swedish Hip Register we can expect the overall survival for a hip replacement at 14 years to be 89% in woman and 85% in men.

Surgical approaches

The hip is usually approached through either a posterior or an antero-lateral approach. Each has its own benefits and risks and usually the choice is based on the surgeon's preference. Minimally invasive surgery is a recent development in the evolution of hip replacement surgery. Two broad categories are practised involving either a smaller incision to the skin but a standard approach to the hip or a two-incision approach to the hip joint with little soft tissue damage. As surgeons become more experienced, the length of incision required to safely approach the hip decreases. In good hands and the correct patient an incision less than 10 cm can safely be made.

The two-incision technique is still controversial and debate exists as to whether any true benefits are offered. This technique has potential soft tissue complications of its own and is not widely practised but may become more widely accepted if surgical technique and instrumentation improves. There is no current good evidence to show that the minimally invasive technique is more beneficial than routine techniques.

Total knee replacement

Knee replacement has followed a similar evolution to total hip replacement, with control of infection a major hurdle to overcome. Where early hinged designs limited movement and failed early, newer designs based on better understanding of biomechanics are aimed at mimicking the replaced joint and restoring movement to as near as possible to normal. Many of the same surgical principles apply and therefore will not be repeated.

Indications are similar, namely:

- Pain uncontrolled by non-operative measures is the main indication
- Night pain is often not as prominent a symptom
- Deteriorating walking distance.

Progressive deformity should aid in timing surgery.

Similar contraindications exist as those mentioned previously for total hip replacement. The evolution of osteoarthritis of the knee joint is such that articular damage may be confined to very specific aspects of the joint such as a single compartment (medial or lateral or the patellofemoral joint). This concept has led to the development of the unicompartmental knee replacement, designed to replace only that part of the joint that is affected by osteoarthritis. Long-term data are available to show the benefits of these designs (Svärd et al. 2001). Progression of this concept has led to the newer patellofemoral joint replacement, which is designed to only replace that part of the joint with osteoarthritis and leave the parts of the joint that are healthy. No long-term studies exist for this prosthesis though and it is not widely performed at this stage, but early results are favourable in certain centres.

Similar materials are used in the manufacturing of the prosthesis and cemented or uncemented designs are available. Long-term studies are not available for all implants and care needs to be taken before using an unproven design.

Complications include:

- Deep infection
- DVT and PE
- Neurological injury
- Stiffness and decreased range of movement
- Persistent pain
- Loosening
- Periprosthetic fractures.

Long-term function for knee replacements is good with 15-year survival rates in the 90% region.

Soft tissue surgery around the knee and knee arthroscopy

The knee is an inherently unstable joint with incongruent articular surfaces. Stability and congruency, however, are afforded by the various soft tissue structures around the knee, which make up a crucial part of the joint. Whereas articular surface degenerative damage occurs typically in the older patient population, soft tissue injuries have a high incidence in the 10–30-year age group. With the development of the fibre-optic light into the arthroscope in 1967, there has been a rapid expansion in the use of arthroscopy for the diagnosis and treatment of knee soft tissue injuries. Knee arthroscopy has become the third most commonly performed orthopaedic surgical procedure. As instruments have advanced, as well as surgical techniques, more procedures can now be performed through this minimally invasive method.

Menisci

The fibrocartilaginous meniscus has load bearing, shock absorption, joint lubrication and joint stabilisation properties. Symptomatic damage to these structures occurs during abnormal movements to the knee. Although this is usually forced, it may also occur during more subtle movements such as rising from the crouched position. The damage may be part of greater structural derangement with other structures being involved or may occur in isolation.

A good history will usually describe a particular movement that resulted in pain. This is followed by knee swelling in the form of a haemarthrosis, which develops over a few hours. The more peripheral the tear the quicker an effusion will develop and it is particularly these peripheral tears that are amenable to repair/ salvage procedures. If the meniscus is unstable it may jam in the articular surface preventing movement and causing characteristic locking of the knee. The patient can often localise the pain to a particular side of the knee and a specific area of tenderness at the joint line may be felt. Plain radiographs are usually normal and magnetic resonance imaging (MRI) is the predominant method of diagnosis if a good history and clinical examination are not conclusive.

Symptomatic tears are amenable to arthroscopic surgery and whereas the majority of tears will require little more than debridement, peripheral tears caught early (within six to eight weeks) may be suitable for arthroscopic repair. Success rates of repair in suitable cases range from 60% to 90%. Enthusiasts operating in ideal circumstances usually perform these and this may not be the experience of the majority of surgeons. If the meniscus is repaired the patient will usually have a period of protected weightbearing in which the cartilage is given a period to heal while maintaining a range of movement. There is little evidence to suggest surgery to asymptomatic tears is of much benefit.

Anterior cruciate ligament injury

Up to 70% of all ligament injuries to the knee involve the anterior cruciate ligament (ACL), and this injury is particularly prevalent among the young sporting population. Patients typically give a clear history of injury and may describe how they felt their knee 'go'. A haemarthrosis typically develops rapidly and they experience difficulty in weightbearing. Once the knee has been given time to settle for a few weeks the patient may describe intermittent giving way or even locking with reduced range of movement. An MRI will usually confirm the diagnosis after history and clinical examination raise suspicion. Two clear methods of treatment exist, namely conservative with a rehabilitation programme or rehabilitation followed by surgery after at least six to eight weeks. A good outcome can be expected in 85% of cases after surgical reconstruction and a number of techniques are described.

The reconstruction is performed using autograft, allograft or synthetic material. Autograft is the principal method and this is typically harvested from the patella tendon, the quadriceps tendon, or the gracilis and semitendinosus (four-stranded hamstring). The technique is performed as an open or arthroscopic technique and when delayed, arthrofibrosis is uncommon (<5%). Patients should be warned that the rehabilitation might take up to 12 months, which is also the time taken for the body to revascularise the graft. A physiotherapist strictly supervises this rehabilitation and the patient should not expect to get back to their regular sport for up to nine months.

The treatment of isolated injuries to the posterior cruciate ligament (PCL) remains controversial but should be considered especially when combined with other derangement inside the knee or when the patient is symptomatic. There is evidence that sport may be undertaken at high level despite a PCL injury and although PCL rupture leads to early patellofemoral joint degeneration, there is little evidence to suggest that reconstruction prevents this.

Common conditions of the foot and ankle

Foot and ankle surgery is rapidly developing as a subspecialty within orthopaedics. The foot is a complex structure, which comprises a number of complex joints, and the subject is too vast to detail all conditions. Some of the more common conditions are described below.

Hallux valgus

This is a complex deformity with multi-factorial aetiology. The basis of the deformity is a lateral deviation of the hallux (great toe) and a bunion on the medial eminence of the metatarsal head. The condition is more common in people with poor fitting footwear and typically occurs in women. There is also a hereditary pattern. When a similar bunion occurs on the fifth metatarsal it is called a bunionette. The treatment is usually conservative with adaptation and correction of shoes. A number of factors dictate when surgery should be considered as well as the procedure best suited, but generally involves correction of the metatarsal deviation and removal of the bunion. Complications of non-union, infection, neurological injury and recurrence should be discussed with the patient and care must be taken before considering surgery purely for asymptomatic cosmetically unattractive hallux valgus.

Hallux rigidus

This condition, as the name suggests, occurs with limitation of movement of the metatarsophalangeal joint of the great toe. The cause is typically degenerative changes within the joint such as occurs with osteoarthritis. Pain occurs when moving the stiff joint, such as with walking. Non-operative intervention involves preventing the movement of the joint with shoes to alleviate the pressure. Local infiltration of the joint with anaesthetic and steroid may offer temporary relief. Operative intervention may involve debridement of dorsal osteophytes (cheilectomy), soft tissue procedures, arthrodesis or joint replacement.

Ankle arthritis

Degeneration of the ankle joint usually follows previous trauma or rheumatoid arthritis but when it occurs, it can be disabling as in osteoarthritis in other load bearing joints. Patients tend to compensate for the painful and stiff ankle joint (responsible for flexion and extension) by rotating the foot externally and walking on the medial border of the foot. As with arthritis in the hip and knee, a trial of non-operative intervention should be considered before contemplating surgery. Non-operative intervention involves:

- Encouraging mobility and range of motion
- Analgesic and anti-inflammatory medication
- Corticosteroid injections
- Orthotic support to off-load the joint.

Operative treatment principally involves:

- Arthrodesis
- Ankle replacement.

Patients do surprisingly well following **arthrodesis/fusion** of the ankle but this may place strain on other joints of the foot and lead to degeneration in these. The procedure essentially involves removal of the remaining joint cartilage and fusion of the bone on either side of the joint. This eliminates not only any mobility but also any pain. This may be performed as an open or arthroscopically assisted operation, with better union rates in those performed arthroscopically. Careful patient selection is important as factors such as smoking may push non-union rates up from 5% to 40%.

Techniques for **ankle replacements** have been improved over recent years, but this operation still has higher complication and failure rates than those expected in total hip or knee replacement (Anderson et al. 2004). In experienced hands survival rates in the medium term are acceptable with better results for unconstrained cementless designs such as the Scandinavian Total Ankle Replacement (STAR). As yet the ideal prosthesis is still to be designed and patients should be made aware of the potential complication rates and potential need for further surgery (Saltzman 1999).

Arthritis of other foot joints

Joints that are commonly affected by degenerative changes especially following foot and ankle trauma are the subtalar, talonavicular, calcaneocuboid and transtarsal joints. Selective injections with local anaesthetic may help differentiate the exact joint causing pain; non-operative intervention is similar to other arthritic joints. Operative intervention is in the form of arthrodesis.

The diabetic foot

Patients with diabetes need to pay particular attention to their feet and have a vascular and neuropathic element in their condition, which may affect the feet in particular. Typically, autonomic abnormalities lead to dry, thin skin prone to trauma. The altered sensation in the presence of these abnormalities means small injuries and repetitive trauma are not noticed and may be neglected. Muscle wasting can lead to deformity and therefore bony prominences liable to trauma. Vascular changes produce ischaemia, and therefore ulceration and poor healing following injury are a risk. These problems along with immunosuppression associated with poor glucose control makes them susceptible to chronic ulceration of the feet and wound deterioration. Interventions include:

- Regular foot care and specialist clinic assessment
- Good control of serum glucose

- Dressing of ulcers with simple dressings
- Relief of pressure to prominent areas with simple dressing or total contact casts
- Early treatment of deteriorating cellulitis or sepsis with antibiotics.

When uncontrolled infection continues, surgical debridement or amputations of affected digits may be necessary. Occasionally this may progress to higher-level amputations. In the initial stages of a Charcot/neuropathic joint, emphasis must be placed on protection and cast immobilisation can be effective. This technique is difficult to perform and is not practised in all centres. If recognised early, limb salvage is a realistic goal.

Summary

Orthopaedic surgical intervention to the lower limb encompasses some of the most commonly performed procedures and joint replacement of the hip and knee joints is still the bench mark to which other joint replacements are compared. Although these procedures are major surgery they can have a profound influence in improving quality of life in many people.

References

Anderson, T., Montgomery, F., & Carlsson, A. (2004). Uncemented STAR ankle prosthesis. *Journal of Bone and Joint Surgery, American Volume, 86*, 103–111.

Berbari, E. F., Hanssen, A. D., & Duffy, M. C. (1998). Risk factors for prosthetic joint infections: case control study. *Clinical Infectious Diseases, 27*, 1247–1254.

Berry, D. J., Von Knoch, M., Schleck, C. D., & Harmsen, W. S. (2004). The cumulative long-term risk of dislocation after primary Charnley total hip arthroplasty. *Journal of Bone and Joint Surgery, American Volume, 86*, 9–14.

Cameron, H. U. (1997). Managing length: the too long leg. *Orthopaedics, 20*, 791–792.

Edeen, J., Sharkey, P. F., & Alexander, A. H. (1995). Clinical significance of leg length inequality after total hip arthroplasty. *American Journal of Orthopaedics, 27*, 347–351.

Klapach, A. S., Callaghan, J. J., Goetz, D. D., Olejniczak, J. P., & Johnston, R. C. (2001). Charnley total hip arthroplasty with use of improved cementing techniques: a minimum twenty-year follow-up study. *Journal of Bone and Joint Surgery, American Volume, 83*, 1840–1848.

Svärd, U. C., & Price, A. J. (2001). Oxford medial unicompartment knee arthroplasty. A survival analysis of an independent series. *Journal of Bone and Joint Surgery, British Volume, 83*(2), 191–194.

Saltzman, C. L. (1999). *Total ankle arthroplasty: State of the Art. Instructional Course Lecture, 48*, 263–268.

Further reading

Greene, W. B. (Ed.). (2001). *Essentials of Musculoskeletal Care* (2nd edition). Rosemont, IL: American Academy of Orthopedic Surgeons.

Ochsner, P. E. (Ed.). Translated by Hinchliffe, R. (2003). *Total Hip Replacement: Implantation Technique and Local Complications*. Berlin: Springer-Verlag.

Chapter 3

Occupational therapy following elective lower limb surgery

Alis Moores

Current practice

The clinical area of elective orthopaedics gives the occupational therapist an opportunity to work collaboratively to facilitate people's return to occupations following a planned, isolated surgical procedure. For people whose functional difficulties may be more long term in nature, the occupational therapist can work with the person to address specific needs, aiming to maximise functional outcomes.

Elective orthopaedics has unique demands for the health care professional. Discharge efficiency is essential for the management of waiting lists, which have historically been lengthy. Responding to the need to maximise bed occupancy, by promoting efficient discharge, is integral to decision making when working in acute settings and can cause conflict if this cannot be achieved (Pethybridge 2004). Despite these challenges, Robertson and Finlay (2007) identified that occupational therapists, when interviewed about their experiences of working in acute physical settings, considered their work to be enjoyable, exciting and rewarding.

Care pathways, usually produced locally, have encouraged the standardisation of efficient practices for the multi-disciplinary team. However, in the UK, and in many other countries, orthopaedics has received limited attention, in terms of guideline development, from professional bodies in the same way that other clinical specialities have. Existing published guidelines (British Orthopaedic Society 1999; National Health Service Modernisation Agency 2002; National Institute for Clinical Excellence 2000) have centred on the medical management of people having a total hip replacement and provide limited guidance for rehabilitation. Therefore, local protocols often determine practice for occupational therapy in the absence of national guidelines (Sorby 2006).

This chapter will present guidance for the occupational therapist working in elective orthopaedics with people who have had, or are due to have, lower limb surgery. It will present the expected functional difficulties people may experience relating to specific surgical procedures. These surgical procedures have been selected as they represent those most commonly seen by an occupational therapist. This information is important when planning assessment and treatment and is therefore presented towards the beginning of the chapter. Ways to ensure that assessments and interventions are tailored will be explored. The issues when choosing outcome measures will also be addressed.

The nature of intervention – theory to guide practice

The aim of the occupational therapist in orthopaedics is to conduct a thorough assessment to facilitate an individual's discharge (Griffin 2002) and to enable them to resume roles and occupations. The rehabilitative frame of reference (Seidel 2003) is one, among others, which can guide occupational therapists when working with people in orthopaedic settings. This frame of reference emphasises the promotion of maximum functional performance in activities of daily living. It acknowledges the need for compensatory methods to counteract disability, the influence of the environment as well as the importance of the teaching–learning process (Seidel 2003). With people commonly needing to adapt the way they perform occupations post operatively, compensatory strategies are commonly adopted and education, in the context of an educative approach (Foster 2002), is essential for these strategies to be incorporated into daily occupations.

An alternative and sometimes complementary frame of reference is biomechanical (McMillan 2002). This frame of reference focuses on restoring motion which relates to the capacity for movement, muscle strength and endurance (McMillan 2002). These sources of motion are likely to be compromised following orthopaedic surgery. In order to be true to the values and beliefs inherent in an occupational paradigm, movement, strength and endurance need to be assessed within the context of the person completing their occupations (McMillan 2002). Therefore a frame of reference which was not specifically designed for the profession can be used to broaden the knowledge base and inform practice (McMillan 2002).

The fundamental beliefs of the profession emphasise the holistic nature of assessment and the importance of a client-centred approach (Duncan 2006). However, the demands in orthopaedic departments can, at times, challenge this philosophy. Treatment is guided by the importance of resuming independence in particular tasks, necessary for safe discharge. These goals are often influenced by the priorities of hospital trusts, which emphasise timely discharge and maximum admission rates. In this environment, occupational therapists must prioritise the most important tasks the individual needs to perform for a safe discharge. The relatively short-term nature of disability in elective orthopaedics must be acknowledged and treatment tailored accordingly. Consistent with the biomechanical approach, a person's independence will improve as an automatic consequence of joint healing (James 2003). In the short term, both the rehabilitation and biomechanical frames of reference incorporate compensatory strategies that can be used to facilitate independence in occupations to enable a person to be discharged home from hospital safely.

A large proportion of joint replacements occur as a result of osteoarthritis. Many people are admitted for an isolated surgical procedure and are expected to regain their previous level of function. However, since osteoarthritis is a prevalent condition in older people (Grant 2005) multiple pathologies, common in the older population may affect the recovery of some people. For example a person who has chronic obstructive airways disease will find mobilisation post surgery particularly challenging due to their preoperative respiratory function, often resulting in reduced exercise tolerance.

Some people may require multiple replacements for different joints over an extended period of time. Alternatively, the need for revision surgery of a particular joint may also necessitate a series of admissions. Surgery may be planned to relieve pain, therefore maximising independence and reducing discomfort. However, in some cases it may not be possible for the person to completely regain their range of movement and function. Peoples' needs will vary and must be assessed using a client-centred approach. Their individual needs must be kept paramount despite demands for efficiency and timely discharge. In such cases a more holistic model such as the Canadian Occupational Performance Model (Law et al. 1994) may be more appropriate.

Functional implications for common elective surgical procedures

Gathering information

It is important that the occupational therapist has adequate knowledge of the surgical procedure that the person has had (see Chapter 2). This scientific knowledge needs to include the aims of surgery, the prosthesis which has been used, any postoperative pre-cautions and the timescale of the expected recovery phase. This theoretical knowledge alone is insufficient to inform clinical reasoning but does serve to inform an understand-ing of function and deficits (Chapparo and Ranka 2000). This scientific knowledge would be expected to be similar for each person having the same procedure. However, therapist should be aware of variations related to age and the disease process.

Patients' home situation, roles and responsibilities, or life context, vary greatly and are fundamental to clinical reasoning (Chapparo and Ranka 2000). It is the occupational therapist's role to work with the person to identify and understand how the precautions and post surgical implications will impact on his/her daily life once discharged. Only then can treatment be planned, which is guided by the person's needs.

Referral procedures vary among wards and hospitals. Occupational therapists on some wards will be responsible for identifying which people they need to assess. On other wards the nursing staff will refer the people who require occupational therapy assessment. This procedure needs to be negotiated and agreed among the multi-disciplinary team. The process needs to be sensitive to the fact that the surgical pro-cedure alone does not dictate whether or not a person will need an assessment by an occupational therapist. A person admitted for relatively minor surgery may need extensive occupational therapy intervention if they have very limited social support and were perhaps having difficulty with occupations prior to admission.

Although not an exhaustive list, people having the following surgical procedures are likely to need to be assessed by an occupational therapist:

- Total hip replacement/revision total hip replacement
- Total knee replacement
- Girdlestone's excision arthroplasty
- Joint fusion.

These procedures will now be discussed in turn relating to the factors that occupational therapist intervention may need to address for efficient discharge. The factors discussed are not intended to be a prescriptive list but to assist in guiding clinical reasoning.

Total hip replacement/revision total hip replacement

Knowledge of precautions

People having total hip replacement surgery or a revision of a total hip replacement will be advised to restrict movement at the hip joint post operatively to limit the possibility of the hip dislocating. These restrictions are commonly referred to as hip precautions (see Chapter 2). It is unknown whether restricting movement can reduce the prevalence of dislocation (Peak et al. 2005). There is a lack of scientific evidence, leading to decisions being made based on practitioner experience and formal consensus (O'Donnell et al. 2006), often decided at a local level. Therefore advice regarding hip precautions will vary between consultants and hospitals. It is important that the occupational therapist is familiar with and is guided by local policies and protocols.

The movements a person will be advised to avoid are usually, although not always, flexion beyond 90°, adduction across the midline and external/internal rotation (Sorby 2006). The timescale for which a person will be advised to follow these precautions also varies depending on individual consultants' preferences. In general terms it is usually advised that precautions should be followed for approximately three months post surgery. It is the occupational therapist's role to problem solve with the person to ensure that precautions are applied to the individual's unique occupations.

The occupational therapist's core skills in occupational analysis are important in assessing the demands of a particular task related to the person's ability to perform it (Duncan 2006; Hagedorn 2001). The role of the occupational therapist as an educator (Foster 2002) is also central to the skills necessary when working with a person to develop their understanding and application of hip precautions. This may be challenging if a person has cognitive or communication difficulties. In this case careful assessment is essential and strategies such as using written information, reinforcement by other staff and family involvement may need to be particularly utilised.

Mobility

The physiotherapist will ensure that an individual is progressing with his/her mobility, using prescribed walking aids. The majority of people will be fully weightbearing post surgery. However, if the prosthesis is uncemented the person will remain partially or non-weightbearing for between six and 12 weeks (Engh and Bobyn 1985). The occupational therapist needs to encourage the person to apply the techniques they have learnt while engaging in activities. The occupational therapist is central to providing the team with information about the person's home environment to ensure that he/she receives the necessary practice in hospital to prepare him/her for discharge. The occupational therapist will need to collect information such as the layout of the person's property, the distances he/she will need to walk regularly and whether there are any unusual slopes or narrow passageways at home. Information about steps, stairs and rails will be necessary. Attention should also be paid to hazards at home. These may include uneven floor coverings, mats, rugs or trailing wires. Ideally the person should be given information about possible hazards before admission so that appropriate adaptations can be put in place (Rivard et al. 2003).

Transfers

A person's minimum sitting height must be calculated to ensure hip precautions are maintained. Sitting on furniture of this height or higher will ensure that the angle at the hip joint is maintained at 90° or greater. To calculate this height, a measurement should be taken from the popliteal fossa to the floor (while wearing normal footwear) and 5 cm should be added. This will ensure that the person's hip is higher than his/ her knee when sitting.

The occupational therapist will need to consider the heights of all furniture the person will need to use on discharge. A supportive armchair is important. This will need to be of adequate height, preferably with arms. The person's bed will also need to be of adequate height. Individuals are usually advised to ensure that they get out of bed with the leg which has been operated on leading. This limits the tendency for the affected limb to go into adduction when getting out of bed. If this is not possible due to the layout of the room the person will need advice on care to be taken when carrying out this transfer. The person's toilet seat is likely to need to be raised for precautions to be followed and to ensure they can rise without difficulty.

In addition to these basic furniture needs, the occupational therapist must also pay attention to other activities that will require the person to sit during the day. This will include where they will eat their meals. A dining chair is usually of adequate height but one without arms may encourage excessive flexion at the hip when rising from sitting to standing. They may need seating upstairs for washing at the sink or for dressing. Stair lifts, electric scooters and bath lifts also need to be taken into consideration. These often involve rotating components that may encourage rotation at the hip, which is not advisable. Such equipment needs to be individually assessed and advice given as to whether the person will be able to use them safely while following precautions. Independence in all transfers will be an important goal for discharge. Supervised practice will promote independence and ensure that precautions are applied and understood.

Self-care

Accessing washing facilities at home can be difficult following a total hip replacement. Getting in and out of the bath requires excessive flexion at the hips. Stepping over the bath side to access a shower is usually discouraged, again due to excessive hip flexion and an uneven base of support. A shower cubicle can offer a safe washing environment provided the step is not too difficult to negotiate. A bath board, placed across the back of the bath, at the same height as the top of the bath, can provide a stable bench on which the person can sit to lift their legs over the bath side. This will only be safe if the person leans back when transferring, to increase the angle at the hip, and stays on the board to use the shower. Strip washing is also a safe alternative but sometimes this is viewed as dissatisfactory.

When following hip precautions, people must be discouraged from attempting to reach their lower legs and feet as this would necessitate excessive hip flexion. An alternative should be negotiated with the person. While some people are willing to accept assistant from a spouse or relative, others are keen to perform this task for themselves, even if help is available. Long handled devices such as a long handled shoe horn, sponge and reacher can be demonstrated and issued for washing, drying and dressing lower legs and feet. The occupational therapist needs to use activity analysis skills to advise on ways that an individual's usual washing and dressing style needs to be modified. For example, a person would be likely to benefit from sitting on a high surface to dress, dressing their operated leg first.

Domestic activities

Accessing food and drink is obviously a basic requirement, which will be essential for discharge. Forward planning will enable the person to have stocked up on 'easy to heat' meals, rather than cooking meals that require increased standing tolerance and endurance. Environmental preparation will allow for most commonly used items to be placed in cupboards that are easy to reach.

A table and chair in the kitchen will be helpful to eliminate the need to carry items while using a walking aid in each hand. If there is not adequate room for a table in the kitchen the person may benefit from a kitchen trolley. This equipment is unsuitable for a person who is not fully weightbearing and safety when using this item therefore needs to be assessed. Alternatively, a perching stool placed at a kitchen work top will often suffice, provided they do not sit sideways to the work top, which encourages hip rotation when turning to face their food.

Automatic kitchen appliances make tasks such as laundry much easier. The occupational therapist needs to ascertain how these tasks are usually completed and whether they require excessive hip flexion. The person will be unable to carry items, such as a washing basket, as they will be dependent on walking aids. It may be necessary to enquire if a friend or neighbour could help with these tasks. Shopping is also a task for which a person will commonly require assistance. However, local supermarkets, the milk man or butcher will often deliver groceries. Alternatively, internet shopping can remedy this difficulty. Any other household tasks that require the person to reach to the floor need to be addressed. It is important that the person helps to identify these, as they will be unique to the individual.

Other life roles need to be addressed and may need to be limited for the period of recovery. Some people may have children, grandchildren and/or pets for which they care. With forward planning the occupational therapist can assist the person to problem solve and arrange a means to address these short-term limitations.

Work and leisure

Return to work and leisure activities are usually determined by the demands of the particular task. In general terms if the task requires movements that are not permitted due to precautions, the person should be advised against it. Only after the period for which the precautions need to be followed can the activities be resumed gradually.

For the period of the precautions the person should be advised not to drive. This needs to be discussed with the person to ensure that alternative arrangements can be made, particularly if he or she is the only driver in the family. Alternatives for meeting friends and attending groups need to be discussed. The person should be reminded that if he or she travels outside the home, during the time, they should consider the height of the chair and toilet which they will need to use. More sedentary past times, such as sewing or drawing can be carried out once discharged. The occupational therapist should explore these, preferably prior to admission so that the person can make preparations. Clearly most people will want to resume a range of different pursuits once discharged from hospital which may include gardening, sports and sexual activity. Specific demands will vary and these need to be analysed with the individual so that appropriate decisions can be made about the extent to which they can be resumed and when.

Revision total hip replacement

The factors identified above are likely to need consideration when planning treatment for a person who has had a revision total hip replacement. It is common for the person to need to follow strict precautions. The consultant may give individual advice concerning particular movements for which the person needs to be careful, and timescales for which precautions need to be followed. Revision surgery often requires bone grafting, which may require the person to either non-weightbear or partially weightbear. Careful attention to medical notes is vital for appropriate goal setting and treatment planning.

It is likely that the person will be familiar with the precautions from their original hip replacement. However, revising precautions are strongly recommended, as primary surgery may have occurred many years ago, and advice regarding precautions will differ depending on where the surgery was performed.

Some people will need to have two-stage revision surgery because of infection. This involves the removal of the hip prosthesis, a course on antibiotic treatment followed by surgery to insert the new prosthesis approximately three months later. How they progress and their home support and the environment will dictate whether discharge between the first and second stage is possible. The aim will be for the person to be discharged in the interim period using walking aids for minimal distances.

Total knee replacement

Precautions

Although people are not required to follow specific precautions after their surgery, advice regarding daily activities is necessary. Treatment is aimed at encouraging full range of movement at the knee joint and avoiding undue pressure through and around the joint while it is healing.

Mobility

People will be dependent on walking aids on discharge. Attention will therefore need to be paid, as for total hip replacements, to environmental factors which may impact on safe, independent mobility.

Transfers

Independent transfers should be encouraged without equipment wherever possible. Raising furniture will make transfers easier, due to the reduced knee flexion necessary. However, people must be discouraged from using high furniture that prevents the knee from flexing.

Self-care

Getting in and out of the bath is unadvisable, due to weightbearing through the knee when it is in an excessively flexed position when standing up from sitting in the bath. Immersing the knee in water is not advisable, particularly before the wound is completely healed. Stepping over a bath side to access the shower can be dangerous, again due to the uneven base of support. A bath board may be useful to access an over bath shower. Alternatively, the use of a shower cubicle or strip washing offer safe solutions. People should be encouraged to wash and dress independently, including reaching their feet. This will promote desirable knee flexion at an early stage during functional tasks.

Domestic activities

As with self-care, flexion of the operated knee should not be discouraged. However, the need to carry items, such as food or a clothes' basket must be addressed, as for total hip replacements.

Work and leisure

The return to work and leisure activities are dependent on the demands of the specific task. The task components should be explored with the individual, related to their progress.

Girdlestone's excision arthroplasty

Various, often long-term, difficulties are likely to be experienced by a person whose management results in a Girdlestone's operation. His or her needs will vary considerably depending on the reason for surgery, preoperative functional ability and likely outcomes. This type of surgery is becoming less common due to advances in revision surgery (Atkinson 2005).

Although precautions will not need to be followed, intervention must address daily activities discussed above for total hip replacement surgery. Peoples' needs must be individually assessed and treatment planned accordingly.

Joint fusion

Fusion of any joint will undoubtedly lead to permanent changes to the way that a person is able to perform particular tasks and engage in occupations. This often involves the compensation of other more mobile joints and the reduction or elimination of pain at the affected joint. It may be possible for the occupational therapist to be involved in analysing the person's occupational performance so that appropriate information can be collected to guide the decision to operate. The implications of having a fused joint when engaging in particular occupations can be assessed by the occupational therapist. Advice can be offered concerning ways in which occupational performance will change as a result of the surgery.

Depending on the joint involved, the occupational therapist will address the necessary daily tasks the person needs to perform post surgery. There are no specific precautions other than that they must not put excessive strain on the joint, particularly while it is in the process of healing in the fused position.

Pathways of care

Integrated care pathways (ICPs) are widely used in orthopaedics. These are also known as care profiles, care protocols, critical care pathways or multi-disciplinary pathways of care (Hammond 2002). These terms can be used largely interchangeably. ICPs have been defined as 'structured multidisciplinary care plans which detail essential steps in the care of patients with a specific clinical problem and describe the expected progress of the patient' (Campbell et al. 1998).

Being multi-disciplinary, ICPs share the professional interventions that each team member needs to contribute in order for the person to progress to discharge. The original design lent itself to beginning with the general practitioner when a referral was made to secondary care and following the person through to post-discharge rehabilitation. However, it is more common for ICPs to be used in secondary care only.

ICPs are condition specific and therefore generally relevant to the needs of a particular group of people. However, if the stages in the pathway are not relevant or a person has particular needs, professional judgement can be used to tailor the treatment accordingly. The pathway includes preset goals for the person to achieve each day, which are aimed at ensuring standardised treatment and timely intervention and discharge.

Clinical reasoning in the area of elective orthopaedics needs to be adapted to accommodate the various needs of the individual. According to Rogers and Massagatini (1982) there are areas of occupational therapist practice that can be standardised due to the predictable elements of a person's response to a specific condition. Assistants and support staff can be effectively utilised to address predicted needs identified by a care pathway that guides a procedural approach. The assistant needs to be able to adequately identify those whose needs or progress are not consistent with a generally recognised norm. The occupational therapist can then use his or her experience and theoretical knowledge with people whose needs are more complex.

Professional guidelines may inform the contents of locally developed care pathways. The American Occupational Therapy Association (1999) produced practice guidelines for adults with hip fractures and hip replacement. These guidelines provide information to support decision making which is quality driven, accessible and cost effective. The information includes assessment, treatment, discharge planning and outcomes. This type of guideline has not been replicated by other professional bodies internationally. However, information from professional bodies can be used to guide practice in an orthopaedic setting. The College of Occupational Therapists (1994) and the Canadian Association of Occupational Therapists (1991) have produced guidelines for client-centred practice which must be central to work in all clinical areas, including orthopaedics.

As well as guidelines from professional bodies, orthopaedic standards of care are commonly produced by governing health departments (Department of Health 2002). They aim to streamline services, guiding particular areas for improvement. Local therapy services or occupational therapy departments are likely to have produced their own guidelines or standards which are related to a specific local need. These may also include invaluable information relating to the surgeon's preferences for treatment post surgery. These guidelines should be reviewed regularly and contributed to by all team members.

Assessment

Assessment in elective orthopaedics can take many forms. This section will address preoperative education and assessment. Factors will then be considered which need to be included in an assessment, whether this is conducted pre operatively or post operatively, in a group or individually.

Preoperative education and assessment

The literature has presented much debate as to the benefits of preoperative assessment and education. Spalding (2005) states that: 'preoperative education is widely used by occupational therapists all over the world to help patients prepare for their impending surgery and postoperative needs.'

The pre-planned nature of elective surgery enables the occupational therapist to be able to forward plan to address the needs of the patient for his or her admission. Government documents have outlined the benefits of preoperative assessment and encouraged its wide utilisation (Department of Health 2002).

The Cochrane review (McDonald et al. 2005) hypothesised that if a person has a full understanding of the operation, including postoperative routines, the person will be less anxious, have a shorter hospital stay and be better able to cope with postoperative pain. However, the review found this not to be the case. Only one study in the review (Crowe and Henderson 2003) concluded that beneficial effects were a direct result of preoperative education. The review did not specifically consider the potential influence of occupational therapy contribution to preoperative education. In contrast, other studies have considered the benefits of preoperative education in terms of empowerment and reducing anxiety (Spalding 2005). Anecdotally benefits appear to include the person not only feeling more prepared but also having the opportunity to make timely arrangements for equipment and other services in preparation for admission.

The Cochrane review (McDonald et al. 2005) included preoperative services which took many forms regarding the professionals involved, the length and location of sessions. Therefore it is with caution that conclusions should be drawn regarding the value of preoperative services generally as they may vary greatly from those included in the study. If a preoperative service is to be conducted, a review of this process needs to be completed regularly. Reviews must include resource implications, the benefits to the person as well as to the service in terms of being able to make preparations in advance of admission.

Timing of assessment

Preoperative assessments are generally carried out four to six weeks prior to admission when a date for surgery has been confirmed. However, particular people will benefit from occupational therapist intervention at an earlier stage prior to surgery. People who are waiting for surgery often experience considerable limitations in terms of occupational performance caused by the symptoms of osteoarthritis. Grant (2005) identifies that the scope of occupational therapy practice in this area is broad and includes a range of assessments and interventions that can assist the individual at this stage. Whether or not a person with osteoarthritis is waiting for surgery, holistic assessment is recommended to include the effect of osteoarthritis on a person's occupations and quality of life (National Institute for Health and Clinical Excellence 2008). Education and self-management techniques are recommended within a team approach to early intervention (National Institute for Health and Clinical Excellence 2008). If the person is due to have surgery, intervention will also encourage familiarity with equipment and advice which will be useful post operatively.

Occupational therapists can assist the person to gain an understanding of the implications of the proposed surgery on their functional performance before being placed on the waiting list for surgery. An assessment, which includes the extent to which they are limited in terms of their daily activities, may also inform the surgeon when deciding if joint replacement is necessary and at the stage it will be most beneficial for the person. Spalding (1999) gives details of a service which involved a priority assessment carried out by an occupational therapist to determine the impact of the degenerative disease on the individual's occupations, self-care, work, rest and leisure. The assessment, which was designed by a surgeon, assisted in providing a need's led service. Spalding (1999) presents a critique of the service, documenting the difficulties encountered by the occupational therapist. However, particular advantages indicate that this type of assessment is worthy of further consideration. Spalding (1999) also identified that the priority assessment system was beneficial to people by facilitating the provision of equipment, advice relating to the forthcoming surgery and access to other professionals as required.

In many services, preoperative assessment or intervention for people who are on the waiting list for surgery may not be possible due to service demands. The associated costs of home visits cannot be ignored (Barras 2005). In these situations it may be helpful to prioritise those who are having particular functional difficulties. A screening questionnaire is a helpful means of identifying such people. A variety of assessment tools could be used for this purpose, an example being the Western Ontario and McMasters University Osteoarthritis Index (Whitehouse et al. 2003). Self-reported tools allow for the information to be sent and returned by post. In addition the benefits include a reduction of potential assessor bias as they are not present when the tool is completed. An assessment tool provides information relating to the person's perceptions of their difficulties. Some tools are designed and extensively validated for a specific client group, such as the Oxford Hip Score (Dawson et al. 1996). Others are generic such as the Mayers Lifestyle Questionnaire (Mayers 1998). Although not specific to a client group, this tool includes a range of occupational performance areas, including leisure.

Content of assessment

Guidance on the wide range of information that should be included in an assessment by an occupational therapist is widely available in texts such as Neistadt (2000). Similarly, in a qualitative study that investigated clinical decision making when making arrangements for discharge in acute care settings, Jette (2003) identified some important factors which need to be considered. These include the context, the person's ability to participate in rehabilitation, the person's wants and needs, their function and their disability.

Guidance concerning factors to include in an assessment, adapted from Neistadt (2000), is discussed below relating to an orthopaedic setting.

Identification of person's priorities in terms of his or her activities

It is important to consider that the benefits of the proposed surgery are consistent with the person's expectations. Informal discussion can reveal the activities a person expects to be able to resume within different timescales. The occupational therapist can provide information to ensure that the person's expectation of the occupations they may resume and the timescales are realistic. Identifying the person's specific needs relating to their home environment, social support and personal priorities is central to effective discharge planning.

A summary of assets and strengths

Discussion with the person will reveal a range of unique strengths which he or she will bring. These may include his or her knowledge of the surgery or disease process, good family support or high levels of motivation. All of these factors, or lack of them, will guide treatment planning following assessment.

Preoperative difficulties with activities of daily living and their related living environment

The person's preoperative functional performance will need to be assessed either pre or post operatively. This may involve observation by the occupational therapist or self-reporting by the person. If the assessment is carried out post operatively then obviously the occupational therapist will need to rely on the person's report of their preoperative functional ability.

Skill level needed for discharge

General discharge criteria for each surgical procedure may be pre-agreed by the multi-disciplinary team and documented in the care pathway. Discharge goals will needs to be adapted to ensure that they address individual needs. These will be dependent on their social situation, previous level of function and environmental factors.

An intervention plan

This will need to be tailored to assist the person to achieve the goals outlined above. The plan will need to be negotiated with the person so that a shared understanding is reached about the achievements that are required prior to discharge.

Standardised assessment tools

Assessment methods and tools used in orthopaedics vary from standardised, formal and structured to observation. Standardised tools have generally been studied for validity and reliability, however, structured non-standardised tools have the benefit of being modified by the occupational therapist (Neistadt 2000). Information collected in a structured format can provide a narrative. This includes the person's general background and priorities and provides helpful information (Neistadt 2000). The assessment process for some people may be predetermined by a care pathway that may or may not include a standardised tool. For others, standardised tools may be used to identify priorities to guide treatment or to measure a baseline from which outcomes can be measured. The following questions need to be considered when choosing an appropriate outcome measure for use in orthopaedics.

Has the tool been designed for use with people experiencing orthopaedic conditions?

Some tools have been designed to be used with a specific population. The Arthritis Impact Measurement Scale (Meenan et al. 1992) assesses the physical, social and emotional well-being of people with arthritis. As it is condition specific, it is expected to address the common difficulties prevalent in this client group. Other tools are not designed to be used with a specific group. An example is the Mayers Lifestyle Questionnaire (Mayers 1998). This tool has not been designed for use in orthopaedic specifically but does have the benefit of enabling the people to identify their own priorities. When choosing a tool it is important to investigate whether it has been tested for validity and reliability and whether these tests were related to a specific client group.

Can it be used as an outcome measure?

The tool may be suitable for use at the assessment stage and repeated following the intervention stage. The changes in functional ability will indicate the outcomes of intervention. An assessment tool which can be used in this way, such as the Oxford Hip Score (Dawson et al. 1996), clearly provides useful comparative data from which to evaluate the effect of intervention on the person's functional performance.

Is it a self-rating scale or does it require the occupational therapist to be present?

The time factor of administration needs to be considered as demands vary between tools. The occupational therapist's presence may influence the answers the person gives. This needs to be taken into account. People's perceptions of their pain will vary greatly, therefore caution needs to be used if data are compared between people.

Will it assist in identifying treatment priority areas?

Some assessment tools identify priority areas from the person's responses, such as the Canadian Occupational Performance Measure (Law et al. 1994). This can guide the occupational therapist and the person to prioritise treatment needs. The difficulty here is that these priority areas may not be in keeping with those determined by the service. For example, a person may prioritise a leisure activity that is not essential for safe discharge from acute services. Robertson and Finlay (2007) identify such tensions as being contradictions between the occupational therapist's holistic ideals and the more reductionist focus of the work context.

Postoperative intervention

People are likely to have preset goals on admission, guided by a care pathway and adjusted to ensure they are specific to the person. People who have more complex needs may still have a care pathway. If this is not the case, treatment goals will need to be documented in a similar format. Those who have more complex needs will require an in-depth assessment, possibly involving an assessment of their home environment, particularly if they are much less mobile than they were prior to admission. The person's performance needs to be assessed in relation to the demands of each task. The person may need to develop particular physical requirements such as exercise tolerance. Alternatively, the occupational therapist may be able to modify the task to accommodate the person's difficulties. The occupational therapist will need to communicate broadly with other agencies who may be involved in supporting the person on discharge. These agencies may include care agencies, home and minor adaptation services, equipment services and voluntary sector groups.

Outcome measurement

Guidance on the selection of an outcome measure can be found in various texts and publications including the College of Occupational Therapists outcome measures information pack (Clarke 2001). Papers also discuss the characteristics of particular measures in relation to validity and reliability. The reader is urged to refer to this information in his or her own evaluation of an appropriate outcome measure to use in a clinical area. Some factors to consider, adapted from the College of Occupational Therapists outcome measures information pack (Clarke 2001), will now be discussed in relation to orthopaedics.

- **Be clear about what is going to change** – The purpose of surgery varies from one person to another. Some people are not expected to reach improved range of movement at their affected joint yet functional ability is expected to improve due to the reduced pain that can be achieved as a result of surgery. Therefore an outcome measure needs to assess the benefits that are included in the aims of surgery.
- **At what stage the measure needs to be utilised** – Careful consideration must be given to the appropriate stage at which an outcome measure is undertaken. A person waiting for elective orthopaedic surgery is likely to have functional limitations. Following surgery, the person will also be limited until the site of surgery heals fully, they regain range of movement and pain subsides. If functional ability is the same after the recovery phase as immediately pre operatively, the outcome is not favourable. If a person is able to regain the functional performance which they had prior to the onset of symptoms, the outcome would be positive. A person may need to use equipment for a period of time after the surgery, for example in order to follow precautions after a total hip replacement. In this case the use of dressing aids and furniture raisers may inaccurately indicate the person is more dependent after than before the surgery. However, this compensatory approach is inevitable and should not be used to evaluate the outcomes of surgery or occupational therapy intervention.
- **Whose outcome is being measured** – It is difficult to confirm which outcomes are direct results of occupational therapy intervention. This may be desirable when justifying the need for occupational therapy in terms of service planning and resource allocation. The person would be expected to have improved function as a result of the surgery alone. In addition to this they will have been treated by other professionals including a physiotherapist and occupational therapist, which will all have contributed towards a positive outcome. Some outcome measures may evaluate the success of the admission on service factors such as length of stay, which the occupational therapist may have directly influenced. While this will account for the success of one aspect of the service, it will not distinguish between the contributions of different professions or consider quality of the person's experience. Figures may be collected on the number of contacts made by an occupational therapist. These often do not accurately evaluate the quality of the intervention.
- **Ease of administration** – Some outcome measures, particularly those incorporating standardised assessments, are costly to purchase and may require specialist training for the administrator. The time the tool takes to complete needs to be considered both in terms of the occupational therapist's time, which is likely to be pressured,

and the person's time. The questions need to be easily understood by the person and the purpose made clear.

Summary

Drivers in elective orthopaedics include efficient, timely discharge planning which aims to maximise bed occupancy and minimise length of stay. Occupational therapists are increasingly required to respond to the needs of people for whom innovative surgical procedures and new ways of working have been utilised. Within this context, people's needs must remain the focus of occupational therapy interventions. With new developments in this area comes opportunity for occupational therapists to become increasingly involved in extending their roles while developing the roles of support staff to carry out more routine, standardised work loads managed by a care pathway approach.

This chapter has presented specific information relating to the functional difficulties which a person is likely to experience post surgery. The occupational therapist needs this information in order to effectively identify people's needs during assessment. Care pathways, which promote standardised approaches, are helpful to guide timely treatment. These need to be appropriately adapted for people whose needs differ from the majority. Occupational therapists need the time, flexibility and support from their colleagues and departments to ensure that their practice addresses the various, diverse needs of people with orthopaedic conditions engaging in their occupations.

References

American Occupational Therapy Association. (1999). *Occupational Therapy Practice Guidelines for Adults with Hip Fracture/ Replacement*. Bethesda, MD: American Occupational Therapy Association.

Atkinson, A. G., Coutts, F., & Hassenkamp, A. (2005). *Physiotherapy in Orthopaedics: a Problem Solving Approach*. London: Churchill Livingstone.

Barras, S. (2005). A systematic and critical review of the literature: The effectiveness of occupational therapy home assessment on a range of outcome measures. *Australian Occupational Therapy Journal, 52*(4), 326–336.

British Orthopaedic Society. (1999). *Total Hip Replacement: A Guide to Best Practice*. London: British Orthopaedic Association.

Campbell, H., Hotchkiss, R., Bradshaw, N., & Porteous, M. (1998). Integrated Care Pathways. *British Medical Journal, 316*, 133–137.

Canadian Association of Occupational Therapists. (1991). *Occupational Therapy Guidelines for Client Centred Practice*. Ottawa: Canadian Association of Occupational Therapists.

Chapparo, C., & Ranka, J. (2000). Clinical reasoning in occupational therapy. In J. Higgs and M. Jones (Eds). *Clinical Reasoning in the Health Professions*. London: Butterworth Heinemann.

Clarke, C. (2001). *Outcome Measurement: Information Pack for Occupational Therapy*. London: College of Occupational Therapists.

College of Occupational Therapists. (1994). *Patient Focussed Care: guidelines for BAOT members*. London: College of Occupational Therapists.

Crowe, J., & Henderson, J. (2003). Pre arthroplasty rehabilitation is effective in reducing hospital stay. *Canadian Journal of Occupational Therapy, 70*(2), 88–96.

Dawson, J., Fitzpartrick, R., Carr, A., & Murray, D. (1996). Questionnaire on the perceptions of the patient about total hip replacement. *Journal of Bone and Joint Surgery, British Volume*, 78(2), 185–190.

Department of Health. (2002). *Improving Orthopaedic Services: A Guide for Clinicians, Managers and Service Commissioners*. London: Her Majesty's Stationery Office.

Duncan, E. A. S. (2006). Skills and processes in occupational therapy. In E. A. S. Duncan (Ed.). *Foundations for Practice in Occupational Therapy*. London: Churchill Livingstone.

Engh, C., & Bobyn, J. (1985). *Biological Fixation in Total Hip Arthroplasty*. New Jersey, Thorofare: Slack.

Foster, M. (2002). Theoretical frameworks. In A. Turner, M. Foster and S. E. Johnson (Eds). *Occupational Therapy and Physical Dysfunction: Principles, Skills and Practice*. London: Churchill Livingstone.

Grant, M. (2005). Occupational therapy for people with osteoarthritis: scope of practice and evidence base. *International Journal of Therapy and Rehabilitation*, 12(1), 7–12.

Griffin, S. (2002). Occupational therapy practice in acute care neurology and orthopaedics. *Journal of Allied Health*, 31(1), 35–42.

Hagedorn, R. (2001). *Foundations for Practice in Occupational Therapy*. London: Churchill Livingstone.

Hammond, R. (2002). *Integrated Care Pathways*. London: Chartered Society of Physiotherapy.

James, A. B. (2003). Biomechanical frame of reference. In E. B. Crepeau, E. S. Cohn, B. A. Boyt Schell, & M. E. Neistadt (Eds). *Willard and Spackman's Occupational Therapy*. New York: Lippincott, Williams and Wilkins.

Jette, D. U., Grover, L., & Keck, C. P. (2003). A Qualitative Study of Clinical Decision Making in Recommending Discharge Placement From the Acute Care Setting. *Physical Therapy*, 83(3), 224–236.

Law, M., Baptiste, S., Carswell, A., McColl, M. A., Polatajko, H., & Pollock, N. (1994). *The Canadian Measure of Occupational Performance*. Ottawa: Canadian Association of Occupational Therapists.

Mayers, C. A. (1998). An evaluation of the use of the Mayers' lifestyle questionnaire. *British Journal of Occupational Therapy*, 61(9), 393–398.

McDonald, S., Green, S. E., & Hetrick, S. (2005). Pre operative education for hip or knee replacement. *The Cochrane Library*. Oxford: Update Software.

McMillan, I. R. (2002). Assumptions underpinning a biomechanical frame of reference in occupational therapy. In E. A. S. Duncan (ed.). *Foundations for Practice in Occupational Therapy*. London: Churchill Livingstone.

Meenan, R. F., Mason, J. H., Anderson, J. J., Guccione, A. A., & Kazis, L. E. (1992). Aims 2: The content and properties of a revised and expanded arthritis impact measurement scales health status questionnaire. *Arthritis and Rheumatism*, 35(1), 1–10.

National Institute for Clinical Excellence. (2000). *Guidance on the Selection of Prosthesis for Primary Total Hip Replacement*. London: National Institute for Clinical Excellence.

National Health Service Modernisation Agency. (2002). *Improving Orthopaedic Services*. London: Her Majesty's Stationery Office.

National Institute for Health and Clinical Excellence. (2008). *Osteoarthritis: National Clinical Guideline for Care and Management in Adults*. London: Her Majesty's Stationery Office.

Neistadt, M. E. (2000). *Occupational Therapy Evaluation for Adults: A Pocket Guide*. Philadelphia, PA: Lippincott, Williams and Wilkins.

O'Donnell, S., Kennedt, D., MacLeod, A. M., Kilroy, C., & Gollish, J. (2006). Achieving team consensus on best practice rehabilitation guidelines following primary total hip replacement surgery. *Healthcare Quarterly*, 9(4), 60–64.

Peak, E. L., Parvizi, J., Ciminiello, M., Purtill, J. J., Sharkey, P. F., Hozack, W. J., & Rothman, R. H. (2005). The role of patient restrictions in reducing the prevalence of early dislocation following total hip arthroplasty: a randomised, prospective study. *Journal of Bone and Joint Surgery, American Volume*, 87(2), 247–253.

Pethybridge, J. (2004). How team working influences discharge planning from hospital: a study of four multi-disciplinary teams in acute hospitals in England. *Journal of Interprofessional Care*, *18*(1), 29–40.

Rivard, A., Warren, S., Voaklander, D., & Jones, A. (2003). The efficacy of preoperative home visits for total hip replacement clients. *Canadian Journal of Occupational Therapy*, *70*(4), 226–232.

Robertson, C., & Finlay, L. (2007). Making a difference, teamwork and coping: the meaning of practice in acute physical settings. *British Journal of Occupational Therapy*, *70*(2), 73–80.

Rogers, J. C., & Massagatini, G. (1982). Clinical reasoning in occupational therapists during the initial assessment of physically disabled patients. *Occupational Therapy Journal of Research*, *2*(4), 195–219.

Seidel, A. C. (2003). Rehabilitative frame of reference. In E. B. Crepeau, E. S. Cohn, B. A. Boyt Schell, & M. E. Neistadt (Eds). *Willard and Spackman's Occupational Therapy*. New York: Lippincott, Williams and Wilkins.

Sorby, K. (2006). Travelling the integrated pathway: the experience of a total hip replacement. In L. Addy (Ed.). *Occupational Therapy in Practice for Physical Rehabilitation*. Oxford: Blackwell Publishing.

Spalding, N. (1999). The assessment of surgical priority by occupational therapists. *British Journal of Occupational Therapy*, *62*(5), 229–231.

Spalding, N. (2005). Reducing anxiety by pre operative education: make the future familiar. *Occupational Therapy International*, *10*(4), 278–293.

Whitehouse, S. L., Lingard, E. A., Katz, J. N., & Learmonth, I. D. (2003). Developing and testing of the reduced WOMAC function scale. *Journal of Bone and Joint Surgery*, *8*(5), 706–711. Available at: www.asd.co.uk/guides/how_to_posters.htm (accessed 27 February 2008).

Chapter 4

Orthopaedic surgery for the upper limb

Oliver Pearce

Introduction

This chapter provides an outline and overview of the anatomy, common presenting conditions and the surgical management of the upper limb. Reference should be made to anatomical texts for more detailed descriptions of the musculoskeletal system.

The key function of the upper limb is to be able to place the hand where one chooses and then to be able to use it to manipulate objects to carry out activities and tasks. As long as the upper limb is capable of doing this, it is described as having good function. Surgical intervention due to injury or disease aims primarily at maintaining or increasing function, and although cosmetic appearance is important, it should never compromise the level of function that may be achievable.

Each component of the upper limb can be subject to disease, but joint disease presents most commonly in clinical practice.

The shoulder

The shoulder comprises two joints (Figure 4.1):

- Glenohumeral joint – this articulates between the head of the humerus and glenoid portion of the scapula.
- Acromioclavicular joint – this articulates between the lateral end of the clavicle and the acromion process of the scapula.

Movements of the shoulder usually occur at the glenohumeral joint and between the scapula and the posterior chest wall that it lies against. This is known as scapulo-thoracic movement.

The glenohumeral joint is described as a ball and socket joint, however, the ball part of the joint is an incomplete sphere and the socket is a very shallow concavity. The joint would be immensely instable without the surrounding structures described below:

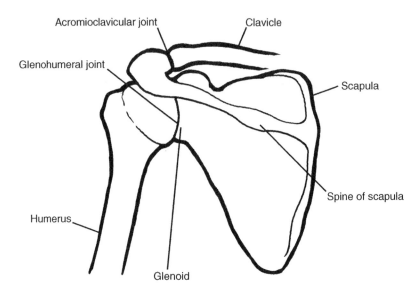

Figure 4.1 Anatomy of the shoulder girdle.

- Glenoid labrum – this is a lip around the glenoid circumference which deepens the socket.
- Humeral head – this has a cuff of tendons known as the rotator cuff attached around it from the muscles of the scapula which pull it with greater force into the socket.
- Shoulder joint capsule – this resists subluxatory movements.

Because of the shallow socket and incomplete humeral head, the shoulder has an impressive range of movement:

- Shoulder forward flexion: 0–180°
- Shoulder extension: 0–45°
- Shoulder abduction: 0–180°
- Shoulder external rotation: 0–90°
- Shoulder internal rotation: 0–90°.

Therefore the shoulder is relatively unstable and is capable of subluxation and dislocation.

The elbow

The elbow comprises two components (Figures 4.2 and 4.3):

- A hinged articulation between the olecranon (part of the ulna) and the trochlea (part of the humerus)
- A rotatory articulation giving pronation and supination at the radiocapitellar joint (the head of the radius and the capitellum (humerus).

Due to its structure, the elbow is a far more stable joint than the shoulder and rarely suffers problems of instability.

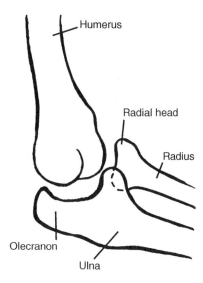

Figure 4.2 Bones of the elbow joint.

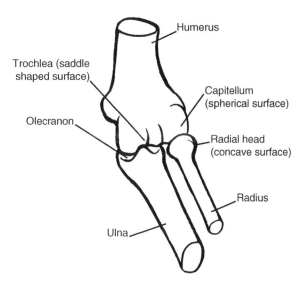

Figure 4.3 Articular surfaces of the elbow joint.

The wrist

The wrist is a joint between the radius and ulna on one side and the carpus. The carpus is the name given to the collection of eight small bones located at the base of the hand (Figure 4.4). The scaphoid, lunate and triquetrum articulate at the wrist, and the others articulate against each other in a series of complex joints.

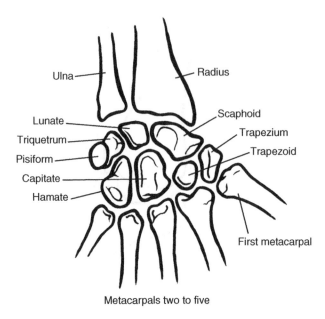

Figure 4.4 Bones of the wrist.

Movements at the wrist include:

- Palmar flexion (also known as volar flexion)
- Dorsiflexion
- Medial and lateral flexion
- Circumduction (a circular combination of the above movements).

The hand

The metacarpal bones articulate with the carpal bones and lead to the digits (phalanges). The hand comprises the following joints (Figure 4.5):

- Metacarpophalangeal: between the metacarpals and digits (phalanges); these are hinge joints
- Two types of joints within the digits (phalanges):
  - Proximal interphalangeal joints (PIPJs)
  - Distal interphalangeal joints (DIPJs).

PIPJs and DIPJs are both hinge joints. The thumb, which has only two phalanges, has only one interphalangeal joint.

The thumb is capable of opposition, which is the movement and manipulation at 90° to the plane of movement of the fingers. The thumb is described as being responsible for 60% of the hand's function. Therefore disabling conditions of the thumb including osteoarthritis or trauma can have a major effect on hand function and activities of daily living.

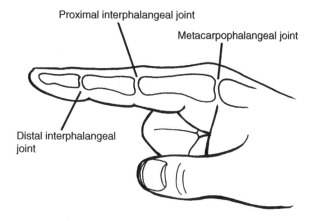

Figure 4.5 View of the finger in extension showing the joints.

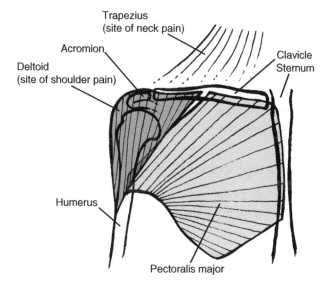

Figure 4.6 Sites of pain in the shoulder.

The shoulder – main conditions, diagnosis and treatment

The shoulder can present as painful, stiff or unstable, or any combination of these signs. The clinician must be wary of mistaking neck pain with shoulder pain, and therefore they must listen carefully to the person's exact description of their pain. If the pain is located on the upper border of the trapezius muscle, particularly if it radiates towards the neck, it is considered as neck pain and not shoulder pain (Figure 4.6). If, however, the pain is located in the deltoid muscle or the patient indicates that the pain is felt deep within the shoulder, this is considered shoulder pain.

Osteoarthritis

Osteoarthritis presents with insidious onset of pain and stiffness within the shoulder, and is generally seen in the older person. There is often no other coexisting joint disease (unlike rheumatoid arthritis where other joint involvement is common).

Treatment

Simple pain killers can keep the symptoms under control for a long period of time. Occupational therapists may be involved in advising people how to moderate their activity by ceasing or changing the way they carry out activities which set off the pain, e.g. gardening, heavy lifting and other heavy manual work.

Physiotherapy can also help to improve the range of movement and muscle strength in those muscles that have atrophied due to lack of use of the painful shoulder. These atrophic muscles can also be painful and therefore strengthening and training them back to normality can alleviate pain.

The next stage of treatment is the use of a steroid injection into the shoulder joint. This injection is a combination of steroid and local anaesthetic. The steroid often known as cortisone or cortisol (although there are many different types of injectable steroids) acts an anti-inflammatory. It does not affect the process which is causing the arthritis (which is poorly understood), but damps down the inflammation which is responsible for some of the pain within the joint.

However, the pain of severe osteoarthritis can be refractory to all these non-operative measures. If this is the case then the person may require a joint replacement. The principles, outcomes, risks and complications of arthroplasty are described in Chapter 2.

Total shoulder replacement

This procedure replaces the humeral head with a metal ball and the glenoid with a polyethylene socket (Figure 4.7). Good pain relief is obtained with this surgical procedure;

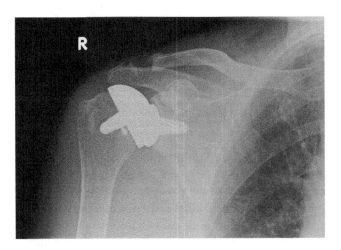

Figure 4.7 Shoulder arthroplasty.

however evidence shows that the glenoid component seems to be prone to early loosening. Thus some surgeons do not use this component and claim enhanced results.

Shoulder hemiarthroplasty

The hemiarthroplasty procedure only replaces half of the joint – the humeral head. This procedure achieves good pain relief without the complications of loosening. The prosthesis is made up of a stem and a head (Figure 4.8). After removal of the humeral head, the stem is cemented into the humeral shaft and the head fits onto the shaft.

The surgical approach is via an incision at the front of the shoulder to avoid nerve and blood vessel damage. The joint capsule and subscapularis tendons must be securely sutured as they provide restraint against anterior dislocation.

Complications include those associated with the general risks of surgery and having a general anaesthetic (these are described in more detail in Chapter 1) and with the actual surgery itself. These include risk to the adjacent structures, including the axillary nerve (deltoid muscle function) and the musculocutaneous nerve (biceps function). There is approximately 1% chance of wound infection. Scar tenderness and neurovascular damage can also occur. The shoulder can also have an abnormal reaction to the surgery and can develop a condition called frozen shoulder; symptoms include pain and stiffness lasting up to 18 months. A small proportion of people undergoing hemiarthroplasty continue to experience pain despite the surgical intervention. The reasons for this are not understood.

A deep-seated infection is a rare but devastating complication, when the prosthesis becomes irretrievably infected and requires removal for antibiotic treatment to have a chance to work. Unfortunately, further surgery involves the risks associated with the ageing process and anaesthesia.

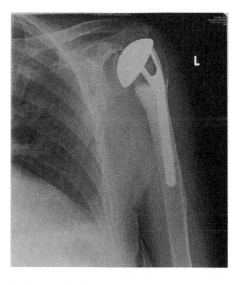

Figure 4.8 Long stem shoulder hemiarthroplasty.

Post operatively, the person is managed in a soft foam sling with a simple dressing over the wound. The dressing is usually removed around 10 days and sutures removed two weeks post operatively. Gentle, supervised mobilisation is encouraged by the physiotherapist. Postoperative regimens will vary from surgeon to surgeon, so the occupational therapist will need to liaise with the team to be aware of postoperative protocols and any contraindications before commencing assessment and activities.

Usually the individual will need to refrain from work or light activities for six weeks and this will be up to three months for those involved in manual and heavy work.

Arthrodesis

This procedure is an alternative treatment for severe osteoarthritis of the shoulder. The procedure is performed less often nowadays due to the success of the arthroplasty. A fusion of the joint involves opening the joint and removing the articular cartilage from the humeral head and glenoid, then using metal work, e.g. a plate, screws and wires to fix one to another to prevent movement. The bony surfaces then 'heal' together, effectively fusing the bone together. This fusing provides good pain relief at the expense of a range of movement.

Rheumatoid arthritis

Rheumatoid arthritis (described in Chapter 1) is a polyarthropathy (disease affecting many joints). The hands are the most commonly affected, but the shoulder can also be involved.

Treatment

Treatment varies from that of the osteoarthritic shoulder with the different medications prescribed, which try to control the inflammation of the synovial lining of the joint. This may take the form of simple pain killers and anti-inflammatories or joint injections of corticosteroid. The main difference is the use of cytotoxics, for example methotrexate, which is toxic to the individual but more toxic to the inflamed synovium, thus reducing the joint disease, and more 'biologic' treatments such as infliximab, which inhibits the hormone 'tumour necrosis factor'. This hormone is a part of the pathway resulting in the disease we know as rheumatoid arthritis. This pathway is still not understood.

The surgical management of the shoulder is very similar to that for osteoarthritis; however there is even greater reason to avoid total shoulder replacement in favour of shoulder hemiarthroplasty due to the relative softness of rheumatoid bone, which is responsible for early glenoid component loosening. Recovery from the surgery may take longer than for people with isolated osteoarthritis. Complications are no different in rheumatoid arthritis but the risk of wound infection may be higher.

Shoulder instability

Instability of the shoulder leads to a tendency for the joint to dislocate repeatedly. The most common cause of recurrent instability is traumatic dislocation of the shoulder.

The younger the individual is at the time of first dislocation, the greater the risk of proceeding to recurrent instability. A teenager is at 75–80% risk of re-dislocation.

Dislocations are generally classified by the direction in which the humeral head has displaced. The commonest by far is anterior dislocation, accounting for 95% of all dislocations. The remaining 5% are posterior dislocations and these are really only ever seen following epileptic seizures and severe electric shocks.

Treatment

The immediate treatment for an anterior dislocation will usually take place in the accident and emergency unit. The shoulder will be relocated under sedation. This requires the use of resuscitation equipment, oxygen mask, monitoring of oxygen saturation with a pulse oximeter, sedative medicine and a skilled practitioner. Many different techniques of shoulder relocation have been described since Hippocrates' traction method. The most commonly used methods are Kocher's and Stimson's manoeuvres. Stimson's procedure is less traumatic and more widely used.

Post relocation, rehabilitation involves immobilising the shoulder by placing the arm in a sling that holds the arm next to the trunk by using a body belt (Figure 5.4, p 79). This is considered the safe position and is helpful in alleviating pain. A graduated therapy regimen will then be carried out to strengthen the muscles of the shoulder. Return to contact sports should be avoided for three to six months.

Stabilisation surgery is usually indicated for those people who continue to have problems with re-dislocation, i.e. shoulder instability. The reason for recurrent anterior dislocation is a weakness in the anterior portion of the shoulder joint. This can take the form of either a tear of the anterior capsule and cartilage labrum from the anterior neck of the glenoid. This is known as a Bankart lesion. Or, it can be the bony equivalent which is a fracture of a portion of the anterior glenoid and is known as a Bony Bankart, which drags the anterior capsule with it, resulting in the same weakness of the anterior restraint of the humeral head. Both versions of the Bankart lesion are commonly seen to coincide with a plastic deformation of the inferior glenohumeral ligament (the tough portion of the anterior joint capsule that lies in the inferior half of the anterior joint.)

Stabilisation surgery therefore must address the Bankart lesion and the laxity of the joint capsule. The surgical approach may be open or arthroscopic. The best results are from open surgery, although arthroscopic stabilisations are improving as technology improves the instruments available. Sutures and screws may be used to make the repairs, which result in a 90–95% success rate. The shoulder is immobilised using a soft sling and body belt (see Figure 5.4, p 79) which helps to prevent external rotation that could damage the surgical repair. A graduated programme of therapy will be required to enable the individual to regain range of movement and to strengthen the muscles of the shoulder.

Complications include:

- Wound infection
- Tender scar
- Restriction of range of movement (if over tightened)
- Painful shoulder
- Frozen shoulder
- Re-dislocation and persistent dislocation despite surgery.

Shoulder impingement

Impingement pain in the shoulder usually occurs from early middle age onwards unless it is post traumatic. It is termed impingement because as the shoulder is raised in abduction, the greater tuberosity of the humeral head is brought into close proximity with the under surface of the acromion. Because the supraspinatus tendon (one of the muscles of the rotator cuff) joins the humerus at the level of the greater tuberosity, it can be 'pinched' (impinged upon) in this position.

People complain of shoulder pain as they attempt movements with their arms above shoulder height. The condition becomes a vicious cycle as the more impingement on the supraspinatus tendon; the more swelling is caused, thus narrowing the amount of space for shoulder abduction and therefore increasing the impingement. This process is repeated and as the condition progresses, the background ache, even when not moving the arm worsens and sleep disturbance ensues. Functional activities and range of movement are also compromised.

Treatment

Simple analgesics can be of help in mild cases, as can rest (for example from heavy lifting). However, the most effective treatment for less mild cases is the subacromial bursal injection of corticosteroid. The steroid acts as an anti-inflammatory and helps to reduce the swelling of the supraspinatus tendon. This intervention breaks the cycle and allows recovery to take place. One and occasionally more injections can actually be curative of this condition. However, in some people, the injections will only give transient relief and the pain keeps returning. In this case, surgery to decompress the acromial space is usually indicated. The thickened tissue of the subacromial bursa is debrided arthroscopically with some burring away of the prominent bone of the under surface of the acromion. Thus the greater tuberosity is no longer restricted in abduction due to the removal of the cause of the impingement.

Post operatively the individual will be immobilised in a soft, simple sling for analgesia and comfort for approximately one week. The postoperative rehabilitation process will then commence with mobilisation of the shoulder. The pain can be slow to disappear post operatively, but usually the person can expect improvement in their symptoms from about six weeks onwards.

Complications of surgery include:

- Wound infection
- Neurovascular damage
- Persistence of pain (despite surgery)
- Frozen shoulder.

Acromioclavicular osteoarthritis

The acromioclavicular joint joins the trunk to the arm, and is mainly involved in movements of the shoulder when the arm is raised above the level of the shoulder. The joint can develop osteoarthritis primarily or as a result of previous trauma to the joint. The pain is usually described as localised on the point of the shoulder, rather than diffuse pain associated with glenohumeral osteoarthritis. The person is able to assist diagnosis as they point a single finger to the top of their shoulder to demonstrate where they experience the pain. Palpation of the acromioclavicular joint will reproduce the pain, as does pulling the arm across the trunk in the cross-over arm test. An X-ray of the shoulder will show loss of joint space and formation of osteophytes at the joint.

Treatment

Treatment commences with simple analgesics, which help some people. If these are ineffective then an injection of local anaesthetic and steroid into the joint is offered. It may take six weeks to resolve the pain, and in many cases the injection may be curative of the symptoms. The injection can be repeated as necessary.

However in some people, the pain remains and surgery is indicated. This is the excision of the acromioclavicular joint and can be carried out as an open or arthroscopic procedure. The most lateral few millimetres of the clavicle are removed where it articulates with the acromion. This procedure is successful at eliminating pain. Post operatively the person is advised to avoid heavy lifting for approximately six weeks and may require therapy to increase and or maintain range of movement.

Potential complications of surgery are the same as described above for shoulder impingement.

Frozen shoulder

The cause of this painful stiffening of the shoulder is the subject of great debate and is still not well understood. There appears to be thickening of the shoulder capsule with infiltration of fibroblast cells, but the synovial lining of the joint is normal. The stiffening may appear after minor trauma to the shoulder, but usually arises de novo.

The disease process is divided into three phases that have a tendency to merge into each other:

- Phase I: painful (pain with gradually increasing stiffness)
- Phase II: frozen (gradual resolution of pain, persistent stiffness)
- Phase III: thawing (gradual resolution of stiffness).

Frozen shoulder is a self-limiting condition and everyone gets better and usually it does not recur, but unfortunately it does take between one to three years to resolve. A small proportion (10%) of people have some residual stiffness.

Treatment

The type of treatment offered is also much debated and generally these are not very effective.

The painful phase should be treated with simple analgesics. Steroid injections are often used but appear not to help in the majority of cases. When the shoulder is stiff and painful, and analgesics are not helping, surgery can be considered. The various operations all have similar results which help some patients, but by no means all, to relieve pain and improve range of motion.

Arthroscopic distension of the joint alone is thought to free up adhesions and stretch the joint capsule, whereas arthroscopic release will free the adhesions. Manipulation under anaesthetic is often used in combination with other procedures, but can be performed on its own. Open release can be used as an alternative and yields similar results.

Mobilisation within the early phase of the condition is not indicated as there is more pain than stiffness at this stage, and the exercise seems to worsen the pain. Mobilisation may be more useful in the thawing stages of the condition.

Complications:

- Increased pain
- No effect on pain or stiffness
- Humeral fracture (post manipulation)
- Capsular rupture.

The elbow – main conditions, diagnosis and treatment

Osteoarthritis

Osteoarthritis affects both components of the joint – the radiocapitellar joint and the ulnohumeral joint. People complain of pain and decreasing range of movement in the elbow. There may also be problems with locking where the elbow gets stuck in a certain position and the individual has to forcefully manipulate their arm to be able to move again. This locking appears to be caused by loose bodies of wear debris from the articular surfaces that are now floating freely and become caught in between them.

Treatment

Simple analgesia is offered with physiotherapy. Joint injections can offer some transient benefit. Surgery has less to offer than that for other joints. This is because the implantation of an elbow replacement in a healthy person with normal levels of activity tends to work loose very rapidly. Loosening leaves a serious bone stock deficiency and a revision elbow replacement is likely to last even less time than the original. The elbow can be washed out arthroscopically, and the synovial lining can be debrided.

In the absence of being able to reliably replace the joint, the final operation for pain relief is the arthrodesis of the elbow (causing the humerus and ulna bones to fuse together). This results in no range of movement in the elbow but does give pain relief. The position and angle the elbow is fused in is vital to get correct, as the person must be able to function in this position (specifically to be able to manipulate objects and grip, but equally importantly to be able to reach their hand to their mouth or to manage personal care). Close liaison with the surgeon, and an upper limb assessment should be carried out by the occupational therapist with the individual to ensure their choices and preferred activities have been taken into account, and that the person is aware of the limitations and impacts the fusion will have upon their daily life and routine.

Fusion will be achieved with the use of bone graft, usually from the person's tibia and internally fixed with screws and or plates. The elbow is usually fixed in 90° of flexion. The arm is protected by the application of a plaster cast for a period of six weeks to protect the fusion until bony union is achieved.

Complications include:

- Non-union (failure of successful bony union)
- Infection
- Malunion (fusion in the wrong position)
- Nerve or blood vessel damage
- Pain from internal fixation hardware.

Rheumatoid arthritis

As rheumatoid arthritis is a polyarthropathy (many joints involved) the day-to-day demands solely on this joint may be less than those on the osteoarthritic elbow, which may be the only joint involved. The consequence is that elbow replacement surgery in the person with rheumatoid arthritis enjoys a far superior result than that in someone with osteoarthritis. It relieves pain reliably and has good longevity.

Treatment

The treatment of the rheumatoid arthritis is undertaken by specialist rheumatologists and their teams, and, like the shoulder involves the use of analgesics, cytotoxics and biological treatments. Joint steroid injections can be very useful for staving off the need for joint surgery.

However, when all non-operative measures have been tried and exhausted, surgery should be considered. Open synovectomy can be useful where marked synovitis (inflammation of the synovial lining of the joint) is present. But, where the elbow is said to be 'burned out', and the problem is really that of long-standing joint destruction with gross erosion of the articulating surfaces, then joint replacement surgery is indicated.

Total elbow replacement

Total elbow replacement involves a posterior incision, and great care is taken to protect the ulnar nerve. The radial head is excised. Total elbow replacement takes the form of a 'sloppy hinge'; one stem located in the humerus and the other in the ulna, which are hinged together allowing minimal side to side angulation (Figure 4.9).

Excessive angulation could lead to loosening of the implant. The canals of the humerus and ulna are reamed and the stems of the implant are cemented in place. The implant acts as a hinge joint and also as the collateral ligaments. So, if there is so much bony destruction that the ligamentous stability of the elbow has been compromised, the hinged prosthesis stabilises the joint in lieu of the normal ligaments.

Post operatively the elbow is placed in a simple sling usually with a waist strap and then the person is encouraged to mobilise gently under supervision. The hospital length of stay is generally short – between two and four days – until the individual is self-caring and safe to be discharged home. Active physiotherapy and occupational

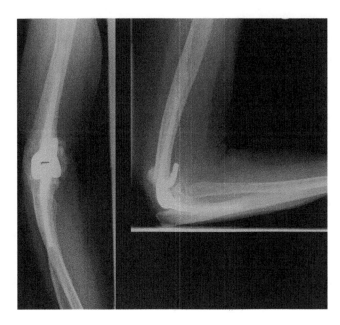

Figure 4.9 Lateral view – total elbow replacement.

therapy assessments and interventions are essential, especially as the person may have many other coexisting impairments and functional problems.

Complications

Possible complications include:

- Neurovascular damage
- Fracture of the soft rheumatoid bone
- Infection
- Early loosening.

It is not always possible to regain the full range of movement back at the elbow, but it is likely to be greater than that prior to the surgery. The main improvement is the relief of pain.

Tennis and golfer's elbow

These conditions are termed 'enthesopathies', meaning pathology of the portion where tendon joins bone. The anatomical organisation of the forearm means there is a 'common flexor origin' and a 'common extensor origin' at the level of the elbow. The wrist flexors have a common origin at the medial humeral epicondyle, the muscles travelling along the volar (palmar) surface of the forearm to the wrist and hand. The wrist extensors have a common origin at the lateral epicondyle, with the muscles travelling along the dorsal surface of the forearm to the wrist and hand.

Tennis elbow

Tennis elbow is an inflammation of the common extensor origin at the lateral humeral epicondyle and is known as a lateral epicondylitis. Characteristically, the person presents with pain in their lateral elbow, following a period of repetitive movements (e.g. painting the ceiling) to which they are not accustomed. The pain is minor at rest, but is exacerbated by activities, even minor ones using that arm.

Treatment

The mainstay of treatment in the first instance is rest. A proportion of people with tennis elbow will therefore not even present to their doctor, as people through their own common sense rest the arm and therefore the pain resolves without further intervention. However, rest alone does not help everyone, particularly in people who have manual jobs, where rest is not an option, and the pain persists. Anti-inflammatories can be prescribed along with using cold, e.g. ice or heat treatments (heat lamp, heat packs or deep heat cream).

Tension through the common tendon origin during the use of the extensor muscles can be relieved by pressure on the muscle bellies just distal to the tendon. This can be achieved through splinting with pressure on this point thus relieving symptoms during use of the arm. The use of this technique can have tremendous effect in some whereas it seems to make no difference in others. In cases resistant to these minor treatments, an injection of local anaesthetic and steroid into the common extensor tendon may cure the condition. Sometimes this injection must be repeated. Some surgeons effectively enforce rest of the arm by using plaster of Paris casting for several weeks.

The final treatment option if none of the other interventions are successful is surgical release of the common extensor origin from its attachment to the lateral humeral epicondyle. A degenerate portion of the tendon is thought to be present in a proportion of people with this condition and identification and excision of this is considered beneficial.

The arm is placed in a sling, and the individual is counselled against any substantial lifting for at least six weeks while the tendon origin heals back to the bone. This procedure relieves the pain in the majority of people.

Golfer's elbow

Golfer's elbow is a similar (although less common) condition to tennis elbow and is due to the inflammation of the common flexor origin at the level of the medial humeral epicondyle.

Treatment

The range of treatments exactly parallels those of tennis elbow described above.

The wrist – main conditions, diagnosis and treatment

Arthritis

The wrist can be affected by both types of arthritis, but rheumatoid is the most commonly presenting. It is possible to get post-traumatic osteoarthritis of the wrist, for example after a missed scaphoid fracture which goes on to develop avascular necrosis and subsequent collapse of the radio-scaphoid portion of the joint. Other forms of arthritis such as the long-term sequelae to septic arthritis or psoriatic arthritis are less common.

Rheumatoid arthritis is highly destructive to the bone in the advanced stages in the wrist. X-rays can show extreme bone loss that results in pain and instability in the wrist.

Treatment

As previously described, the treatment for rheumatoid arthritis is concentrated on analgesics, anti-inflammatories, splintage, joint injection and biological treatments. It is when these have failed to control the symptoms of pain or when instability occurs, that surgery is indicated.

Various surgical procedures are now available to help. In the case of severe flare up of synovitis over the wrist dorsum before any joint destruction has occurred in the wrist itself, there is much benefit to be had in performing a synovectomy. This is an excision of the inflamed synovial tissue through a linear incision through the wrist dorsum. Less commonly, this can also be carried out for the flexor tendons. Because the wrist has the tendency to drift into radial deviation as rheumatoid arthritis progresses there are tendon transfer operations to re-dress the balance. For example, the tendon of extensor carpi radialis longus can be transferred from its normal radial side insertion to the ulnar side of the wrist.

However, when the wrist degenerative change has progressed to severe levels, there is only arthroplasty or arthrodesis left as surgical options to treat the pain and improve the function. Different surgeons vary greatly in their preference of one over the other, as both have advantages and disadvantages. Arthrodesis has a good record in terms of pain relief, but it is obviously at the price of sacrificing range of movement and there is also a non-union rate. Arthroplasty has a reasonable track record for pain relief, but is more technically more demanding and there is a finite lifespan of the prosthesis itself which may go on to loosen.

Arthrodesis and arthroplasty

Wrist arthrodesis is generally undertaken with some form of internal fixation.

The two main methods involve the use of either an intramedullary pin or a dorsal plate. Both procedures have in common the need for exposure of the joint so that the surfaces can be debrided to congruent flat surfaces in a desirable position for function. The position is usually a small amount of dorsiflexion for the best power of grip and neutral in terms of lateral flexion in either direction. It should be noted that if both wrists require fusion, one should be in dorsiflexion but the other should be in palmar flexion, otherwise personal hygiene would prove impossible. Some surgeons advocate fusion for one wrist and arthroplasty for the other. In all cases, the occupational therapist should be involved as part of the multi-disciplinary team to advise the surgeon and the individual regarding the best outcome, and which considers the individual's lifestyle, choices and priorities.

There are many more designs of arthroplasty than fixation systems for arthrodesis but at present there is no consensus as to which provides the best outcome for the individual being treated. As the wrist joint is not one single joint, but a series of complex articulations between numerous small bones, none of the arthroplasties are able to take this into account. The procedure is further complicated by the abnormal tissue balancing around the joint by the time surgery is performed. However, the advantage of arthroplasty systems is that some movement is preserved and a good proportion of patients achieve pain relief.

In arthrodesis, the wrist is maintained in a splint or plaster cast for six weeks or until bony fusion is seen on X-ray. Hand therapy to increase range of movement of the digits can now commence, and the occupational therapist can assist the patient in compensatory movements and techniques to overcome the loss of movement at the wrist. In people who have wrist arthroplasty, hand therapy will increase range of movement both at the wrist and the digits.

Complications

- Infection – of the wound or of the implant itself
- Fracture of the bones
- Loosening of the implant
- Nerve or vessel damage
- Persistent pain despite technically successful surgery.

Tendon rupture

Two obvious causes of tendon rupture are:

- Traumatic
- Degenerate/attrition.

Traumatic tendon ruptures are described in Chapter 12. In this chapter, we shall describe degenerate/attrition ruptures that are seen most commonly with rheumatoid arthritis.

Rheumatoid arthritis is a condition that affects the synovial tissue lining the joints and tendons throughout the body, and these tissues become highly inflamed. This inflammation results in the secondary damage to the articular cartilage of the joints, and can also damage the integrity of the tendons. Also, bony prominences can be instrumental in rubbing against the overlying tendons and gradually wearing through them.

While tendon rupture can technically occur anywhere in the body, it is most commonly seen to affect the tendons of the wrist as they go to the hand. One reasonably common exception to the ruptures seen in people with rheumatoid is the rupture of extensor pollicis longus tendon in people who have had Colles' type of fracture of the distal radius. With time, a sharp edge of bone over the dorsum of the distal radius can cause attrition rupture of even healthy tendon tissue.

Treatment

Surgical repair usually cannot be managed by simply repairing the damaged ends together, and it is often necessary to perform a tendon transfer, from another muscle, to the distal portion of the ruptured tendon, and to weave onto it, or to perform a tendon graft from another muscle's tendon between the ruptured ends for strength. The ruptured tendon ends are generally of poor quality (without well defined cut ends) as they are damaged over a variable distance proximally and distally to the point of rupture.

Extensor tendon ruptures are far more common than flexor tendon ruptures.

Complications

- Wound infection
- Neurovascular damage
- Re-rupture of the tendon
- Reflex sympathetic dystrophy.

Peripheral nerve compression syndromes in the upper limb

Cubital tunnel syndrome

Cubital tunnel syndrome is compression of the ulnar nerve as it swings round the posterior aspect of the medial humeral epicondyle in the elbow. The soft tissue tunnel around it at this level is termed the cubital tunnel. This can become tight, exerting pressure on the nerve. Also, as the nerve passes round the bony corner in the elbow, it can be subject to damage by the persistent traction as a result. Both compression and traction are thought to be implicated in the damaging process.

The person does not complain of symptoms at the level of the elbow, but at the destination of the ulnar nerve – the hand. The person feels an irritating sensation of tingling (paraesthesia and, or dysaesthesia) in the little finger, and on the ulnar border of the ring finger. The ulnar nerve also supplies motor innervation to the hand, and in severe cubital syndrome, results in weakness of abduction and adduction of the digits, and poor control of fine movement of the fingers. Over time, muscle wasting occurs, leading to hollowness between the metacarpal bones.

Treatment

Cubital tunnel syndrome can be mild, moderate or severe. In its mildest form, the individual may simply experience tingling at night when they lie with their medial elbow resting on the bed while asleep. They then wake up in the morning with numbness in the little and ring fingers that rapidly resolves. No active treatment is required here, however, if the individual is bothered by this, then a bath towel or other soft padding can be wrapped around the elbow at night to prevent the pressure on the nerve. As the severity of the symptoms and pain increases, the need for treatment also increases.

Surgery forms the mainstay of treatment in more severe cases. Many surgeons prefer to arrange nerve conduction studies to obtain evidence of compression on the ulnar nerve at the level of the elbow before undertaking surgery to decompress the cubital tunnel. In some cases, the nerve will also be transposed anteriorly and subcutaneously (under the skin), which is the commonest procedure, or submuscularly (under the muscle) to the epicondyle, Sometimes the medial epicondyle is removed completely (known as an epicondylectomy).

Unfortunately in the case of the ulnar nerve, the damage that has occurred through traction and compression does not tend to be fully reversible, even after decompression. Therefore surgery is effective at preventing further deterioration of the symptoms, and resolving the symptoms to a varying extent in some people. Post operatively, a bandage is applied to the elbow for two weeks until removal of the sutures. Movement of the elbow is permitted, but heavy lifting or manual labour is best avoided for six weeks.

Complications

- Damage to the ulnar nerve
- Bleeding and haematoma formation
- Infection
- Painful and sensitive scar.

Carpal tunnel syndrome

Carpal tunnel syndrome refers to the compression of the median nerve as it passes beneath the flexor retinaculum (also known as the transverse carpal ligament) into the hand. The carpal tunnel is the space between the transverse carpal ligament and the bones of the carpus, and it contains the flexor tendons from the forearm into the digits, as well as the median nerve. The function of the transverse carpal ligament is thought to be to stop the flexor tendons from bowstringing when the wrist is pulled into flexion.

The symptoms felt by the person are of numbness and tingling in the thumb, index, middle and radial border of the ring finger. These are known as the radial three digits of the hand. The symptoms are often exacerbated at night and can wake people from their sleep, forcing them to shake their hand to rid themselves of the symptoms.

Driving or holding an object for long periods of time, e.g. telephone, can also set off the symptoms. There is often wasting of the muscle bulk of the thenar eminence, with weakness of grip and a tendency to drop objects.

Often, there is there is no clear identifiable cause or reason of the nerve compression, but any swelling of the wrist can raise pressure on the nerve in this part of the body. This can occur with rheumatoid arthritis, hypothyroidism, pregnancy or trauma, e.g. a wrist fracture.

Clinical tests used to diagnose carpal tunnel syndrome are:

- Tinel's sign: tapping the median nerve on the volar surface of the wrist elicits tingling in the fingers and thumb.

- Phalen's test: holding the wrist in flexion for a minute (thus raising the pressure in the carpal tunnel) elicits tingling in the fingers and thumb.
- Observing wasting of the thenar eminence.
- Testing for loss of sensation in the radial three digits.
- Carrying out nerve conduction studies (particularly where the presenting symptoms are not classical for carpal tunnel syndrome).

Treatment

As the symptoms of carpal tunnel syndrome increase in severity so do the indications for treatment. Treatment takes the form of using a night splint that prevents the person curling their wrist at night. This is known as a self Phalen's splint; it assists in keeping the pressure in the carpal tunnel from rising at night.

The carpal tunnel can also be injected with steroid and local anaesthetic. This form of treatment is effective as a cure for a minority of people and can relieve the symptoms for a variable amount of time for others. If a combination of injection and splinting are unsuccessful, then carpal tunnel decompression surgery is indicated.

Carpal tunnel decompression is a straightforward operation that can be performed under local anaesthesia, depending on the individual's and surgeon's preferences. The use of a local anaesthetic is certainly less of a risk to the person if they can tolerate it. The transverse carpal ligament is incised along its length, thus relieving pressure on the median nerve. The skin is simply closed with interrupted sutures leaving the ligament open.

Post operatively, the wrist and hand will be in a bulky dressing for two weeks until the sutures are removed. There is usually no need for active therapy involvement. Individuals will find that finger movements are not particularly uncomfortable, even when in the dressing, but that gripping objects hard is painful as it involves placing pressure on the wound. This difficulty is the last thing to resolve and can take anything between six and 12 weeks.

Complications

- Wound infection
- Damage to the palmar cutaneous nerve branch
- Damage to the median nerve (rare)
- Ongoing pain on firm gripping
- Development of reflex sympathetic dystrophy – a painful stiffening, setting of the hand and fingers of unknown cause that is quite resistant to treatment.

The hand – main conditions, diagnosis and treatment

Dupuytren's contracture

This is classically named after Baron Von Dupuytren, who employed a coachman with this condition. It is a flexion contracture in the palm of the hand, most commonly affecting the little and ring fingers (Figure 4.10). The contracture is located in the tough tissue of the palm of the hand – the palmar fascia.

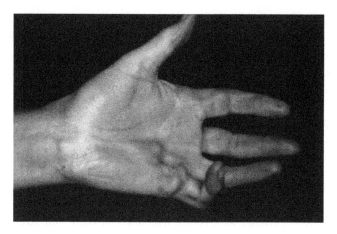

Figure 4.10 Dupuytren's contracture.

The only other anatomical location that contains this specific type of fascia is the sole of the foot and hence this is also susceptible to the same disease process.

It is not known why this condition develops, but the cellular constituents of the contracted tissue have been shown to contain myofibroblasts, which are cells that make scar tissue with contractile tissue. These cells react to tension, and those parts of the palmar fascia that are under tension are associated with the flexor tendons. Thus, the contracture occurs along the line of the flexor tendons, and because the palmar fascia is normally loosely connected to these tendons, the contracture tethers the tendons, pulling the fingers into fixed flexion. This is generally not a painful condition, but the contracted fingers are affected both cosmetically and, as the contraction worsens, functionally. The exception to the painless nature of this disease is the formation of Dupuytren's nodules, which are painful for their first few months of existence; although the nodules themselves do not resolve, the pain resolves as part of the natural history.

Treatment

Treatment for Dupuytren's contracture is primarily surgical. Non-operative treatments have been tried with little proven benefit. This includes injection of the thickened contracted tissue with steroid or collagenase, a chemical that breaks down the major protein constituent of scar tissue. Splinting the fingers does not appear to change the tendency to ongoing contracture progression. Simple analgesia is helpful during any painful phases of nodule formation, until it resolves.

Surgery is reserved until the contracture has progressed to the point where it affects function. The crucial point in the management of Dupuytren's contracture is the identification of the right time to operate. The reason for this is that while surgery can excise the contracted tissue, it cannot affect the disease process itself; in other words, the person will continue to form Dupuytren's tissue even after surgery. They will therefore eventually recur in terms of contracture. Revision Dupuytren's surgery is technically much harder than the first time. Thus, delaying surgery in the first instance will delay the consequent need for revision surgery later. The balance must be reached so as not to let the contracture become so bad that the surgery becomes too difficult to perform. The person is usually requested to contact their doctor when the contracture starts to interfere with their normal day-to-day activities as opposed to being solely cosmetically unpleasant.

Surgery may be performed under general anaesthesia or with a regional block and is usually performed under a tourniquet. The skin is incised over the Dupuytren's tissue in a zigzag fashion over the palm, and linear fashion over the finger. The Dupuytren's tissue is then exposed and dissected off the flexor tendons, which is known as a fasciectomy. Great care is taken not to damage either the digital nerves or the digital arteries which can both be encased in this tissue.

The finger can be seen to straighten considerably as the tissue is removed from the tendon, however, joints that have been contracted for some time may develop a degree of degenerative change as a result, and will not come out straight despite the removal of adequate amounts of contracted tissue. This is particularly true of the PIPJs of the little and ring fingers, which are frequently improved but not completely straightened by Dupuytren's surgery. Metacarpophalangeal joints however, frequently have complete correction of their contracture.

Zigzag palmar incisions are used to prevent contracture of the skin as it heals itself by scarring, which could otherwise cause a contracture similar to that which has just been corrected. The linear incision on the fingers uses a lengthening technique called Z-plasty for the same reasons.

Post operatively, the hand is wrapped in a padded bandage and splinted in the 'position of safety'. This is also known as the 'duck bill's position' and involves the interphalangeal joints being placed in extension, the metacarpophalangeal joints flexed to 90° with the wrist extended. This splint helps to prevent the fingers stiffening in unwanted flexion.

After the sutures have been removed at two weeks, the hand is placed in a thermoplastic splint, and an extensive programme of hand therapy is commenced to maximise the regained range of movement, eventually culminating in a period of night splintage before the person is able to manage without any splinting. It has been demonstrated convincingly that the intensive postoperative rehabilitation phase is at least as important as the surgery itself in order to achieve a successful outcome.

Complications

- Wound infection
- Haematoma
- Skin necrosis
- Damage to the digital nerve or artery causing numbness, or at worse digital necrosis needing amputation
- Reflex sympathetic dystrophy
- Painful swelling of the fingers (lasting over a year)
- Inability to completely straighten the fingers.

Revision carries the same risks, but to a considerably greater extent. The procedure can only be repeated a finite number of times (usually a maximum of two to three times) before it proves impossible. At this point the affected digit will be left severely contracted or an amputation of the finger could be considered as the finger that gets in the way can be worse than an absent finger.

Trigger finger

When a finger gets stuck in flexion, usually with some pain felt over the palm, it is said to be triggered. This is a common condition, becoming more common with advancing age. It is due to a rucking up of the flexor tendon at the level of the palm, getting caught in the A1 pulley as the finger is pulled into flexion. The A1 pulley is a hoop-like structure at the level of the metacarpophalangeal joint that the flexor tendons pass through. There is an A1 pulley for each finger and the thumb. It is not properly understood what causes the tendon to ruck up, but what ever the initial cause of this broadening of its diameter, the repeated passage (effectively a form of repeated trauma) of the rucked up section results in inflammation, causing even more swelling in this area of the tendon. This forms a cycle of events causing a persistence of the problem of triggering.

Treatment

This cycle of trauma and then swelling can be broken by injecting an anti-inflammatory (steroid) in the region of the tendon and the A1 pulley. This is effective in a large proportion of people, although a second injection may be needed. In those, whom an injection does not help, a surgical release of the A1 pulley is required. This is performed through a small incision over the palmar aspect of the metacarpophalangeal joint. A vertical incision through the pulley releases the flexor tendon and its cycle of getting caught in the pulley, thus curing the condition. Only a few stitches are required and these are removed at two weeks. The hand is dressed in a simple bandage. There are no real restrictions on activity, as the discomfort allows. Hand therapy is rarely necessary post operatively.

Complications

- Incomplete release of the pulley leading to persistent triggering
- Infection
- Discomfort
- Neurovascular damage
- Reflex sympathetic dystrophy.

Hand infections

Different parts of the hand are subject to different types of infection, with varying management. The infections are classified by their anatomical location, and range from simple infections which require only antibiotics to abscesses requiring surgical drainage.

Paronychia

This is an infection of the nail-fold (the skin on either side of the nail). Mild cases are usually resolved by antibiotics; however, more severe infections develop into abscesses that need a lateral incision to drain the pus.

Pulp space infection

This refers to pus in the finger tip pulp. It is commonly caused by a minor penetrating wound, e.g. a thorn prick when gardening. This causes intense pain until the pus is released and this is usually carried out by an incision from the lateral side of the digit, thus avoiding a tender scar over the sensitive part of the finger pulp.

Flexor tenosynovitis

This is pus located inside the sheath which surrounds the flexor tendons to the finger or thumb. Again, this generally occurs after a minor penetrating injury, but can also appear *de novo*. The finger develops a characteristic group of signs (as described by Kanavel):

- Swelling
- Tenderness along the anterior finger border
- Held in flexion at rest
- Pain on attempted extension.

There is no place for non-operative management in this condition. The treatment is to surgically release the pus through two incisions and by flushing sterile fluid through the sheath to remove the pus. The wounds are left open to allow any infected fluid to drain, preventing re-formation of the pus collection, and the individual is prescribed antibiotics.

Palmar space infections

There are three potential areas for pus to collect in the palm:

- The thenar space
- The mid palmar space
- The hypothenar space.

Infection can occur in these spaces *de novo*, or secondary to penetrating trauma, or secondary to spread from flexor tenosynovitis. The thumb and index flexor tendon sheathes communicate with the thenar space, the middle and ring finger with the mid palmar space, and the little finger with the hypothenar space.

The management of palmar space infections is essentially surgical (as for flexor tendon sheath infections), followed by a period of time on antibiotics. Antibiotics alone will not successfully treat the infection due to the presence of pus.

Cellulitis of the hand

Simple cellulitis is a skin based infection that can spread elsewhere on the body. It causes pain, erythema, swelling and pyrexia. Treatment is by administration of antibiotics orally if mild and intravenously if severe.

In severe cellulitis, elevation of the hand and splinting in a position of safety is advisable. The elevation reduces the swelling, and splintage prevents joint contractures occurring as a result of the swelling. It also helps with pain relief during the acute phase.

Most of the severe hand infections have in common a propensity to causing swelling and pain on movement of the digits. Severe swelling causes the hand to drift into a sort of clawed position. If left in this position for any length of time, it can stiffen up and require a protracted programme of hand therapy. This is why splintage in the position of safety is recommended. The position of safety refers to metacarpophalangeal joint flexion, proximal interphalangeal joint and distal interphalangeal joint extension by the use of a volar slab of plaster wrapped in crepe. This places all the collateral ligaments of the joints mentioned under maximum stretch so that they do not contract in shortened form.

Hand therapy is usually required after a severe hand infection due to the inevitable post-infection stiffness that develops.

Summary

The upper limb is a complex structure and can be affected by many conditions and injuries. These can have a profound effect on the individual by causing pain and loss of independence in essential everyday activities. Some of these conditions are well understood with established treatment methods, whereas the cause of others is less well known with treatments less well developed. In this chapter we have reviewed the anatomy of the upper limb and how common diseases or injuries can be managed either by non-operative interventions or surgical procedures. In all cases, along with pain relief, the maintenance or re-establishment of the person's functional ability is critical.

Further reading

Bulstrode, C., Buckwalter, J., Carr, A., Fairbank, J., Marsh, L., Wilson-Macdonald, J., & Bowden, G. (2001). *Oxford Textbook of Orthopaedics and Trauma*. Oxford: Oxford University Press.

Hoppenfeld, S., & de Boer, P. (2003). *Surgical Exposures in Orthopaedics: The Anatomic Approach* (3rd edition). Philadelphia: Lippincott Williams & Wilkins.

Miller, M. D., & Carcel, M. (2008). *Review of Orthopaedics* (5th edition). Philadelphia: W.B. Saunders.

Chapter 5

Occupational therapy following elective upper limb surgery

Julie Upton

Introduction

Although hand therapy is a well established specialty within occupational therapy, few occupational therapists would claim to be a specialist in the treatment of shoulder and elbow conditions. This is somewhat strange, as without the shoulder and elbow functioning effectively to place the hand appropriately, we would not be able to use the hand to its full potential or for such a wide range of tasks (Souter 1997).

The elbow is often seen as a simple hinge joint, but the combination of flexion and extension with the supination and pronation it achieves from the wrist allows us to easily complete so many daily tasks, such as putting food in our mouths. The shoulder can achieve such a variety and range of movement that the science is only just beginning to explain how it is achieved and the role of all the structures involved.

Pain and weakness in either of these joints can have a profound effect on an individual's ability to maintain their level and range of daily activities and so occupational therapy has much to offer. This chapter will focus on the occupational therapy intervention following joint replacement of the shoulder and elbow. However, it is worth noting that the underpinning knowledge of the anatomy and functional biomechanics of these joints can inform the therapist when working with people following other procedures or presenting with other pathologies of the upper limb. For occupational therapy following surgery to the wrist and hand please refer to Chapter 13.

The chapter will aim to give an overview of the subject, providing practical information to guide evidence based therapeutic interventions. It is acknowledged that to date, there is little or no published literature regarding the efficacy specifically of occupational therapy for patients with shoulder and elbow conditions. The anecdotal evidence referred to in this chapter comes from within a specialist shoulder and elbow unit and following consultation with colleagues in other specialist centres. The wider evidence base is now very large and contains much useful information that the occupational therapist can use to inform their practice.

Preoperative assessment for shoulder and elbow surgery

The evidence to support the benefits of preoperative assessment and education is far from conclusive. However, anecdotal evidence from expert practitioners is that apart from any benefits for the person, it allows additional time for the therapist to make arrangements for any care, equipment and rehabilitation that may be required post operatively. As hospital length of stay gradually decreases, this preparation time can be very advantageous.

It is acknowledged that working practices can vary and it may not be possible for the occupational therapist to provide comprehensive assessment, education and interventions at the preoperative stage of the pathway. What is important is that the assessments and interventions occur in a timely way and this may mean these are completed during the early stages of the inpatient stay.

Ideally, the occupational therapist should become involved in the preoperative process in the six weeks prior to surgery. The decision to proceed to surgery is often taken some time before, but in cases where there are doubts as to whether surgery is appropriate or not, the occupational therapists' skills in assessment of function can provide vital information in the decision-making process. The majority of people requiring joint replacement will have either multi-joint pathology or co-morbidities that will affect their occupational performance. It may be that the suggested surgery will not bring about a sufficient increase in their quality of life for them to undergo what can be a painful procedure. They need to make an informed decision about whether they want the surgery, being fully aware of the predicted outcome, their potential level of function and the postoperative limitations and rehabilitation required.

Although the postoperative protocols following total elbow or total shoulder replacement vary, they frequently involve a period of immobilisation of the arm. Although the person may have already adapted their daily tasks to accommodate any limitations their joint disease has caused, they may require additional support to manage at home with their arm immobilised in a sling. The occupational therapist can give clear advice about what to expect post operatively and facilitate people to problem solve any difficulties they may experience with their daily activities at home. Education can help the person plan ahead, enabling them to manage their daily life in the short term following their discharge from hospital. Simple advice given could include topics such as choosing clothing that is loose and can be fastened one handed, pre-planning help with domestic chores and planning easy to prepare meals.

Another factor to consider is whether the person needs to use their affected upper limb to assist their mobility. This may include pushing up from furniture and/or using a walking aid. If they will be unable to continue with this in the short term following surgery, liaison with physiotherapy colleagues is indicated to look at alternative walking aids or transferring their walking stick to the other hand. Furniture raises may also be appropriate to aid independence during the recovery and rehabilitation period if the person has relied on their arms to push or pull themselves from sitting into standing.

The goal of upper limb joint replacement surgery is to reduce pain and enable people to return to or maintain their level of function, whether that is for self-care, caring for others, work or leisure. It must be acknowledged at this point that although much progress has been made over recent years in the effectiveness and longevity of joint replacement, the person is gaining an artificial joint, which will be never be the same as an original, normal joint. As occupational therapists, our focus is on helping people to achieve their functional goals, but we may have to temper this with advice regarding the appropriate use of their joint in the long term. Gaining the surgeon's understanding and expectations of the joint replacement is crucial, as is working closely with physiotherapy colleagues when planning treatment regimens, to enable the person to set themselves realistic and achievable goals.

Rehabilitation of the shoulder

When we think of the shoulder, we must always take into account the whole of the shoulder girdle and not just concentrate on the glenohumeral joint. The complexity of the shoulder girdle and its extensive movements make it a challenge to rehabilitate. Like other joints, we must understand the anatomy and the biomechanics if we are to be successful with our treatment and interventions. By providing treatments that aim to restore as closely as possible the 'normal' patterns of movement, we will give the person the best chance of recovering their function. It is easy to adopt compensatory movements in the shoulder girdle and although in the early stages of rehabilitation this may cause problems, in the longer term it enables many people with severe restrictions to maintain a reasonable level of function. Therefore, we will look at how the shoulder functions and the contribution of the different structures to that function before considering surgical procedures and the role of the occupational therapist.

Biomechanics of the shoulder

The scapulothoracic articulation provides the basis for all shoulder movement. For the glenohumeral joint and its musculature to operate effectively, the scapula has to be in the optimum position (Figure 5.1). It must be noted, at this point that the scapulae sit at approximately 30° to the coronal plane (Kelley 1995). Therefore, the plane of the scapula is at this angle, meaning that this is where true abduction occurs and not with the arms out to the side of the body.

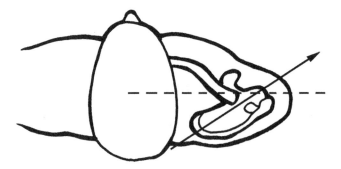

Figure 5.1 Superior view of the shoulder joint – the dotted line represents the coronal plane and the solid line represents the scapular plane, i.e. neutral between flexion and extension of the glenohumeral joint.

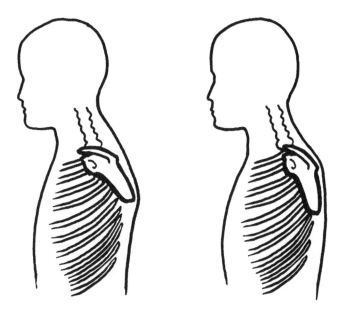

Figure 5.2 From left to right the scapula is shown in an anteriorly tilted position and neutral position.

Controlling the scapula as it glides across the thoracic wall are the serratus anterior and trapezius muscles. They create a force couple that maintains the congruence of the scapula with the chest wall as it moves. It is essential that the serratus anterior and the lower fibres of the trapezius provide a posterior tilt to the scapula, to prevent it remaining in an anteriorly tilted position (Figure 5.2), reducing the size of the subacromial space (Kelley 1995).

The muscles of the rotator cuff are:

- Subscapularis
- Supraspinatus
- Infraspinatus
- Teres minor.

These muscles originate on the scapula and are pivotal in the function of the glenohumeral joint. If the scapula is not in the optimum position, then these muscles cannot function at their most effective.

The large humeral head on the small and relatively flat glenoid surface allows for a very large range of movement but provides no stability. The rotator cuff not only provides the movements of external rotation and internal rotation of the humerus, but it also acts as a dynamic soft tissue stabiliser of the glenohumeral joint. The four muscles of the cuff work together to compress the humeral head against the glenoid. They also counteract the upward pull generated by the deltoid during elevation of the arm, depressing the humeral head to prevent superior migration and impingement on the acromion.

Another key role of the rotator cuff muscles is to rotate the humerus during elevation to prevent impingement (McClure et al. 2001). Impingement in the shoulder is when the contents of the subacromial space are squeezed between part of the coracoacromial arch (most frequently the acromion) and any part of the proximal humerus (usually the greater tuberosity). Around 30° of external rotation is required to allow full elevation of the arm (Kelley 1995) as this causes the greater tuberosity to move away from the acromion (mainly posteriorly), therefore preventing the two bony prominences from making contact and compressing the soft tissues. This fact plays an important part in the rehabilitation process, as people will want to aim for elevation and the function it brings, but to achieve this they must first work on gaining rotation. The therapist will need to explain the biomechanics to the person to help them engage with their rehabilitation.

There is a rhythm to the movement of the shoulder girdle, usually referred to as the scapulohumeral rhythm. Many studies over the years have sought to define what this rhythm is (McClure et al. 2001). It has been established that normal covers a large variation. However, as a general guide during rehabilitation, we should be aiming for the glenohumeral joint to initiate movement with the scapula starting to contribute significantly to elevating the arm when it has moved between 40° and 60°. Both the glenohumeral joint and the scapula will continue to move until full elevation is reached. When lowering the arm, the process is repeated with the scapula reaching its resting position before the arm reaches the side of the body.

These basic biomechanical principles should form the basis of any shoulder rehabilitation programme (Rubin and Kibler 2002). Surgical procedures will bring restrictions and guidelines of a postoperative protocol, but these should be worked into the biomechanical principles if we want to maximise the person's functional outcome.

Shoulder arthroplasty

Shoulder replacement, whether total or hemiarthroplasty, is most commonly used as a treatment for arthritic conditions. Just as with the hip, hemiarthroplasty of the shoulder is sometimes the treatment of choice for a proximal humeral fracture.

When planning the occupational therapy interventions for a person having a shoulder replacement, the therapist needs to be aware of the differing postoperative regimens for trauma and elective procedures. A history of trauma will have more of an influence on the postoperative care than whether or not a glenoid component is used. Likewise, the presence of trauma or an inflammatory joint disease is likely to dictate a less favourable outcome than would be expected from an elective procedure for osteoarthritis.

Assessment

As discussed previously, the assessment should ideally begin preoperatively. Specific assessment tools designed to measure shoulder function are available, e.g. the Oxford Shoulder Score and the Constant-Murley Score (Conboy et al. 1996; Constant and Murley 1987). Other tools such as the Disabilities of the Arm, Shoulder and Hand assessment (DASH) (Hudak et al. 1996; see Chapter 13) also have a role. However, these scores are most useful for measuring change and evaluating outcomes. The occupational therapist's assessment needs to provide a wider range of information to guide the clinician.

When considering the content of an assessment, the pattern of movement used during activities should be considered and not just the range of motion. Many people with an arthritic glenohumeral joint that is becoming increasingly stiff and painful find the easiest way to maintain their daily activities is to increase their use of scapular movements. They may lift, or 'hitch' their shoulder, effectively using the whole shoulder girdle when attempting to raise their arm, in order to avoid pain and increase their reach. This movement can become a habit and may continue to be employed post operatively, instead of the original pattern of movement the surgery is trying to restore. Any treatment that is aiming to restore movement should initially focus on a 'normal' pattern of movement (Rubin and Kibler 2002), and only use the ability of the shoulder to compensate when further progress will not be made.

Most people will return to the ward from the operating theatre with their arm in some form of sling. The surgeon will guide the length of time the sling is used for. The postoperative protocol varies between surgeons and can be for as little as one day to as long as six weeks. The surgical approach used by the surgeon and the viability of muscle repairs are usually the highest influencing factors, though the use of bone graft, type of prosthesis and the stability of the joint are all important. Reading and understanding the operation notes is essential before commencing any interventions.

Acute phase rehabilitation

In the acute setting, the primary role for the occupational therapist will be to facilitate a safe and timely discharge. For most individuals, the priority will be to manage self-care tasks while their arm is immobilised in the sling. This starts with the person learning how to remove and reapply their sling. A useful technique is to employ the pendular position that is frequently used as part of an exercise regimen. The pendular position allows the arm to effectively hang away from the body and early movement to begin. By adopting a similar posture and using the thigh as a support for the elbow, the arm can be supported and access to the axilla is possible. The sling can be removed and applied in this position. It also provides an option for dressing and undressing the operated arm (Figure 5.3). This technique can be modified depending on the person's general level of fitness and function. It also provides the opportunity for the person to combine their physiotherapy exercises with a functional task as they begin gentle pendular movements for their glenohumeral joint and can also extend their elbow.

For people with multi-joint pathology, wearing a sling can have a negative effect on their wrist and elbow joints. It is important to be able to maintain the mobility in these joints as much as possible. This is especially important in the early postoperative stage, when bruising and oedema in the whole arm and hand can occur. If the pendular position is not appropriate, the person can support their forearm on a pillow placed on their lap while they complete self-care activities and remove and reapply their sling.

Bathing can be an issue if the sling must be retained at all times, unless a second sling can be provided so that one can be used specifically for bathing or showering. There is also the difficulty of accessing a bath and managing to wash one-handed. Provision of items such as a bath board and long handled sponge may provide solutions. One suggestion is to use of a towelling bathrobe, to help get dried after bathing, which will reduce the need to reach the back and opposite shoulder. Other aids such as long

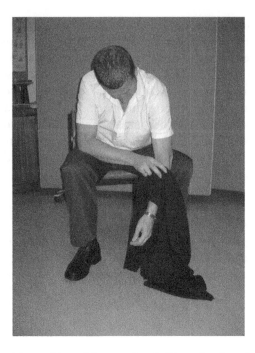

Figure 5.3 Using the pendular position while seated to facilitate dressing of the upper limb.

handled combs and dressing sticks also have their place while active movement is not allowed, but should be discouraged once the person moves into the rehabilitation phase.

Depending on their general level of function and the range of movement in their other joints, some people will not be able to manage their self-care independently while in a sling. If they live alone, they may need help from carers with their personal care and domestic tasks. An appropriate preoperative assessment should identify people who may have such difficulties, giving sufficient time for care to be arranged.

It is important to consider the person's mobility prior to discharge. Difficulties may arise due to the person needing to use their operated arm to hold their walking aid or push up from furniture for transfers. The sling holding their arm so close to their body may also affect their balance. Liaison with physiotherapy colleagues may produce solutions such as the use of alternative walking aids. Reviewing techniques and practice may make rising and sitting more manageable but if required, toilet and furniture raises should be considered.

Pain relief

Pain relief will clearly be an issue in the early postoperative phase and medication will play a major role in helping the person to manage their pain levels. The occupational therapist can also contribute to the pain management process by teaching the person what positions can promote comfort and sleep in sitting and in lying positions. If the shoulder is held or supported in a neutral position (Kelley 1995) that does not put strain on any of the structures of the surgical wound, pain can be minimised and comfort improved.

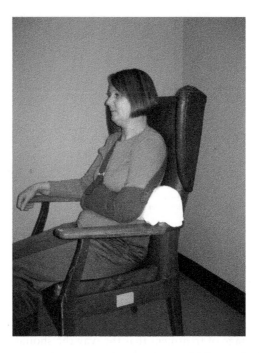

Figure 5.4 The elbow is supported to prevent the glenohumeral joint moving into extension whilst seated.

The ideal position will differ slightly between individuals, but is essentially with the shoulder in neutral or slight flexion, with the scapula allowed to relax and forearm supported. This position is quite easy to achieve in sitting, especially if wearing a sling. Some additional support behind the elbow will prevent the humerus moving into a more extended position, which can occur as people relax (Figure 5.4).

It is more difficult to maintain a good position when sleeping. Most people lie on their back post operatively, and if the elbow is allowed to rest on the bed, effectively in extension, the new humeral head is pushed anteriorly against the surgical wound. The use of a pillow or folded towel to support the elbow, holding the arm in neutral or in slight flexion, combined with ensuring that the scapula is free to relax onto the bed will promote a comfortable position (Figure 5.5). Once the early post operative period is over, should the person want to lie on their non-operated side, a support will again prevent the more extremes of movement, though in side lying this is likely to be protraction. A pillow placed behind the person will allow some movement during the night, but will discourage the person from lying on their affected shoulder. It can take a number of months before people feel able to lie on their operated shoulder again.

Long-term rehabilitation

Once the person is allowed to remove their sling and commence active movement, treatment can move to the long-term rehabilitation phase. Outpatient treatment should be based upon the individual's occupational needs at the same time as following the later stages of the postoperative protocol.

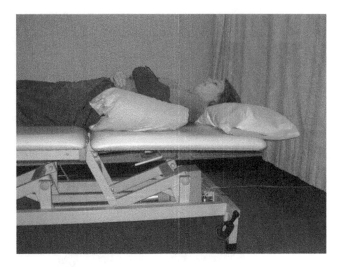

Figure 5.5 Sleeping – the upper arm is supported in the sling to position the glenohumeral joint in neutral in the scapular plane.

It is at this stage of treatment that the way the shoulder moves is as important as the range of movement achieved. People will be anxious to resume their daily tasks and may revert to a 'hitch' movement to compensate for their poor shoulder function. The occupational therapist has an important role to play in advising people regarding how much activity is appropriate as strength and stamina gradually return. Guidance on how to use an optimum movement pattern is also essential and can supplement a physiotherapy exercise programme. Activity analysis skills should be utilised when working with the person to establish what tasks they need to complete and how they will achieve this.

Shoulder impingement can be a problem following shoulder replacement, as the rotator cuff is weak and unable to work effectively to centralise the humeral head on the glenoid. Therefore, encouraging the person to use a movement pattern with the optimum amount of external rotation, maximising the subacromial space, is beneficial. This also has the additional benefit of working the external rotators in a functional way as an adjunct to any physiotherapy exercise. The combination of working through a pattern using external rotation and initiating movement at the glenohumeral joint, as opposed to with the scapula, will promote an optimum movement pattern during function. The person should be encouraged to use this movement pattern each time they move. Practical ideas such as putting notes up around the home in key positions as prompts, can be helpful.

In addition to working with the person to formulate a home programme using optimum movement patterns during daily tasks, treatment sessions utilising a range of occupational therapy treatment media may be used. Remedial games and other activities can be used to practise movements and strengthen muscles. However, in the early stages of rehabilitation when active movement against gravity is not possible or is still limited, but passive movement is being achieved, traditional occupational therapy rehabilitation equipment can be a useful aid to treatment.

The Overhead Balance Help Arm (OB help arm; Figure 5.6) is an example of a free-standing overhead frame that uses slings, a pulley system and counterbalance

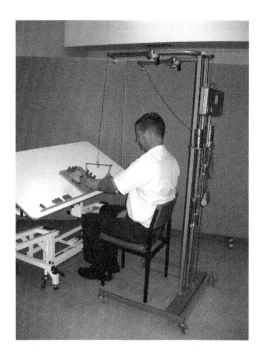

Figure 5.6 The counterbalance weight of the OB Help Arm promotes active assisted functional movement.

weights to allow the person to move their arm in an active assisted way through all planes of movement. Although not practical in a home environment, the OB help arm can be used in the outpatient setting in conjunction with a variety of activities (Turner 1981).

The weights provide a counterbalance to the weight of the arm and can be adjusted as treatment progresses. The system means the person is using active assisted movement, which physiotherapists may achieve by laying the person prone or by using the buoyant effect of water in hydrotherapy. The advantage of the OB help arm is that the person can sit or stand and practise movements and tasks such as reaching to their head. As the person's arm is supported in the slings, the occupational therapist has both hands free to demonstrate and guide movements using physical prompts. This particular model is no longer manufactured, but some occupational therapy departments have continued to use this useful item of equipment and its principles of treatment. Although Turner et al. (2002) describe the demise of some traditional rehabilitation equipment, the overhead sling support system still has a place in facilitating purposeful upper limb rehabilitation. Occupational therapists should ensure they remain up to date with the emerging computer aided rehabilitation technology that will inevitably replace the traditional mechanical equipment.

The use of a mirror so that the person is able to see their own movement pattern is also a useful tool. If they have an unaffected shoulder, they can complete a movement or task and then try to replicate the good movement with their operated arm. This can be especially useful if the person is having difficulty 'feeling' and differentiating between scapular and glenohumeral movement.

The OB help arm reduces the amount of strength needed to move, allowing the person to concentrate on gaining range of movement and controlling the movement pattern. If the occupational therapist does not have access to an OB help arm, some active assisted work is possible by choosing activities where the person can slide their hand over a surface. By the use of a cloth to prevent friction, a range of movements can be achieved, especially if a height adjustable table and a surface that can be positioned at an angle can be used. Simple activities such as rolling out some therapeutic putty are useful as a starting level activity. Working in elevation is harder to achieve and it may require some 'hands on' support from the occupational therapist to provide some of the strength required to lift the arm against gravity.

As external rotation is an essential component of any elevation of the arm, this must be a priority for rehabilitation. In isolation, external rotation is not a functional movement, but must be a key element in any rehabilitation programme. Another practical step in regaining movement is that flexion is easier to control and therefore quicker to gain than abduction and so should be worked on first. The therapist may have to continually educate their patient as to why certain movements need to be achieved first, to maximise the long-term outcome.

The later phases of rehabilitation should continue to be client centred. The focus will shift from the essential activities of daily living to those that bring a richness of experience to the person's life and may centre around family, work or leisure activities. At this stage of treatment, options such as the Baltimore Therapeutic Equipment (BTE; Figure 5.7) Work Simulator and the use of computer games such as the Wii can provide variety in the treatment programme. The BTE work simulator can be set to simulate a large range of tasks and becomes particularly useful when starting to build strength.

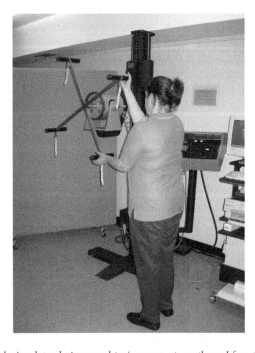

Figure 5.7 The BTE work simulator being used to improve strength and function.

The amount of force the person needs to apply can be graded by varying the amount of resistance required to move the chosen handle.

Strengthening work should only begin when the person has gained their optimum range of active movement and they have control of this movement. Guidance may be required from the consultant as to how much strength work is appropriate. This will vary between individuals depending upon their physical condition, their individual functional requirements and the surgery performed.

Computer games such as the Wii can be an excellent way to improve stamina, exercise tolerance and a smooth, co-ordinated movement pattern without adding resistance. The games chosen can provide a graded programme of movements and time spent exercising. The potential to continue such computer games, as part of a home programme, will be available to some people and advice should be given about appropriateness of the activities and the amount of time to be spent.

It is acknowledged, however, that the availability of resources will be the major influencing factor in how much occupational therapy in the outpatient setting can be provided.

Other shoulder conditions and procedures

Impingement

Impingement is one of the most frequently seen shoulder problems and in many cases can be treated simply (see Chapter 4). In cases where there is a mechanical component to the cause of the impingement and injection alone is not enough to break the cycle of impingement and inflammation, occupational therapy can provide a valuable treatment often in conjunction with physiotherapy.

Impingement is caused when the structures of the subacromial space are 'pinched' between the acromion and greater tuberosity of the humerus. Different movements of the arm change the size of the subacromial space, so if we can help the person to learn what these positions are and avoid them, the amount of impingement will decrease. As discussed in the section regarding the biomechanics of the shoulder, we know that at least 30° of external rotation is required to avoid impingement during elevation (Kelley 1995). We also know that the scapula needs to be in an optimum position and with some posterior tilt to raise the acromion (McClure et al. 2001). These two factors in combination will maximise the size of the subacromial space. If we can teach the person how to incorporate these movements into their daily tasks, they will minimise the amount of impingement caused.

Assessment and treatment

The occupational therapy assessment should begin with identifying the tasks the person completes during their day. A thorough activity analysis of each task, preferably by observing the person either actually performing it or through simulation, will give the therapist a clear picture of the person's usual movement patterns. It may be helpful to begin with the tasks that cause the person the most pain, though it is important that all tasks are covered. By working together, the person and the occupational therapist should identify achievable movement patterns using a good scapular position and the optimum amount of external rotation, they can use when completing their tasks.

Repetitive micro-trauma has been identified as a cause of impingement so every movement can be contributing to the problem. The person effectively needs to change their habitual movement patterns, which requires a large commitment from them. Treatment should therefore include education to help the person understand this aetiology and that every movement that they make could be contributing to their symptoms and not just those that immediately cause pain. To help start this process, treatment using simulated tasks or remedial activities using the optimum movement pattern may be appropriate as a large number of repetitions can be achieved. This approach to treating impingement very much puts the responsibility onto the person; the therapist's main role is to educate and then support and facilitate this process. A physiotherapy programme that aims to strengthen the external rotators and the stabilising muscles of the scapulae is also indicated to support this treatment approach.

Rotator cuff tears

The size and extent of rotator cuff tendon tears can vary greatly. The smallest would be a small area of damage to one surface of the tendon, a partial thickness tear, with a full thickness tear that is large and retracted at the other end of the scale. This can be a degenerative process, as part of the normal ageing process and in some people does not cause symptoms. However, for some people a rotator cuff tear can cause severe pain and muscle weakness and have a negative impact on their daily lives. In some instances the surgical option of a rotator cuff tendon repair is possible but the benefits of surgical repair are not clear.

A large multi-centre trial (UKUFF) hopes to identify which techniques are successful for the various clinical presentations of rotator cuff tears. If surgery is the treatment option chosen, the postoperative protocol usually dictates several weeks of immobilisation, followed by a graduated programme of physiotherapy, starting with active assisted movement. Treatment should aim to restore movement and an optimum movement pattern with strength work commencing when the tendon repair is well healed, possibly as late as three months after surgery. As with a shoulder replacement, occupational therapy can work alongside a physiotherapy programme to help the person regain the function of their operated shoulder. The use of the OB help arm can facilitate early active assisted functional movement when muscle weakness is still a barrier to using the arm for daily tasks. If facilities exist, a return to work programme may be indicated in the later stages of rehabilitation, especially if the person intends to return to a manual occupation. It can take as long as 12 months for the full benefits of a rotator cuff repair to be felt by the person.

Conservative treatment is usually the treatment of choice and research has shown the benefits of a deltoid strengthening programme for people with large irreparable tears (Ainsworth 2006). Anecdotal evidence from experienced therapists indicates that the treatment options advocated here for impingement can have benefits for people with small tears without severe symptoms. More commonly our role should be based on the compensatory approach to facilitate independence and the opportunity to return to or continue with work and leisure activities.

Instability

Instability is commonly divided into two categories: recurrent and traumatic. Recurrent instability following a traumatic dislocation or subluxation can be treated either conservatively or surgically. The majority of people who sustain this type of injury are young, as this is an injury often seen as a consequence of participating in sport. After treatment, they should be able to return to a very high level of function in a relatively short time and are unlikely to require the assistance of an occupational therapist.

The other group of people are those who have traumatic instability. This may be an element of a hypermobility syndrome or a collagen deficiency as seen in Ehlers–Danlos syndrome. Alternatively, the person may have specific problems with one shoulder and no specific medical diagnosis, just a much larger degree of laxity of the joint than the average person. Whatever the aetiology, these people are often described as having multi-directional instability (MDI). This in fact, is somewhat of a misnomer as while they may have laxity of the joint in multiple directions, they usually only have instability (the inability to maintain the normal congruence of the joint) in one. They may dislocate or sublux their glenohumeral joint during activity and some people can learn to do this as a party trick. Due to the joint laxity, they are usually able to relocate the humeral head themselves and indeed some people experience this dislocation and relocation on multiple occasions during one day.

A commonly seen feature of MDI is pseudo winging of the scapula, where the lateral border and inferior angle of the scapula lift off the chest wall rather than gliding around it during movement. If the person is not experiencing any pain or functional difficulties, it is suggested that no treatment is given, as this is normal movement for them. If treatment is required there are surgical options including a capsular shift or plication where some of the 'excess' joint capsule is tightened.

Treatment

Conservative treatment would be the first option. This traditionally consists of physiotherapy, although in specialist shoulder units occupational therapy forms part of the rehabilitation package. Treatment is based on the premise that although laxity is normal for that person, they have, for some reason, lost the normal control mechanisms and are using a different pattern of muscle activation when moving. The therapy aims to change the movement pattern used by the person (Kibler and McMullen 2003) to one that offers more control and stability and is based on the known 'normal' biomechanics of the shoulder.

The elbow

Biomechanics of the elbow

The elbow provides a key link in the chain of upper limb movement. The range of flexion and extension is large; full extension allows for carrying of heavy loads with the arm by the side and flexion means we can wash our face and feed ourselves. A classic study (Morrey et al. 1981) investigated the ranges of movement required to complete a range of daily activities. A range of 100° of elbow flexion (from 30° to 130°) and 100° of forearm rotation (50° of pronation and 50° of supination) allowed all of the activities attempted to be completed by the subjects.

This information is valuable when making decisions regarding what surgery to proceed with and what functional goals are achievable. If full movement is not going to be possible, the aim should be to provide movement within this functional range. If a splint is required after surgery, knowledge of this functional range of movement will also guide the surgeon and occupational therapist in their decision making regarding the position for the splint, especially if it is a static splint and is to be worn for an extended time. Stiffness in the mid range, although far from ideal, is preferable to having the elbow fixed into extension. Ankylosis in full extension is probably the most disabling of all elbow dysfunctions (Souter 1997).

The combination of supination and flexion is a commonly used movement pattern for self-care activities and so should be a priority in rehabilitation, as soon as the postoperative protocol allows. However, pronation with mid range flexion is essential for table and desktop activities such as kitchen tasks and office work, including computer use. If the person is unable to achieve this position, the compensatory movement most commonly utilised is elevation of the shoulder girdle and internal rotation of the humerus (Souter 1997). However, this is a difficult position to maintain as the shoulder will fatigue quickly and in reality it will not adequately provide the function required. It is therefore essential that a full assessment of the individual's functional goals is completed prior to the commencement of surgery and treatment, to establish realistic expectations for the person and plan the rehabilitation.

Elbow replacement

Total elbow replacement is not as widely performed a procedure as other joint replacements. It can provide excellent pain relief and improved function when used appropriately, most commonly for people with rheumatoid arthritis, osteoarthritis and following fracture around the joint. However, the very fact that the person having the surgery has multi-joint pathology brings issues for the person and the team. The person needs to be assessed and treated holistically and any other limitations taken into account when planning treatment.

As with all orthopaedic procedures, there can be a wide variation in postoperative protocols. These will depend on the prosthesis used, surgical approach, and the person's individual health and physical status. The occupational therapist's first responsibility is to become fully informed about the details of the surgery and the postoperative plan before moving on to their assessment of the individual.

Assessment

The occupational therapist must use a range of assessments prior to the commencement of a treatment programme. Goniometry is a useful tool for assessing flexion and extension, but supination and pronation can be harder to measure accurately. These biomechanical measurements are clearly an indicator of any progress but identifying the person's individual goals is essential. The therapist may prioritise an activity such as feeding, but the person may be more interested in personal grooming tasks such as shaving or applying their makeup.

Acute phase rehabilitation

Some form of immobilisation in the very early postoperative period is common; whether this is a sling, collar and cuff or a splint will be dependent on the postoperative protocol in use.

The main indication for immobilisation is to allow initial tissue healing. The surgical wound, situated posteriorly, is very vulnerable to infection as it is in an area where the skin is thin, often of poor quality and there is little tissue between it and the bone. It is immediately under tension as soon as there is any amount of flexion of the elbow joint. This close proximity of the joint to the skin increases the risk of a skin infection tracking to the joint, which is a serious complication. To limit this infection risk, some surgeons require that occupational therapy intervention to regain flexion be delayed until initial wound healing is complete. The occupational therapist may be required to splint the elbow in extension or a plaster back-slab may be used. As a general rule once the wound is healing, movement is encouraged but weightbearing and load carrying through the arm should usually be avoided until six weeks post operatively.

In common with other conditions, the occupational therapist's role in the acute setting will often be to facilitate a safe discharge, with any rehabilitation aimed at returning to a previous or higher level of function taking place on an outpatient basis. Exploring the person's needs on discharge will ideally have been initiated at the preoperative stage, but further assessment will be required as an inpatient following surgery. Once an assessment of the person's essential activities of daily living for discharge is completed, a programme of interventions can be agreed with the person.

One of the occupational therapist's main roles will be to teach the person one-handed techniques to help them maintain independence with daily activities, such as self-care, while their arm is immobilised. In some cases, dressing aids such as dressing sticks may be useful in the short term particularly if the person has pain or stiffness in other joints. Although using this compensatory approach may aid independence initially, the medium and long-term goals are around the person using their arm and new elbow joint to complete these tasks, and so dependence on them is discouraged.

Long-term rehabilitation

Once the period of immobilisation is complete and active rehabilitation has begun, there is much that occupational therapy can offer. Rehabilitation programmes based on the biomechanical frame of reference (Hagedorn 2002) are appropriate in the field of orthopaedics. They aim to improve function through maximising active range of movement, restoring a functional level of muscle strength and gaining an appropriate level of stamina and exercise tolerance.

One factor that can increase the difficulty in achieving this for people who have had an elbow replacement is that there is a lack of balance between the flexors and extensors of the joint (Morrey et al. 1981). Biceps and the other flexors are by necessity stronger than triceps as they have to work against gravity. Additionally, the surgical approach used during elbow replacement is posterior, involving the triceps to some extent and the surgical repair may need some protection. This combination of factors can often lead to people finding it easier to achieve flexion than extension. Some surgeons advocate the use of a night extension splint to help support the person in maintaining the extension gained during the day by preventing the flexed position that most people adopt during sleep.

While the initial emphasis may be on regaining flexion and extension of the elbow, the rotational movements must not be forgotten (Souter 1997). The amount of pronation and supination achieved in the forearm is dependent on both the elbow and wrist. If we accept that most people having an elbow replacement have rheumatoid arthritis and that the wrist joint is commonly affected by this disease they are likely to have a painful and stiff wrist. Wrist pain may limit the amount of exercise and activity the person can tolerate during rehabilitation of their elbow. If there are any limitations of movement at the wrist, improving rotation at the elbow by surgery may not be enough to improve the person's supination and pronation.

The occupational therapist has a range of treatment media available to them to assist a person regain movement, strength and stamina following an elbow replacement. A planned and guided programme of increased daily activities can give confidence to those who are anxious about overworking their new joint and limits for those who may wish to work too hard, too soon. Additionally, the traditional remedial activities used in hand therapy settings can be employed to practise and improve each of the ranges of motion and combine them into more functional movements.

Activities such as solitaire provide scope for practising a wide range of movements. For example, if the person passes the removed pieces to the therapist, the therapist can vary their hand position from near the person's head, axilla or ear. Another good example is bringing the hand to the mouth, flexion alone is not sufficient to feed oneself, there has also to be some supination; this can be simulated using the game pieces.

The level of pain relief and range of movement achieved following elbow replacement will cover a wide spectrum; the person themselves can only measure the success of the surgery. If they are able to return to the range of activities that bring them the quality of life they wish for, the surgery has had a successful outcome.

Other elbow procedures

Distal biceps repair

Ruptures of the distal biceps can be repaired surgically, but do involve the careful postoperative protection of the repair, common to other tendon repairs. Like other procedures, the postoperative care will vary according to surgical technique, surgeon's preference and the person's individual circumstances (Cheung et al. 2005).

A common approach is to use a hinged elbow brace that is progressively adjusted to allow an increasing range of movement over the first six weeks after surgery (Funk and Roney 2007). There are some preformed hinged elbow braces on the market, but a custom-made brace is likely to be used in most cases. This will require the occupational therapist to provide advice regarding activities of daily living while the brace is worn, as even though some minimal movement is allowed, the person will be limited and should not carry any loads in that arm. There will also be a requirement for outpatient appointments to monitor the fit of the brace, as the postoperative oedema settles, and adjustment to the hinge as more movement is allowed. Following removal of the brace, outpatient treatment to improve the range of movement and strength can be offered. The brace will have allowed flexion and extension but no more than a minimal amount of supination and pronation probably leading to some level of stiffness.

Treatment options include the use of the BTE work simulator and the FEPS (flexion, extension, pronation, supination) machine. They have functions for working on supination and pronation and are widely used by hand therapists. Occupational therapy workshops may also offer useful treatment media such as the use of a screwdriver, in particular, which requires a high level of forearm rotation. Return to previous levels of function will be the goal following this type of surgery and occupational therapy can provide work rehabilitation that may be required.

Elbow debridement or release

The problem of a stiff and painful elbow can be caused by a variety of conditions including osteoarthritis and following trauma. A debridement or release performed either arthroscopically or as an open procedure, can provide a level of pain relief and improvement in movement.

There are various surgical techniques described in the literature including the Outerbridge–Kashiwagi procedure (Forster et al. 2001), although rarely is the postoperative rehabilitation regimen given. This appears to be decided on by individual surgeons, based on their personal experience, but should be aimed at maximising movement and preventing the stiffness from reoccurring. Splinting, favoured by some surgeons (Funk and Roney 2007), should be combined with a physiotherapy mobilisation and exercise programme. An extension splint at night and a flexion splint for short periods during the day aim to maintain the full range of movement gained surgically. Close liaison is required between the occupational therapist and surgeon to ensure that the splints achieve the appropriate position and that the person will tolerate the wearing regimen.

Anecdotal evidence also tells us that some surgeons prefer the use of continuous passive motion (CPM) machines during the day in the acute postoperative period, sometimes combined with a splint at night. The CPM machine not only provides movement throughout the range of flexion and extension but also has a supination and pronation element. Occupational therapy outpatient treatment to maintain an active range of movement and increase strength and stamina may be offered if required. Once again, the therapist should work with the person to establish what their priority occupational needs are and plan a treatment programme accordingly. There are a variety of treatment media that can be used as described above for distal biceps repair.

Summary

The shoulder girdle plays a fascinating role in human functioning with its role in positioning the hand enabling us to undertake a vast range of movements and tasks. The combination of complex scapulohumeral rhythm, anatomy, wide range and planes of movement contribute to its instability. This complexity and range of presenting problems provides interest and challenge to the occupational therapist.

Research into all aspects of shoulder pathology and treatment has expanded rapidly in the past 15 years and will continue to do so as we strive to understand and manage shoulder disorders. The elbow seems, by comparison a much simpler joint and yet too has an essential role to play in our daily activities. If occupational therapists bring their wide range of skills to this clinical area, they can become specialists in this interesting field and provide a valuable contribution to the team management for people whose lives are affected by a shoulder or elbow condition.

References

Ainsworth, R. L. (2006). Physiotherapy in patients with massive, irreparable rotator cuff tears. *Musculoskeletal Care*, 4(3), 140–151.

Cheung, E. V., Lazarus, M., & Taranta, M. (2005). Immediate range of motion after distal biceps tendon repair. *Journal of Shoulder and Elbow Surgery*, 14(5), 516–518.

Conboy, V. B., Morris, R. W., Kiss, J., & Carr, A. J. (1996). An evaluation of the Constant-Murley shoulder assessment. *Journal of Bone and Joint Surgery, British Volume*, 78, 229–232.

Constant, C. R., & Murley, A. H. (1987). A clinical method of functional assessment of the shoulder. *Clinical Orthopaedics, 214*, 160–164.

Forster, M. C., Clark, D. I., & Lunn, P. G. (2001). Elbow osteoarthritis: prognostic indicators in ulnohumeral debridement, the Outerbridge–Kashiwagi procedure. *Journal of Shoulder and Elbow Surgery*, 10(6), 557–560.

Funk, L., & Roney, K. (2007). Distal biceps repair rehabilitation protocol. Online. Available at: www.shoulderdoc.co.uk (accessed October 2008).

Hagedorn, R. (2002). *Foundations for Practice in Occupational Therapy*. Churchill Livingstone.

Hudak, P., Amadio, P. C., Bombardier, C., & Upper Extremity Collaborative Group. (1996). Development of an upper extremity outcome measure: the DASH (Disabilities of the Arm, Shoulder, and Hand). *American Journal of Industrial Medicine, 29*, 602–608.

Kelley, M. J. (1995). Biomechanics of the shoulder. In M. J. Kelley & A. C. Clark (Eds). *Orthopaedic Therapy of the Shoulder*. Philadelphia: J.B. Lippincott.

McClure, P. W., Michener, L. A., Sennett, B. J., & Karduna, A. R. (2001). Direct 3-dimensional measurement of scapular kinematics during dynamic movements in vivo. *Journal of Shoulder and Elbow Surgery*, 10(3), 269–277.

Morrey, B. F., Askew, L. J., An, K. N., & Chao, E. Y. (1981). A biomechanical study of normal functional elbow motion. *Journal of Bone and Joint Surgery, American Volume*, 63, 872–877.

Rubin, B., & Kibler, W. B. (2002). Fundamental principles of shoulder rehabilitation: conservative to post operative management. *Arthroscopy, 18*(suppl), 29–39.

Souter, W. A. (1997). The contribution of the elbow joint to upper limb function. In S. Copeland, N. Gschwend & A. Landi (Eds). *Joint Stiffness of the Upper Limb*. London: Taylor and Francis.

Turner, A. (1981). *The Practice of Occupational Therapy: An Introduction to the Treatment of Physical Dysfunction*. Edinburgh: Churchill Livingstone.

Turner, A., Foster, M., & Johnson, S. E. (2002). *Occupational Therapy and Physical Dysfunction: Principles, Skills and Practice*. Edinburgh: Churchill Livingstone.

UKUFF Trial. *British Elbow and Shoulder Society*. Online. Available at: www.bess.org.uk (accessed October 2008).

Further reading

Dawson, J., Hill, G., Fitzpatrick, R., & Carr, A. (2001). The benefits of using patient-based methods of assessment: medium term results of an observational study of shoulder surgery. *Journal of Bone and Joint Surgery, British Volume, 83*, 877–882.

Gross, J., Fetto, J., & Rosen, E. (2002). *Musculoskeletal Examination*. Oxford: Blackwell Science.

Kibler, W. B., & McMullen, J. (2003). Scapular dyskinesis and its relation to shoulder pain. *Journal of the American Academy of Orthopaedic Surgeons, 11*, 142–152.

Morrey, B. F. (2000). *The Elbow and Its Disorders* (3rd edition). Edinburgh: Elsevier.

Chapter 6

Spinal conditions: management and occupational therapy

Heather McDowell

Introduction

This chapter explains basic treatment approaches for degenerative and progressive disorders of the spine in children and adults, including assessment, treatment and evaluation by occupational therapists.

The approaches can be grouped as follows:

- Education
- Rehabilitation
- Management
- Compensation.

A brief description, aetiology, overview of occupational therapy intervention and guidance for further reading is given for a range of disorders, loosely grouped according to the treatment approach (although some fit into more than one group). Spinal fractures are not covered within this book; persons presenting with a spinal fracture and no neurological impairment should have any functional problems addressed by the occupational therapist in the same way as any other injured person. Damage to the spinal cord as a result of accident and injury is outside the scope of this book and transfer to a specialist spinal injuries unit best meets these patients' rehabilitation needs.

What are we aiming for?

As the centre of the skeletal system, the spine is involved in all functional activities to provide mobility, stability and shock absorbency for effective head and limb movement. A healthy back requires a buffer of flexibility and strength in each plane of movement, beyond the demands of daily activities to enable it to cope with changes in routine and less frequent, more demanding tasks. This needs to extend to the shoulders, hips and ribs to be effective.

Damage to the spine is often cumulative so in activity analysis the frequency and duration of each task needs to be considered as much as the degree of strain or movement required. Deformities are often progressive. From experience, the key to good management of spinal conditions is to restore balance and reduce cumulative damage wherever possible. Sometimes this will require surgery and/or medication; for other individuals, a graded programme of activity is more effective and occupational therapy should be central to that programme.

Degenerative disorders of the spine

Degenerative disorders of the spine often start with disc problems. Degeneration starts soon after skeletal maturity is reached. Desiccation of the disc with age means less shock absorbency and flexibility in the spine, hence less of a buffer against damage.

Degenerative disorders that the occupational therapist is likely to see can be grouped as follows (Lucas 2000):

- Low back pain – acute
- Low back pain – chronic/recurrent
- Sciatic/radicular pain – herniated/prolapsed disc
- Stenosis
- Discitis
- Tumour/infection
- Low back pain.

Low back pain is defined as pain and discomfort, localised below the costal margin and above the inferior gluteal folds, with or without leg pain (van Tulder et al. 2004). Simple low back pain (i.e. without a specific pathology) is commonly divided into three sub-sets:

- Acute (lasting less than six weeks)
- Sub-acute (lasting 6–12 weeks)
- Chronic (lasting more than 12 weeks) (Lucas 2000).

These are arbitrary cut-off points on a continuum of pain and disability, but can be useful to occupational therapists when treating dysfunction caused by pain rather than a specific condition.

Acute low back pain is usually self-limiting (recovery rate 90% within six weeks) but 2–7% of people develop chronic pain. Recurrent and chronic pain accounts for 75–85% of total workers' absenteeism in Europe. Over 70% of people in industrialised countries report back pain at some point in their lifetime. This peaks between ages 35 and 55. Symptoms, pathology and radiological appearances do not always add up; about 85% will have no pathology or neurological encroachment. About 4% of people seen with low back pain in primary care in Europe have compression fractures, 1–3% per cent have a prolapsed intervertebral disc and 1% have a neoplasm. Ankylosing spondylitis and spinal infections are rarer.

Risk factors for back pain are poorly understood. The most frequently reported are heavy physical work, frequent bending, twisting, lifting, pulling and pushing, repetitive work, static postures and vibrations. Psychosocial risk factors include stress, distress, anxiety, depression, cognitive dysfunction, pain behaviour and job dissatisfaction (van Tulder et al. 2004).

'Red flags' are risk factors associated with serious disorders causing low back pain. If any of these come to light during the occupational therapist's interaction with the individual, they should be reported back to the referring physician for further investigation. Red flags (van Tulder et al. 2004) include:

- Age of onset less than 20 years or more than 55 years
- Recent history of violent trauma
- Constant progressive, non-mechanical pain (no relief with bed rest)
- Thoracic pain
- Past medical history of malignant tumour
- Prolonged use of corticosteroids
- Drug abuse
- Immunosuppression, human immunodeficiency virus (HIV) infection
- Systemically unwell
- Unexplained weight loss
- Widespread neurological symptoms (including bladder or bowel dysfunction)
- Structural deformity
- Fever.

'Yellow flags' are psychosocial factors that increase the risk of developing, or perpetuating chronic pain and long-term disability, including work-loss associated with low back pain. Screening for 'yellow flags' should occur early in the person's journey and be repeated if the individual is not responding to treatment. Examples of 'yellow flags' are (adapted from van Tulder et al. 2004):

- Negative attitudes and beliefs about back pain (e.g. belief that back pain is harmful or potentially severely disabling or high expectation of passive treatments rather than a belief that active participation will help)
- Excessive pain behaviour (e.g. fear-avoidance behaviour and reduced activity levels)
- Work related problems or compensation issues (e.g. poor work satisfaction)
- Emotional problems (e.g. depression, anxiety, stress, tendency to low mood and withdrawal from social interaction).

Acute and sub-acute low back pain

Assessment of this client group is likely to be limited to screening for selection criteria, which should exclude red flags, obvious yellow flags and pain lasting longer than six weeks. The aims of treatment for acute low back pain are:

- To relieve pain
- To improve functional ability
- To prevent recurrence and chronicity (van Tulder et al. 2004).

    Relevant outcomes for acute low back pain are:

- Pain intensity
- Overall improvement

- Back pain specific functional status
- Impact on employment
- Generic functional status
- Medication use.

Education

The individual needs adequate information and reassurance, along with regular medication (e.g. simple analgesia or non-steroidal anti-inflammatory drugs) in order not to take bed rest but to continue normal daily activities and work. This can be provided in a 'back school', probably in conjunction with a physiotherapist, involving a session or series of group demonstrations, illustrated talks, discussion and handouts to a group of people and should include the topics listed below under 'Rehabilitation'.

In the UK, the Health and Safety Executive produces some excellent leaflets on reducing risks, illness and injury in all kinds of work, of particular interest for this client group: 'Working with VDUs', 'Getting to grips with manual handling', 'Handling the news' (also about manual handling) 'Understanding Ergonomics'. These are available at: www.hse.gov.uk/pubns/leaflets.htm (accessed 27 February 2008).

Rehabilitation or management?

If the individual has been off work for four to eight weeks or has been referred two to 12 months post surgery, rehabilitation programmes offer a more supportive route back to normal routines than a back school and may be offered as closed groups, rolling groups or one to one sessions.

Chronic low back pain covers a wide range of levels of impairment, disability and duration. Chronic problems are multidimensional therefore treatment approaches need to be comprehensive, flexible and consistent. It is vital that all members of the treatment team, the individual and significant others are 'onside' (Airaksinen et al. 2004). The person's expectations of the outcome need to be managed as part of a multi-disciplinary pre-admission assessment for a treatment programme. In the absence of yellow flags, a rehabilitation programme is likely to be effective, with elements such as goal setting, pacing and relaxation techniques added for participants to use as required. In rehabilitation, the person may expect physical gains – strength, range of movement, overall task performance and reduction of pain. In a management programme, gaining some control over pain and activity cycles and being able to fulfil desired roles should be the priority.

For chronic pain management, systematic reviews and international guidelines support the use of cognitive behavioural therapy, supervised exercise therapy, brief educational interventions, and bio-psycho-social treatment but note that the effects of any treatment are likely to be small when the client group is considered as a whole (Airaksinen et al. 2004). However, the author and colleagues at other pain management programmes have observed significant improvements in quality of life for many individuals.

Back schools and short courses of manipulation/mobilisation produced only short-term improvement for such complex conditions. Transcutaneous nerve stimulation (TENS) and physical therapies (heat/cold, traction, laser, ultrasound, short wave, interferential, massage, corsets) have not been proven to be effective (Airaksinen et al. 2004).

Assessment and goal setting

Functional goals should be agreed as part of an initial interview with the person and the rest of the multi-disciplinary team. In order to break down activities for themselves, SMART (specific, measurable, agreed, realistic and time limited) goal setting can be taught and practised on the programme, using the person's own examples. Goal setting as an intervention has been shown to be effective where lifestyle change is the main outcome of treatment.

In a cohesive, client-centred, multi-disciplinary team, any member of the team can set goals with the person on behalf of the others if trained in the use of a tool such as Goal Attainment Scaling (GAS) (Becker et al. 2000; Kiresuk et al. 1993). For a multi-dimensional treatment programme, between three and five goals would be appropriate. Progress on the goals is assessed through discussion with the person, e.g. at the end of the programme and at follow-ups.

The occupational therapist makes a baseline assessment of function appropriate to the goals. A multi-dimensional assessment tool such as the Assessment of Motor and Process Skills (www.amps-uk.com) or Valpar VCWS9 or VCWS19 (www.valparint. com) can be used if a standardised assessment tool is required. Otherwise, the use of video can be a very effective tool in demonstrating change to the person over a period of time and is quick to administer. However, the occupational therapist must remember to obtain written consent.

A simple sequence could include:

- Walking 5 m to a chair
- Sitting down
- Taking off shoes
- Getting up
- Walking up and down a small set of steps
- Reaching down to a low shelf to pick up an object to waist height and then shoulder height
- Returning to the chair to put shoes on.

Any activities relevant to the individual's goals may be substituted. If the patient is being weaned off a corset, orthosis or walking aids, the occupational therapist should review dynamic and static postures, in sitting, standing and mobilising, with and without the aids.

Treatment

The treatment plan will depend on the person's goals but group education, supported by functional activity should include the following elements:

- **Normal movement** – Individuals are encouraged to graduate from adaptive equipment and return to normal movements as soon as appropriate after injury or surgery (timescales will need to be checked with the referring physician/surgeon), even if this means an increase in pain in the short term. The person can be encouraged to manage this with appropriate analgesia/anti-inflammatory, relaxation and breathing techniques and pacing (see below).

- **Posture and core stability** – Adjustments to seating and standing positions should be made to encourage neutral lordosis and kyphosis and lateral symmetry and enable efficient head and limb movements appropriate to the task. The occupational therapist should check that strong muscle groups (such as psoas, levator scapulae, upper trapezius and the dominant arm) are not compensating for weaker muscle groups or creating asymmetry in posture. An individual core stability programme should be incorporated into daily activities. The use of a variety of shaped back cushions, seat wedges, gym balls, perching stools and office chairs to provide a balance of rest and activity for all muscle groups is recommended. Leaflets and fact sheets are available to download with clear diagrams and tips on improving posture for seated work tasks (Advance Seating designs 2002/2003). A simple internet search will produce a wide range of companies supplying cushions.

- **Sleep posture** – The same principles apply as for other postures. The mattress needs to be firm enough to support the body without sagging but soft enough to mould to the contours of the body supporting the spine in the optimal shape. Pillows can be found which accommodate both side lying and supine while keeping the cervical spine neutral. A pillow between the knees in side lying or under the knees in supine can position the spine to relieve some people's pain while asleep. Materials may vary according to personal comfort. The need for these supports may reduce as the individual becomes fitter.

- **Manual handling** – Individuals should be prompted to use core muscle groups, quadriceps and gluteals to support and carry out tasks. (see the Health and Safety Executive leaflets, p 95). For high functioning individuals, the occupational therapist can encourage the individual to try carrying out some tasks with a mobile base of support such as seated on a gym ball or standing on a wobble board.

- **Stretches** – Loss of mobility (including surgical fusion) in the spinal column or one section of it, places extra strain on surrounding structures. During an unusual task (or after many repetitions of a familiar task) damage is likely to occur at the weakest point, so a stretch programme needs to be started gradually, especially for post-surgical patients. With the physiotherapist, the occupational therapist will ensure that the patient is stretching with optimum intensity and time limits for their needs and is achieving a balanced programme over each day. The occupational therapist should familiarise themselves with a global programme of stretches. Some of these can be incorporated into everyday activities, particularly during self-care (e.g. put socks on by placing the ankle on the opposite knee, instead of bending down to the foot) or used as essential breaks during static tasks (e.g. neck movements as a break from using a visual display unit.) Once tasks have been practised in a supervised functional setting, an individual home programme can be set up.

- **Pacing** – The aim of pacing is to even out the cycle of over and under-activity experienced by people with chronic pain. Repetitive or static tasks need to be time limited (a stopwatch or egg timer can be used), built up gradually, sometimes starting with as little as a few seconds if the posture is difficult or painful to maintain and alternated with other tasks. In general, the individual should start with two minutes activity with correct posture and two minutes in a good resting position, i.e. one which is not contraindicated. The furniture may need to be moved around to facilitate this. Twenty minutes is a generally accepted target for repetitive work tasks and once this is achieved the individual is likely to be able to continue the programme themselves.

- **Stress management:** Stress is a significant factor in the way pain is experienced. Encouraging the individual to identify stressors and gain some control over these is likely to assist their progress. Achieving balance between life roles is an important element of occupational therapy intervention.
- **Return to work:** Occupational therapists have a key responsibility in supporting people back towards work (College of Occupational Therapists (COT) and National Social Inclusion Programme (NSIP) 2007). People need to explore their rights and options for return to work in conjunction with their employer (if they have one), JobCentre Plus and charities such as the Shaw Trust in the UK. For many people, a programme focused on return to work seems more relevant than a medical model.

Try reading this section again, this time assuming you are seeing the person only in their work environment. Is there anything that suddenly becomes irrelevant? Are there sections which make more sense? What implications does this have for your practice as a whole? For more information, see the references and further reading list at the end of this chapter.

Evaluation and discharge

At the end of the rehabilitation or pain management programme, discharge goals should be set and follow-up planned. At follow-up (e.g. at three months, six months, one year and two years), the occupational therapist will be repeating baseline assessments, reviewing the goals, providing positive reinforcement for goals achieved and offering coaching points and encouragement, reframing or re-grading goals not achieved.

Other conditions that may benefit from rehabilitative or management approaches

Coccydynia

Coccydynia is chronic pain of the coccyx, without significant effect on the surrounding structures. It is exacerbated by sitting, and may be caused by coccygeal instability in sitting with hypermobility (greater than 25°) or subluxation (Maigne et al. 2000a). Causes include (Maigne et al. 2000b):

- Trauma
- Childbirth
- Obesity
- Idiopathic.

There is no universal treatment protocol, but non-steroidal anti-inflammatory drugs, steroid injections and coccygectomy (high rate of infection) are the three main treatments (Hodges et al. 2004). Manipulation is still considered to be experimental (Maigne and Chatellier 2001).

People referred to occupational therapy should be assessed holistically and a judgement made about what type of treatment approach will fit the duration of condition and functional deficits of the individual.

Osteoarthritis

Osteoarthritis can be considered more of a process than a disease, involving loss of the articular cartilage in synovial joints and growth of bony spurs or nodules in response. This leads to a cycle of pain in the joints, reduced activity, loss of range of movement and muscle weakness. In the spine, bony spurs can cause spinal stenosis (see below).

Osteoarthritis is frequently a secondary process to developmental deformity, trauma, obesity or sepsis. Genetic factors play a strong part in the development of primary osteoarthritis. In addition to the lumbar spine, the hip, knee and distal interphalangeal joints of the fingers are commonly affected (Williamson and Wordsworth 2000).

Occupational therapy management needs to be person centred in order to be effective. In a functional activity programme, tasks involving (mostly isometric) strengthening and non-weightbearing range should be used, as cartilage wear is accelerated by repetitive ranging and weightbearing exercise. A rehabilitative approach (see above) should be encouraged in preference to compensatory strategies (see below) as the benefits are likely to be broader and longer lasting. However, if the person is awaiting surgery (or trying to delay surgery) and wants to increase their independence in the short term or is unable to carry out an exercise programme for any reason, adaptive equipment may meet these requirements. A rehabilitative approach could be introduced at a later date.

Rheumatoid arthritis

Eighty per cent of individuals with rheumatoid arthritis have involvement at C1–2 (Whitesides 2000). Destruction of the transverse ligaments leads to anterior subluxation and destruction of the vertebral arches and facet joints, which can lead to compromise of nerve roots and spinal cord. The occupational therapist should be vigilant for signs of cervical nerve root and cord compression (such as paraesthesia in limbs or bladder/bowel dysfunction) and should not assume that clumsiness is as a result of disease in the limbs.

Decompression and spinal fusion at this level may be supported by a hard collar for eight weeks or more and compensatory strategies (see below) will be needed during this phase. A rehabilitative approach (see above) can be a positive step when the disease is in remission, but joint protection principles, appropriate use of adaptive equipment and splints need to be incorporated into the regimen. Pain management strategies (see above) need to be used during flare-ups.

Ankylosing spondylitis

Ankylosing spondylitis is an inflammatory disease of the spine and pelvis, which progresses from the sacroiliac joints upwards. Ossification leads to fusion between the vertebrae and costovertebral joints, limiting chest expansion. The bone becomes osteopenic, therefore the individual is at risk of fractures from falls. Exaggerated kyphosis is common, along with shoulder and hip involvement. As with other progressive spinal deformities, exercise and orthotics are ineffective at preventing progression (Whitesides 2000), although participation in exercise programmes does contribute to the 'buffer' of strength and flexibility and can be an advantage in general health and post-surgery rehabilitation (see above).

Total hip replacements (see Chapter 2) are used to release fixed flexion deformities and wedge osteotomies of the vertebrae can correct up to 60% kyphosis, which may be treated as per spinal fusions (see below), taking into account individual factors for each person. The individual may also experience symptoms and bony changes in the hands.

Osteoporosis

Apart from falls, multiple compression fractures in the vertebrae often occur insidiously as a result of this condition. This leads to a range of symptoms similar to other degenerative conditions: no symptoms; pain due to muscle spasm; pain and/or loss of neurology with nerve root or spinal cord compression and deformity, normally a kyphosis.

Depending on co-morbidity (a significant factor in this older client group) and bone quality, surgical methods, described later in this chapter, may be employed to relieve symptoms otherwise treatment will be conservative.

Severe kyphosis may impair lung function and it may be appropriate to perform a release and fusion to correct this as per scoliosis. The risks in this client group, however, will be much higher for any surgery and the period of recovery likely to be longer. The occupational therapist may be able to offer assessment and advice about current and desired functional levels and, in conjunction with the multi-disciplinary team, look at non-surgical ways of meeting these goals, giving the patient more choice about their treatment.

Whether surgery is indicated or not, a goal-centred rehabilitative approach is needed to gradually restore confidence and independence in valued activities. Wherever possible, the person should be encouraged to use appropriate regular analgesia and any recommended brace or corset to increase mobility and engage in functional tasks, rather than staying on bed rest after an acute exacerbation of symptoms. The techniques described earlier in this chapter for pain management can also be used to manage poor respiratory function and ergonomic principles can be adapted for severe deformities. Delegation of the riskiest tasks (those involving risk of falling, lifting, twisting and impact) is advisable unless bone density improves through exercise or drug therapy.

Sciatic/radicular pain

Prolapsed/herniated intervertebral disc

This is defined as bulging of the nucleus pulposus through the annulus of the intervertebral disc. Symptoms are likely to be caused by impingement of nerve roots or spinal cord and will indicate the level of the lesion. Symptoms may persist even after apparently successful surgical removal of the protrusion (discectomy – see p 102). This is thought to be due to nerve memory or scar tissue but in many cases the symptoms may not appear to correlate with the physical findings. Some individuals also seem to have higher levels of pain chemistry than others.

Spinal stenosis/neurogenic claudication

Spinal stenosis refers to narrowing of the spinal canal, nerve root canal or intervertebral foramen within the spine due to bone overgrowth, normally at the facet joint, sufficient to cause spinal cord or nerve root symptoms. There may also be hypertrophy of the lamina and soft tissue, including the ligamentum flavum and capsule of the facet joint. It is common in people over the age of 60, experienced at L4/5 or diffused along the spine. It may be of congenital origin, especially in individuals with achondroplasia or the end result of degenerative changes, e.g. spondylolysis or scoliosis.

Spinal stenosis may be called neurogenic claudication as the pain can be mistaken for vascular claudication. It can be differentiated from vascular claudication as these persons find relief from standing still, whereas neurogenic claudication is more likely to be relieved by sitting or stooping. The cauda equina is more susceptible to compression due to the lack of myelin sheathes.

To relieve symptoms, surgical decompression is required via laminectomy or foraminotomy if there is no deformity or instability present. Otherwise correction and spinal fusion will be required. Discectomies normally increase problems by creating instability. See pages 106–7 for occupational therapy intervention for laminectomy and spinal fusion (Lucas 2000).

Spinal tumour

The majority of spinal cord tumours are extrinsic and benign. For example, a neurofibroma, for which nerve root pain is an early symptom, has a good prognosis if surgically removed (Matthews 2003). Rehabilitation is as per an incomplete spinal cord injury.

Malignant tumours are most commonly metastatic lesions in the vertebral body from lung, breast or prostate primaries. Treatment is likely to include large doses of chemotherapy (e.g. dexamethasone), localisation and staging (assessment of size and state) of the tumour, then radiotherapy. Radical surgery to remove the lesion normally has only temporary success. These individuals present with back pain rather than paraesthesia or nerve root pain. Occupational therapy treatment is as per spinal fusion if the lesion is removed and the vertebrae reconstructed. The occupational therapist will also need to take into consideration the fact that this is a cancer, involving pain, co-morbidity (e.g. other tumour sites), fatigue (which can vary from hour to hour), malaise (often depending on chemotherapy cycles), different prognoses and often a fragile psychological state of the individual and carers.

Spinal infections

Spinal infections have high potential for morbidity and mortality therefore they need prompt diagnosis and treatment (Reiter and Heller 2000). The team need to know whether bacteria or mycobacteria or a fungus is responsible, which structures are affected (vertebral bodies, discs, epidural or soft tissues), the route of infection and the age of individual.

- **Osteomyelitis** – Most commonly from methicillin resistant *Staphylococcus aureus* (MRSA) infection. Pain is unrelated to activity. Associated with fever and feeling unwell. The rehabilitative occupational therapy approach should be taken once the individual is off bed rest.
- **Epidural abscess** – This is a surgical emergency. The site is debrided, decompressed and reconstructed with bone graft or instrumentation. Occupational therapy treatment is as per spinal fusion.
- **Postoperative infection** – Occupational therapy treatment will depend on the type of surgery undertaken.
- **Tuberculosis/Potts disease** – Immunosuppressed individuals are most at risk and barrier nursing is essential. Neurological problems are more likely with tuberculosis than other spinal infections. Abscesses are formed slower than with *Staphylococcus aureus* infection, but more bone is destroyed. The individual may or may not feel unwell. Many clinical signs are similar to other infections, therefore an aspiration biopsy is required to differentiate. Immobilisation may be required to halt the spread of infection throughout the body, and therefore a compensatory occupational therapy approach should be used. Surgery will be required if the neurological problems worsen. This consists of debridement, decompression and reconstruction. Occupational therapy intervention is as per spinal fusion.

Decompression

Decompression surgery refers to the restoration of normal spaces for spinal cord and nerve roots to pass through. The foramen may have become narrowed by abnormal growth of bone, tumour, or scar tissue and may be restored by removal of the growth and no specific occupational therapy treatment is required. However, if the spinal cord or nerve roots are at risk due to collapse of a vertebral structure, this will normally need to be supported with instrumentation and/or bone grafts, resulting in fusion of two or more vertebrae and should therefore be treated as a spinal fusion.

Discectomy

Discectomy involves the removal of a part or whole of the intervertebral disc from between the vertebrae to remove impingement on the nerve root or spinal cord. Advice should be taken from the surgeon regarding postoperative precautions. These are normally not essential, but may be useful for pain relief and to help reduce muscle spasm during the initial postoperative phase, leading to better compliance with exercise programmes, normal movements and better outcomes.

If the reason for the disc prolapse was occupational, education to prevent recurrence is advisable. See pages 94–5 on acute low back pain.

Better results have been obtained from microdiscectomy; the same surgery through a much smaller incision or two small incisions, reducing damage to soft tissue. It is possible for the hernia to reoccur following partial discectomy due to the loss of integrity of the disc.

Laminectomy

This refers to the removal of the lamina and spinous process from a vertebra, leaving the body and transverse processes intact. This removes pressure on the spinal cord and nerve roots. A laminotomy leaves the spinous process intact and just makes a hole in the lamina leaving the muscle and ligament attachments intact, allowing earlier return to normal activities. Post operative precautions are not normally recommended for a straightforward laminectomy.

Prosthetic intervertebral disc replacement

Artificial intervertebral discs consist of two metallic endplates separated by a more pliable inner core. The implantation of the prosthetic discs involves a major operation through an incision below the umbilicus. The diseased disc is partially or fully excised (depending on the prosthesis used). The vertebral endplates and surrounding spinal ligaments are preserved and help to maintain implant stability. Single or multiple discs can be replaced during the same operation (National Institute for Clinical Excellence (NICE) 2004).

NICE (2005a) advises that lumbar prosthetic intervertebral disc replacement (PIDR) is a viable alternative to discectomy and spinal fusion in persons with herniated intervertebral disc, degenerative disc disease, post-laminectomy syndrome or back pain, which has not responded to conservative treatment for more than six months. Cervical PIDR is indicated for acute disc herniation or cervical spondylosis as an alternative to discectomy, with or without fusion, as fusion of one segment causes increased strain at consecutive segments and further fusions being required in the future. By replacing the disc with a biomechanically similar prosthesis, the aim is to maintain proper kinematics and load sharing properties and reduce the need for further intervention (NICE 2005b). The main limitation of this procedure is the level of expertise required for an anterior approach to the spine as most of the traditional procedures would take a more straightforward posterior approach.

NICE encourages the collection of long-term safety and efficacy evidence as data are currently only available for two to three years. In the studies reviewed by the author, no postoperative restrictions were placed on the individuals and they were encouraged to return gradually to daily activities on discharge. The outcome measures used in studies to date have been variable in validity, reliability and relevance to functional status. This should encourage occupational therapists to get involved in studies, providing relevant, standardised, functional outcome measures to compare multi-disciplinary treatment including PIDR versus traditional and conservative treatments.

Spondylolysis

This is disruption in the vertebral arch at the inferior/superior interarticular surface (pars interarticularis), sometimes due to a stress fracture from hyperextension in children and adolescents (Emans 2000). The reported incidence of symptomatic defects is much higher in young athletes than the general population. Treatment depends on severity of symptoms and the sporting activity.

Conservative treatment may include cessation of sport and restriction of other activities, with or without bracing and core stability exercises. Surgery is reserved for those who do not respond to conservative treatment. It involves fusion of the fractured elements of the vertebra, using screws or wires, but as it does not require fusion of more than one segment, movement is preserved. Occupational therapy management is therefore likely to be minimal. Success rates were difficult to compare in the studies reviewed, as they used small sample sizes, athletes (practising different sports) versus general population and postoperative regimens used any combination of the conservative treatment methods. Compensatory strategies may be useful for some people if braced (Debnath et al. 2003; Iwamoto et al. 2004).

Spondylolisthesis

Spondylolisthesis describes the displacement of one vertebra on top of another, which develops gradually rather than being present at birth. It can be genetic, developmental, of unknown cause or from the traumatic rupture of connective tissue, with the risk of damage to the spinal cord or nerve roots. If asymptomatic, strengthening of core muscles and using good lifting and bending techniques will be beneficial as for a 'normal' back (see 'back school', p 95). If the condition is symptomatic and progressing or there is greater than 50% slip, surgical correction and fusion of the two vertebrae is required (Emans 2000). See below for occupational therapy management of spinal fusion.

Scoliosis

Scoliosis is a curvature of the spine in the coronal plane. Axial rotation, translational deformity and excessive kyphosis and lordosis of the spine may combine with scoliosis to produce complex spinal deformities. The changes may be of unknown cause (idiopathic), as with many adolescent cases or may be attributed to malformation of a vertebra as an embryo, muscle tone imbalance, such as in cerebral palsy or lack of muscle strength against gravity as in muscular dystrophy.

Many deformities deteriorate with growth but some spontaneously improve. Untreated, severe spinal deformity can lead to pain, difficulty with sitting balance, respiratory problems and even spinal cord impingement as well as cosmetic distortion which can have a significant psychological impact on adolescents and young adults.

Curves are described by their aetiology, direction, apex and Cobb's angle (formed between the top of the uppermost tilted vertebra in a curve and the bottom of the lowermost tilted vertebra) as these elements will inform treatment decisions. Curves will tend to progress quickest during a growth spurt, which starts about a year after menarche or voice breaking, and children will be closely monitored from this time until they reach skeletal maturity to choose the best time for surgery. Thoraco-lumbar spinal orthoses (TLSOs) may be used to slow down progression of mild curves and support but have limited effectiveness depending on the size, shape and compliance of the wearer and have little corrective effect on fixed curves.

If the curve is causing significant functional problems, spinal fusion surgery is likely to be indicated and the occupational therapy should use compensatory strategies (see below).

Spinal fusion

The purpose of spinal fusion is to restore symmetry and strength to the spinal column. However, by fusing two or more vertebrae into a solid column, the flexibility of that section of the spine will be lost and more strain placed on the movable joints either side of the fusion.

If only two vertebrae are to be fused, for example to correct a spondylolisthesis at L4/5, the joints at L3/4 and L5/S1 and beyond will have to flex and twist more to enable the individual to bend to tie their laces. If a whole section from S1 to T2 is to be fused, we may expect that the individual will have to become much more flexible at the hips and shoulder girdle to reach their feet. We should also expect the shock absorbing properties of the spine to be diminished in proportion to the size of fusion, so high impact activities, such as horse riding would be less tolerable the more vertebrae were involved.

Compensatory strategies

Adaptive equipment and techniques compensate for temporary or permanent loss of range of motion and strength. They can be helpful in protecting spinal structures immediately post surgery to allow fusion to occur (this takes from about three months in early childhood to 12 months or longer in adulthood) and to avoid exacerbating inflammation, muscle spasm and spread of infection. Some surgeons will be confident enough in the instrumentation, bone quality and compliance of the person not to impose restrictions on movements 'as long as you are careful', however, people often need help to interpret this and equipment can offer reassurance. Others may be placed in plaster jackets or orthoses and need these strategies to retain independence during this phase.

Assessment

Occupational therapy assessment for elective surgery should commence before admission. This should include a holistic initial interview and an outline of possible restrictions with adequate time to allow the person and carers to prepare for admission.

Intervention

It is important that only the necessary postoperative restrictions are applied, maintaining quality of life, strength and flexibility as far as possible. The frequency and duration of each task should be taken into account as much as the degree of strain or movement required, as damage to the spine can be cumulative.

Written guidelines (patient information leaflets) with clear illustrations offer a valuable starting point for explanations, which can be customised for the individual with some 'fill in the blanks' sections. These need to be age appropriate with discretion shown for sections on work, driving and sex for young people. The surgeon needs to advise when they may recommence more demanding activities. As the rate of healing is dependent on many individual factors, people should be advised to wait until their follow-up appointments with the surgeon where it can be checked through radiographs, rather than making early predictions. If they are having difficulty resuming daily activities or returning to work, a referral for a rehabilitation programme is indicated (see above).

If the person has multiple disabilities the occupational therapist is likely to be the main person liaising with the individual's key worker in the community as well as the person, parents, and carers who will be providing care immediately on discharge to set goals for occupational therapy intervention. For an example of best practice in communication see the Complex Disability Exemplar, National Service Framework for Children, Young People and Maternity Services (Department of Health 2005).

Short-term goals for this complex client group are likely to be minimising disruption to daily activities in activities of daily living, vocation/study and leisure. Long-term goals could be improving posture for respiration, feeding and communication to improve quality of life in all areas. Manual handling, positioning in bed and wheelchair/ other seating, toileting, bathing, washing hair, feeding, accessing transport, and school and other outings may all be affected by the fusion process.

In order to protect the fusion, carers will need to handle the person, supporting their spine as a single fused shape – log rolling to carry out self-care activities and position hoist slings. The sling should support the weight through the ischial tuberosities, sacrum and spine as a whole, including head support, with the hips no more than 90° flexed, rather than creating a curved 'hammock' shape with pressure under the thighs and shoulders. The position and length of straps as well as the size of the sling is important in achieving this. Battens to stiffen the sling are also useful. Unless the occupational therapist has significant experience with assessment for hoist equipment, it can be helpful to ask a renowned company for a demonstration/assessment with the individual. If in doubt between two sizes of sling, the smaller size should be used, or a custom-made sling chosen depending on availability of funding.

Special seating systems where a custom moulded seat is attached to a powered or attendant propelled base will need to be adjusted to suit the new shape of the spine and early review by the area Special Seating Service is recommended. Temporary provision of a manual reclining wheelchair with adequate lateral and head support allows graded sitting tolerance at different angles prior to sitting in their own chair.

Case study 6.1

Diagnosis – Spinal fusion

Ellie – female, aged 15 years

Ellie lives with her parents and younger brother in a two-storey house and attends mainstream school. Her mother first noticed a slight rib hump when, aged 11, Ellie was getting changed for ballet class. Following diagnosis with adolescent idiopathic scoliosis, she has been monitored by the orthopaedic surgeon and, due to the recent progression of the curve, the decision is taken to carry out a spinal fusion.

Six weeks prior to surgery, Ellie is sent a patient information booklet and a form to complete the heights of her furniture and lower leg length (42 cm), which she returns to the occupational therapy department. From these measurements, the occupational therapist can see that her bed and toilet are too low (both 40 cm) but there is a chair of suitable height (47 cm). On contacting the family, they decide that Ellie can swap beds with her brother in the short term as his bed is 50 cm high. The occupational therapist advises that they will loan out a raised toilet seat to use at home and gives more direction on how to measure the bath for a bath board.

On admission, consent for occupational therapy intervention is confirmed and the remainder of the initial interview is conducted on postoperative day two with Ellie's mother present. Questions are answered, prompted by the patient information sheet, in particular with regard to not being able to take the bus or cycle for six months and being reliant on parents for lifts again. Ellie's mother also asks about carrying school books and an advice sheet is given for her to pass on to school to arrange to borrow an additional set of textbooks to keep at home. She is also advised to carry minimal coursework around in a small A4 folder. The sheet also includes ergonomic advice for school work. A plan is made to carry out a functional assessment of bathroom transfers on day five post op, pending discharge that evening if all is well. Bath measurements are confirmed.

Day five post op: Ellie has been practising sitting out of bed in her brace and is still a little unsteady on mobilising but manages to walk to the bathroom unaided. Transfers are demonstrated then practised with the raised toilet seat and bath board with Ellie's mother present. The appropriate equipment is loaned (with fitting instructions) for six months. Ellie and her mother agree that her mother will dry her feet and put her socks on and a Helping Hand is purchased for other reaching tasks. Ellie is discharged from occupational therapy on day five post op and goes home that evening, having practised stairs safely with the physiotherapist.

On returning the equipment six months after surgery, Ellie and her mother have a brief conversation with the occupational therapist about graded return to activities, as the consultant has given her the go ahead but she is nervous of activities such as cycling.

Case study 6.2

Diagnosis – Chronic low back pain

John – male, aged 55 years

John is 55 years old and has a nine years' history of back problems, which started when he was lifting paving slabs from his driveway. This episode caused him to take three weeks off work as a lorry driver and he underwent a partial discectomy at L5/S1. This helped the symptoms radiating down his right leg but he has had numerous further episodes of back pain, with different triggers and becoming longer in duration, until it is now 'constant, with good days and bad days'. He has tried physiotherapy and osteopathy and has recently had to stop taking non-steroidal anti-inflammatory due to a suspected stomach ulcer. He continues to work but has to space out jobs to be able to cope, which has considerably reduced his income. His wife says that he has lost interest in life but is looking forward to the birth of their first grandson. John says he would like to be able to kick a ball about with his grandson when he is old enough and get back to some DIY as his house is 'going to pot'.

At pre-admission assessment, conducted by the health psychologist, John says he is fairly convinced that more surgery will not help so he just wants to 'make the best of it'. He agrees to a three week inpatient self-management programme. John's goals at the beginning of the programme are:

- To be able to work more often, without being flat on my back in between
- To be able to exercise more, doing something I like
- To enjoy a holiday in four months' time
- To be able to pick my grandson up and not worry about dropping him
- To paint the front of the house.

During the programme, John covers the recommended sessions and at the end he sets three month goals to:

- Use pacing, stretches and relaxation techniques to build up driving tolerance to one hour comfortably
- Buy and use seat and back cushions in the lorry and while sitting at home
- Go swimming once a week
- Walk to the paper shop ten minutes each way every day, instead of driving
- Practise lifting the cat with good posture and technique.
- Get help from son to paint the front of the house, starting in two months time and finishing before holiday.

Summary

The spine is the body's central structure and is affected by both degenerative and acute disorders. Spinal disorders can cause tremendous pain, deformity and disability, leading to loss of functional ability, and can affect all areas of occupational performance. The psycho-social impact of these conditions is well researched, with evidence demonstrating the effectiveness of the different treatment approaches. The common conditions and their non-operative or surgical management have been described along with evidence based management and rehabilitative approaches.

With over 70% of people in the industrialised nations experiencing back pain at sometime during their life, it is certain that occupational therapists as part of the multidisciplinary team will continue to actively support this client group.

References

Advance Seating Designs. (2002/2003). The ideal posture (2002); How to sit correctly (2002); Using a mouse (2002); How posture affects disc pressure (2003). Online. Available at: www.asd.co.uk/guides/how_to_posters.htm (accessed 27 February 2008).

Airaksinen, O., Brox, J. I., Cedraschi, C., Hildebrandt, J., Klaber-Moffet, J., Kovacs, F., Mannion, A. F., Reis, S., Staal, J. B., Ursin, H., & Zanoli, G. (2004). European guidelines for the management of chronic non-specific low back pain. European Commission, Online. Research Directorate General. Available at: www.backpaineurope.org (accessed 13 June 2006).

Becker, H., Stuifbergen, A., Rogers, S., & Timmerman, G. (2000). Goal Attainment Scaling to measure individual change in intervention studies. *Nursing Research*, 49(3), 176–180.

College of Occupational Therapists & National Social Inclusion Programme. (2007). *Work Matters: Vocational Navigation for Occupational Therapy Staff*. COT and NSIP. Online. Available at: www.cot.co.uk/public/publications2/categoryshow.php?c=7 (accessed 27 February 2008).

Debnath, U. K., Freeman, B. J. C., Gregory, P., de la Harpe, D., Kerslake, R. W., & Webb, J. K. (2003). Clinical outcome and return to sport after the surgical treatment of spondylolysis in young athletes. *Journal of Bone and Joint Surgery, British Volume, 85*, 244–249.

Department of Health. (2005). Complex disability exemplar. *National Service Framework for Children, Young People and Maternity Services*, pp. 46–50.

Emans, J. B. (2000). Paediatric and adolescent spinal deformity. In P. J. Morris & W. C. Wood (Eds). *Oxford Textbook of Surgery* (2nd edition). Oxford: Oxford University Press.

Health and Safety Executive. (2004). *Working with VDUs. Getting to Grips with Manual Handling. Handling the News. Understanding Ergonomics*. Online. Available at: www.hse. gov.uk/pubns/leaflets.htm (accessed 27 February 2008).

Hodges, S. D., Eck, J. C., & Humphreys, S. C. (2004). A treatment and outcomes analysis of patients with coccydynia. *Spine Journal, 4*(2), 138–140.

Iwamoto, J., Takeda, T., & Wakano, K. (2004). Returning athletes with severe low back pain and spondylolysis to original sporting activities with conservative treatment. *Scandinavian Journal of Medicine & Science in Sports, 14*(6), 346–351.

Kiresuk, T. J., Smith, A., & Cardillo, J. E. (1993). *Goal Attainment Scaling: Application, Theory, and Measurement*. London: Psychology Press.

Lucas, P. R. (2000). Degenerative disorders of the spine. In P. J. Morris & W. C. Wood (Eds). *Oxford Textbook of Surgery* (2nd edition). Oxford: Oxford University Press.

Maigne, J. Y., & Chatellier, G. (2001). Comparison of three manual coccygeal treatments: a pilot study. *Spine, 26*(20), E479–483.

Maigne, J. Y., Lagauche, D., & Doursounian, L. (2000a). Instability of the coccyx in coccydynia. *Journal of Bone and Joint Surgery, British Volume, 82*(7), 1038–1041.

Maigne, J. Y., Doursounian, L., & Chatellier, G. (2000b). Causes and mechanisms of common coccydynia: role of body mass index and coccygeal trauma. *Spine, 25*(23), 3072–3079.

Matthews, W. B. (2003). Spinal cord. In D. A. Warrell, T. M. Cox, J. D. Firth & E. J. Benz (Eds). *Oxford Textbook of Medicine* (4th edition). Oxford: Oxford University Press, pp. 1264–1265.

National Institute for Clinical Excellence. (2004). *Prosthetic Intervertebral Disc Replacement*. London: Department of Health.

National Institute for Clinical Excellence. (2005a). *Prosthetic Intervertebral Disc Replacement in the Lumbar Spine*. Online. Available at: www.nice.org.uk/Guidance/IPG100/Guidance/pdf/ English (accessed 26 June 2006).

National Institute for Health and Clinical Excellence. (2005b). *Prosthetic Intervertebral Disc Replacement in the Cervical Spine*. Online. Available at: www.nice.org.uk/Guidance/IPG143 (accessed 26 June 2006).

Reiter, M. F., & Heller, J. G. (2000). Spinal infections. In P. J. Morris & W. C. Wood (Eds). *Oxford Textbook of Surgery* (2nd edition). Oxford: Oxford University Press.

van Tulder, M., Becker, A., Bekkering, T., Breen, A., Gil de Real, M. T., Hutchinson, A., Koes, B., Laerum, E., & Malmivaara, A. (2004). European guidelines for the management of acute non-specific low back pain in primary care. European Commission, Research Directorate General. Online. Available at: www.backpaineurope.org (accessed 13 June 2006).

Whitesides, T. E. (2000). Inflammatory disorders of the spine. In P. J. Morris & W. C. Wood (Eds). *Oxford Textbook of Surgery*, (2nd edition). Oxford: Oxford University Press.

Williamson, L., & Wordsworth, P. (2000). Osteoarthritis. In J. G. Evans, T. F. Williams, B. L. Beattie, J. P. Michel, and G. K. Wilcock (Eds). *Oxford Textbook of Geriatric Medicine* (2nd edition). Oxford: Oxford University Press.

Chapter 7

Paediatric orthopaedic surgery

Andrew M. Wainwright

Introduction

Paediatric orthopaedics is a subspecialty of medicine that involves the prevention and treatment of musculoskeletal problems in children. This encompasses a wide variety of conditions, in a group of individuals who are very varied, and who are changing rapidly with age.

Children are different from adults in many ways and respond to disease in a different way to adults. In particular, children are different from adults in their musculoskeletal system. Throughout childhood, the skeleton is growing at an incredible rate. There are many conditions that affect growth, and have an impact on a child that would not affect an adult (who has stopped growing). Conversely, on occasions, it is necessary to manipulate growth to help a child for example if they have limb length inequality. A child's skeleton is also more flexible than that of an adult. This means that they sustain different patterns of injury compared with adults with the same types of trauma; major trauma may cause injuries to the soft tissues but without breaking the bones.

Any medical problem in childhood affects not only the child but will usually have an impact on their parents, brothers and sisters. However, a family is also able to offer support and is used to looking after them; if they need extra help, it is usually available. Children are also very adaptable; if they have restrictions placed on them because of an illness, or its treatment, they will find another way of coping with activities. Children are also developing in lots of areas; socially, educationally, as well as physically and it is increasingly acknowledged that one goal in the management of children's physical problems is to minimise the impact on the rest of a child's development.

This chapter covers many of the common musculoskeletal conditions that affect children. Some less common conditions are also included because they may have a significant impact in terms of the amount of support that they need from health care professionals. These have been organised into three sections:

- Conditions that children are born with, that affect an individual from the day that they are born. Examples:
  - Congenital talipes equinovarus
  - Developmental dysplasia of the hip (DDH)
  - Cerebral palsy
  - Leg length discrepancy
  - Bone dysplasias.
- Conditions in which they will have a predisposition to having a problem later in life. Examples:
  - Perthes' disease
  - Scoliosis.
- Problems that can affect people at any age but result in particular problems for children while they are growing up. Examples:
  - Infection
  - Tumour
  - Trauma
  - Non-accidental injury.

Conditions that manifest themselves in childhood

Congenital talipes equinovarus/clubfoot

Clubfoot (Figure 7.1) is a common foot deformity that develops in a baby in the womb. The most common form of clubfoot is congenital talipes equinovarus (CTEV). Literally, this translates as the *talus* (ankle) and *pes* (foot) are in *equinus* (as a horse's foot, pointing downwards) and *varus* (pointing inwards).

Clubfoot affects about one in 1000 babies in the UK and now is most often diagnosed on antenatal ultrasound scans. This means that parents can discuss and prepare for their baby's treatment during the later stages of pregnancy, although treatment

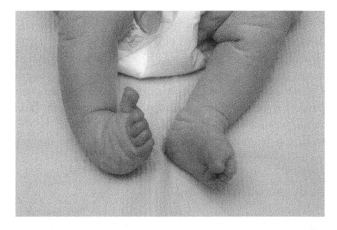

Figure 7.1 Baby with clubfoot (CTEV).

cannot start until the baby is born. It may be associated with other conditions, that affect muscles and nerves, such as spina bifida or arthrogryposis, but most often it is an isolated problem and the cause is still not known fully.

CTEV occurs in boys more often than girls and affects only one foot in half the cases. Not only are the ankle and foot abnormal but the whole calf is involved. Even with good correction of the foot deformity, the underlying imbalance of muscles remains and many children cannot hop on the affected leg owing to calf weakness. The aim of treatment is to correct the deformity while preserving mobility in the foot, so that the foot does not cause pain and so normal footwear can be worn.

If a true clubfoot deformity is left untreated, the foot will not correct itself and the child will be left walking on the outer border of a deformed foot. Although this is seldom seen in the Western world now, it remains a big problem worldwide. An untreated clubfoot is difficult to fit into a normal shoe, making walking difficult, it may lead to pressure areas breaking down, and may be painful.

The deformity can be classified by severity according to how deformed the foot is and how correctable that deformity is.

Treatment

There have been several forms of treatment proposed since Hippocrates first described manipulation of the foot over 2000 years ago. By the late twentieth century, treatment with manipulation lost favour and many children had operations before their first birthday to lengthen tight ligaments and tendons, and to realign bones. This operation was usually preceded by manipulations and plasters and was followed by plasters and splints to maintain the correction. Getting the required amount of correction may be difficult, and many feet become very stiff after an extensive operation around the hindfoot and midfoot.

Recently there has been a resurgence worldwide for treatment by manipulation after Ponseti reported good results from his technique. Using his method of treatment, a newborn with a clubfoot problem is assessed and treatment started as soon as possible after birth. With a series of casts (Figure 7.2), changed on a weekly basis, the deformity is gradually corrected, firstly correcting the forefoot cavus, then the midfoot adduction, supination, and finally the hindfoot equinus. The heel cord usually needs lengthening to allow the heel to come down into the heel pad – often the heel cord is cut under local anaesthetic in the outpatient clinic.

Once the deformity is corrected with serial plasters, the feet are placed in (Dennis–Brown) boots fixed on a bar. According to Ponseti these need to be worn by the infant for three months, full time once the plasters have stopped and then at night-time only until the age of 4 years. This presents a challenge to many families. Some children still need some surgery following this, particularly to transfer the over active tibialis anterior tendon to stop it from continually pulling the foot into inversion.

Developmental dysplasia of the hip

DDH (Figure 7.3) is a spectrum of conditions where the developing hip can be shallow or unstable. Included in this spectrum are:

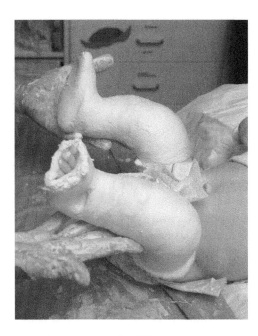

Figure 7.2 Child in plaster casts for treatment of clubfoot.

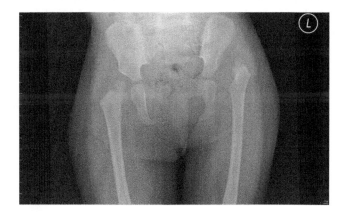

Figure 7.3 X-ray showing a child with a dislocated hip (DDH).

- A hip that is found to be dislocated and cannot be reduced
- A hip that is dislocated but will relocate with careful positioning
- A hip that is located but will completely, or partially, dislocate
- A hip that is shallow and the femoral head tends to lie at the edge of the socket.

There are particular risk factors for having DDH including:

- Breech positioning in the womb
- Positive family history (in a first degree relative having had DDH)

- Cramped conditions in the uterus such as experienced by twins, firstborn children
- Other moulding deformities such as torticollis and metatarsus adductus.

The condition is sufficiently common and has serious implications so that screening programmes are often used to assess all babies with these risk factors, involving a clinical examination and an ultrasound by an experienced clinician.

Treatment

For those children who have dislocated or dislocatable hips, treatment is usually very effective with a splint such as a Pavlik harness (Figure 7.4).

Most babies use one of these for six weeks until their hips become stable. They need to be closely monitored to ensure that the harness fits well to avoid complications such as nerve palsy and avascular necrosis of the femoral head (where the blood supply to the femoral head is obstructed, which may lead to severe deformity of the femoral head).

A few children fail treatment with a harness, or are not picked up at an early enough stage to use a harness. In this situation a closed reduction is attempted. This involves the infant coming into hospital for a general anaesthetic so that the hip can be examined while they are relaxed. As the femoral head is mainly composed of cartilage, an arthrogram is used to outline the ball-and-socket joint with a radio-opaque dye. This helps to show whether there is an obstruction to the femoral head being reduced into the socket and also assesses how snugly they fit together.

If the hip can be reduced safely a plaster 'spica' (Figure 7.5) is used (*spica* means 'ear of corn' and refers to the criss-cross appearance of plaster bandages that is supposed to look like an ear of corn). The baby is placed into the plaster in a position that maintains the hip in joint. The hips need to be kept flexed and abducted; too little abduction risks the hip falling out of the joint, but excessive abduction risks the blood vessels being

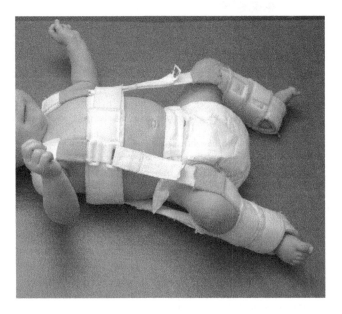

Figure 7.4 Baby in a Pavlik harness.

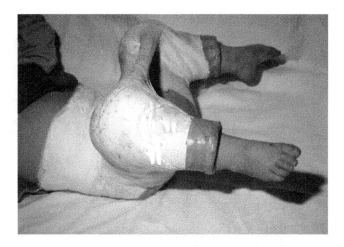

Figure 7.5 Baby in a 'human' hip spica after closed reduction of the hip.

squashed, leading to avascular necrosis of the femoral head. This safe position is usually with the hips flexed up to 90–100° and abducted to about 40° and is maintained for two to three months, usually with a plaster change halfway through, as a day case procedure. This position can make it difficult to find a pushchair or car seat for the infant.

Some children's hips cannot be manipulated into position by closed reduction and require an open operation. At this operation the hip joint is explored, to open the joint capsule and remove the obstructions that are keeping the hip out of joint. After an open operation a plaster spica is used to hold the hip in joint while the capsule heals to keep the femoral head securely in the socket. If this has been done via an anterior approach the anterior part of the hip is opened and it is important for stress to be taken off the repair of this part of the capsule. In this case the plaster is applied with the hip internally rotated, slightly flexed to about 30°, and abducted 30° (Figure 7.6). This makes it slightly easier to sit or lay a child and find appropriate seating for the weeks when the infant is in a plaster spica. In the older child it may be necessary to reinforce this with a cross-bar to stop the spica from breaking at weak points where the legs join onto the trunk.

Some of these children will continue to have a shallow acetabular socket, even though the hip is located in the joint. If the socket remains shallow the femoral head tends to put a lot of pressure on the lateral part of the acetabulum rather than having the forces spread evenly across the socket. This tends to lead to arthritic changes at an early age, requiring hip replacement surgery at a young age – often in the twenties and thirties. There are several operations used to help deepen the socket. The most commonly used osteotomies in childhood are the Salter osteotomy, the Pemberton osteotomy, and the Dega osteotomy. These all have the effect of making the roof of the acetabulum more horizontal to make the hip more secure and spread the forces more evenly across the joint. This is done by adding an extra wedge of bone above the socket to lever it down.

After these operations it is usual to protect the osteotomy, until the bone has healed, with a plaster cast or brace for six weeks. This means that the child is usually dependent on a wheelchair for six to eight weeks, but can usually transfer safely.

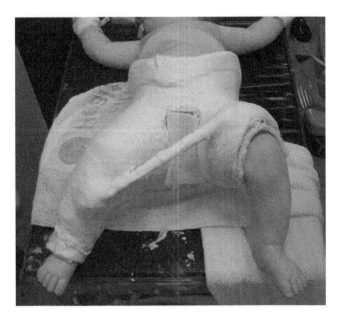

Figure 7.6 Baby in a 30-30-30 spica after an open reduction of the hip.

Cerebral palsy

The term cerebral palsy includes a number of conditions that all result from an injury to the developing brain (this is usually defined as being a brain injury in children less than 2 years). Although the brain injury is not progressive, the musculoskeletal effects do become more marked with time. Overall, this affects 2 in 1000 live-born babies in the UK.

The most common form of cerebral palsy causes spasticity, where there is increased tone in the muscles of the affected part of the body. The type of involvement has commonly been described in terms of the parts of the body that are affected, i.e.:

- Monoplegia – one limb
- Hemiplegia – one half of the body, usually more severely affecting the upper limbs
- Diplegia – affecting predominantly both lower limbs
- Quadriplegia – or total body involvement cerebral palsy.

More recently classification systems have been used that focus more on the functional ability of the child (which is compared with other children of the same age) such as the Gross Motor Function Classification System (GMFCS).

Treatment

The increased tone in muscles results in the joints being stiff or held in abnormal positions at a time when a co-ordinated motion (such as walking) requires a joint to be in a specific position. While the child is still young enough this tightness can be managed with physiotherapy and stretching. Often this is done in combination with splints, to hold the joints in a functional position, or with medications that reduce muscle tone, such as baclofen or botulinum toxin injections.

As a child with cerebral palsy gets older, some of the joints that have been pulled into abnormal position (by overactive muscles) become fixed in that position. This may be due to tendons that have become short, joint capsule that has become contracted or bones that have not been able to grow in the usual way. To correct this fixed deformity often requires surgery to lengthen short tendons and reshape bones (Figure 7.7). The concept of one-stage multi-level surgery has become the preferred method of treatment

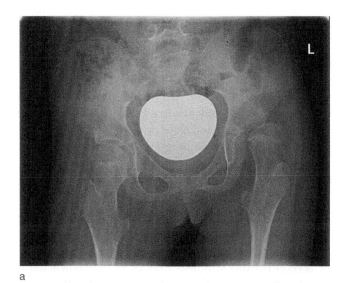

a

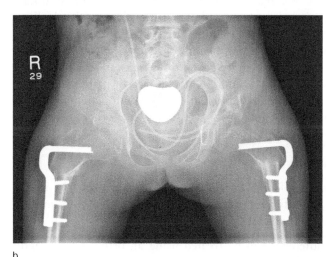

b

Figure 7.7 X-ray of a child with dysplastic hips because of cerebral palsy: (a) before, and (b) after a femoral and pelvic osteotomy to stabilise the hips.

to avoid 'birthday syndrome' (where a child has a series of operations throughout their growing years and seems to spend every birthday recovering from another operation).

In many centres three-dimensional gait analysis is used to assess the pattern of walking in a gait laboratory. A combination of video cameras, force plate measurements, dynamic electromyography and three-dimensional, computer assisted motion analysis system is used to produce a list of problems that need to be addressed at the time of surgery. It is also possible to repeat this assessment after surgery to audit the results of treatment. After surgery there is a prolonged recovery period of many months, initially in, and later, out of hospital to regain strength and function.

In some children the forces that are across the hip joint are so unbalanced that the femoral head is driven out of the socket. Surgery is usually performed to release the tight tendons that are driving the hip out of joint. If the hip is already becoming deformed, surgery to the femur and the acetabulum is required to make the hip more stable. This usually requires a period of six weeks in a brace to hold the hips securely while the bones heal (as in the osteotomies used in older children with DDH).

In children with total body involvement cerebral palsy, the spine can also become progressively deformed. This can lead to difficulties with standing and sitting requiring the intervention of posture, independence and mobility specialists. It may be possible to accommodate the deformity and slow progression with custom-made seating and sleep systems. However, children with progressive deformities often require treatment to fuse the spine in a straighter position. This is a major, specialised operation using rods to hold the spine attached to the front and/or the back of the spinal column.

Leg length discrepancy

There are several reasons why legs may be of different lengths. These are most commonly due to congenital problems where part of a limb does not grow normally, such as congenital short femur, fibular hemimelia or Ollier's disease. As a result the limb grows at a slower rate than the unaffected limb. In hemi-hypertrophy one side of the body grows too fast and one limb becomes longer than the other.

There are other acquired conditions that can result in a difference in leg length. This may be because of trauma, where a growth plate may be injured and stop growing, leading to a bone that is too short. A growth plate may also be affected by a bacterial infection and cease to grow new bone while other growth plates are still active.

Treatment

When the leg length difference is small, particularly if it has been static throughout growth, no intervention is required. If there is a more marked leg length discrepancy then there are several options for treatment.

- The difference can be treated using an orthosis, i.e. building up the height of the shoe on the shorter limb.
- During the growing years it is possible to surgically stop the growth of the longer leg. With planning, it is possible to estimate how much growth is left in the shorter

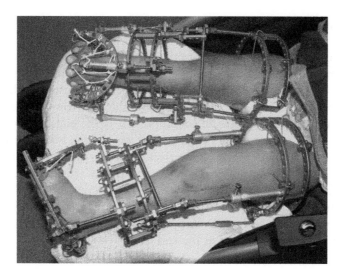

Figure 7.8 Child with Ilizarov frames *in situ*.

leg. Knowing this, the growth in the longer leg can be stopped at a point where the shorter leg can catch up with it. Growth is stopped using staples or screws that are placed across the growth plate to hold back the growth. Alternatively the growth plate cartilage can be removed.
- The longer leg can be shortened, by removing a segment of bone and then fixing the shortened bone back together (like a fracture).
- The bone may be lengthened using different techniques; a Russian doctor called Ilizarov described the most effective method for doing this. He reported a method of cutting the bone and gradually pulling it apart as it was trying to heal. The bone is held with an external fixator or frame (Figure 7.8), which can be adjusted several times a day to lengthen the healing bone by a millimetre per day. Once the correct length is achieved, the bone is held at the corrected length until the bone is strong enough to remove the fixator. Although this is a powerful surgical technique, it can take a long time for the process to finish.

There are usually several problems that are encountered by patients during the course of treatment. These include:

- Infections developing in the pins that hold the bone
- Problems with tightness of muscle and nerves that are also being stretched
- Mechanical problems with the fixator breaking or locking
- Adjacent joints becoming stiff or being pushed out of joint.

Despite this most people are able to perform most activities of daily living while they are being treated, taking weight through their frame to walk. Splinting is often required in order to treat for the resulting tightness in muscles across joints.

The technique is also successful at correcting angular deformities, which can be associated with length differences.

Bone dysplasias/hormonal imbalances

There are many conditions where the complex processes involved in growth of bones and cartilage do not occur in the normal way. As a group these are called bone dysplasias. There are also conditions that affect the musculoskeletal system where the hormones that control the growth of tissues do not work properly, such as in rickets.

There are a large number of conditions where the building blocks that make up connective tissue are not made in the normal way by the body, particularly the collagens. Examples such as osteogenesis imperfecta, result in the bones being weak and deformed. Another example is achondroplasia or classical dwarfism where bones do not grow to the usual length. Each individual form of dysplasia is associated with specific problems including deformity, educed stature and premature arthritis. Further details can been found on websites such as Online Mendelian Inheritance in Man (www.ncbi.nlm.nih.gov) or in the reference list at the end of this chapter.

Conditions that some individuals may be prone to

Perthes' disease

Perthes' disease (Figure 7.9) is a condition, in a primary school child, where the epiphysis of the femoral head loses its blood supply, becomes weakened, collapses and flattens. As the blood supply returns to the bone it is able to re-grow and remodel so that the situation may improve over several years during growth.

Perthes' disease commonly affects boys more than girls, usually between the ages of 4 and 7 years. This causes the child to limp and affects 1 in 10 000 children in the UK. The condition varies in severity, but the outlook is better if only a small part of the

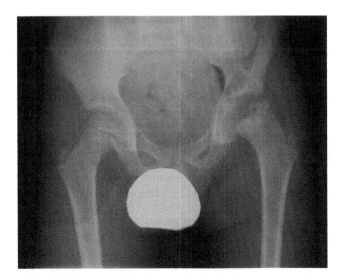

Figure 7.9 Perthes' disease of the hip.

femoral head is involved, if there is only a little collapse and if it starts when the child is younger, there is more chance for remodelling to occur if there is more growth left.

Treatment

The principle of treatment is to prevent collapse and flattening of the femoral head as much as possible while the bone is soft and deformable. This can be difficult to attain, as many of the children who are prone to Perthes' disease are usually very active. However, if they can be encouraged to use crutches, avoid contact sport and reduce impact on the hip, in theory this can lessen the amount of collapse.

Once the remodelling has started the principle of treatment is to allow the femoral head to remodel as spherically as possible. This is best achieved when the head is contained well within the acetabular socket and children maintain a good range of movement. In some children this does not occur and the femoral head lies with part of the femoral head outside the acetabular socket. It then becomes necessary to do something to hold the femoral head within the socket.

Historically, children were treated in bed for many weeks during their childhood and then treated with braces that held their legs apart so that the femoral head remained located within the socket. More recently there has been a trend to performing an operation to achieve the same result. This can be done with an osteotomy at the top of the femur that points the femoral head within the socket (effectively doing the same thing as an abduction brace). The other option is to do an operation on the socket to redirect it over the top of the femoral head with an operation such as a Salter osteotomy. If this is not possible then another option is to build on an extra shelf of bone on the outside of the femoral head to keep the femoral head covered with bone and remain spherical.

After these operations, children are often in a brace for six weeks to allow the bone to heal. Although they are able to transfer from bed to chair, they often rely on a wheelchair for longer distances.

Scoliosis

Scoliosis (Figure 7.10) refers to a deformity of the spine that is apparent in the frontal plane (i.e. it can be seen as a side to side curvature when looking at someone's back from behind). In reality it is a three-dimensional deformity that also involves a rotational deformity. This may result in the chest wall also being more prominent on one side compared with the other.

There are several causes for scoliosis to develop; for example it may be due to the shape of the individual vertebrae that can be partially fused together, or can be due to uneven muscular forces on the spine causing it to twist, such as those that develop in neuromuscular diseases such as cerebral palsy. The most common form is adolescent idiopathic scoliosis, which as the name implies is first seen around puberty, but the cause has not yet been discovered. Girls are more likely than boys to have a significant curvature.

The curvature once present has a tendency to become greater, particularly through the adolescent growth spurt. Not surprisingly there is more risk of the curve becoming worse with curves that are bigger when they are first noticed and in those that are

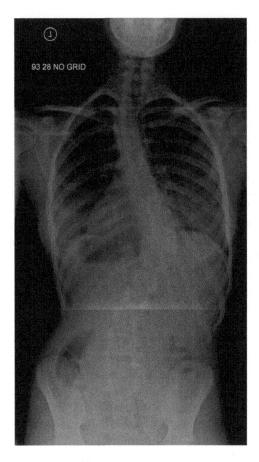

Figure 7.10 X-ray appearance of a scoliosis.

first noticed at a younger age, when there is more growth left. Although the deformity is three-dimensional, the amount of curvature is most often judged on the basis of a two-dimensional X-ray of the spine. From this it can be assessed how much of an angle there is between the two most angled vertebrae of the spine. This angle is called Cobb's angle. Other important factors that can be assessed from the radiograph are how much rotation of the spine is involved and at which level the spine is curved abnormally.

Treatment

The most common form of adolescent idiopathic scoliosis is centred in the thoracic region of the spine, and convex to the right. Treatment is based on the likelihood of the curvature causing further deformity. For a curve that is less than 30° and particularly for an older patient, the curve is commonly monitored but no treatment is recommended unless there is progression. For a curve that is greater then this, or for younger girls, treatment with a brace is recommended in many units. Braces can be worn beneath clothes and are often advocated for use 23 hours per day. There may be problems with compliance, particularly at an age when image and self-esteem may be fragile.

For greater degrees of curvature and curves that are progressing rapidly, surgery may be recommended. The surgery involves fusing segments of the spine to prevent further curvature and to correct some of the deformity. This has inherent risks, particularly that of paralysis, which is a very infrequent, but significant risk. For this reason, during surgery the functions of the nerves that run in the spinal cord are monitored. If there is seen to be loss of signal transmission during the correction of deformity, then correction is lessened until normal signals are monitored. If there is no problem with the nerve signal transmission, metal rods are attached to levels of the spine using hooks and screws, and the spine can be straightened and fused using bone graft.

Surgery may also be performed from the front of the spine (which is in fact anterolateral). The spine is approached through the chest and/or abdominal cavity. Intervertebral disc material is removed from between the vertebral bodies, and a fixation device can be inserted to help fuse the spine from the front. Newer techniques have been developed to perform this surgery though a keyhole approach (thoracoscopically) with specially devised telescopes and instruments.

After such major surgery children often need care in a high dependency unit for a short time and then may also need a brace to protect the correction. Some people with scoliosis may also have deformity of the chest wall and rib prominences. These can also be treated with surgery to cut the ribs and reshape the chest wall.

Conditions that may develop during the growing years, after birth

Infection

One of the most significant events in the twentieth century was the development of antibiotics, which meant that infections could be effectively treated. Despite this, infection still affect the bones and joints of children and can lead to major problems resulting in destruction of a joint or, even death in severe cases, if left untreated.

Acute infections can reach bones and joint via the blood stream in children. *Haemophilus* infections were a leading cause of infection until the HIB (*Haemophilus influenzae* B) vaccine was routinely given to children; the most common cause of infection is now *Staphylococcus aureus*. In North America, there has been a rising incidence of methicillin resistant *Staphylococcus aureus* (MRSA) (multiple drug resistant bacteria) that have been acquired in the community, and which are harder to treat, with more frequent complications.

A child who has an infection in a bone or joint will not want to move the limb; in infants this can appear to be a paralysis. They may also be generally unwell from the effects of an infection, with a fever, and may also have local signs of tenderness, warmth and swelling of the affected area. Suspicions based on clinical signs are supported by investigations such as blood tests, looking for evidence of infection, and by imaging tests such as ultrasound and magnetic resonance imaging. However, X-rays often do not show any changes in the early stages until an infection has been present for over a week.

Treatment

If a joint is infected (septic arthritis) this can cause destruction of the joint owing to the enzymes that are generated by the body to fight off the infection and to the pressure of fluid in the joint. This may also lead to dislocation of the joint. It is vital to release the pressure and washout the infection as soon as possible, before destruction of the joint occurs. This urgent operation may be done with an open or arthroscopic technique and may need repeating if there is no improvement. Antibiotics alone cannot eradicate an infection once a collection of pus has developed, as they cannot penetrate in sufficient strength to stop the infection. However, they are important to treat the rest of the infection once the majority has been cleared by surgery. Antibiotics may be needed for several weeks.

A child who has a washout of a joint in good time with appropriate antibiotics can go onto have no further problems; however, delays in treatment may lead to destruction of the joint, which may lead to chronic problems and deformity pain and stiffness of the joint.

When an infection affects the bone this is termed osteomyelitis. In the early stages this may present in a similar way to septic arthritis and the two may occur together. Initially this may be effectively treated with antibiotics; however, collections of pus may develop, as an abscess. This is often located under the periosteal lining of the bone. Once a collection of pus develops the antibiotics cannot penetrate into the collection to stop the bacteria and surgery is needed to drain the pus and wash out the infection. Subsequently, antibiotics can be used to treat the residual infection.

A child who has had timely and effective treatment of an acute osteomyelitis can have no further problems, however, a delay in treatment may lead to death of the bone, and this can harbour infection that can flare up as a problem many years later, throughout life. If the growth plates are affected by an infection this can lead to abnormal growth patterns which may lead to deformity or limb length differences; this may then lead to chronic problems and deformity pain and stiffness.

Tumours

The Latin term for a swelling is *tumour*. Many tumours that affect children occur because the bone is growing so actively, and these types of tumour are rarely, if ever, seen in adults. Tumours may be benign, if they do not have a tendency to grow outside of the area that they started, or malignant, if they invade into surrounding structures or spread distantly.

Benign tumours can result in deformities and cause functional problems even though they do not invade into neighbouring tissues. Some, such as osteoid osteomas cause intense pain, even at rest, that require treatment such as surgical removal, or more modern X-ray guided techniques (such as radiofrequency ablation) to stop the cells from growing.

Some benign tumours, such as unicameral bone cysts, can cause weakness of the bone, which may result in fractures. These are cysts within the bone where the bone is replaced by a fluid filled cyst. They are found close to growth plates and only occur in growing bones, but may be resistant to treatment aimed at obtaining healing with bone. If they are causing frequent fractures, they may require protection with plates to bridge the bone or rods inside the bones to splint them until the end of growth.

Other benign tumours can cause pressure on other structures around them, although they do not invade into the substance of those structures. An example is seen in osteochondromas, where a spur of bone with a cartilage cap can grow away from the growth plate along the outside of a bone. This can interfere with the function of tendons, nerves and other bones that are displaced by the extra bone. Such cases may require surgery to remove the spur and correct any deformity.

There are a few malignant tumours that may affect bones in childhood. Leukaemia is the most common form of childhood malignancy affecting bone that can result in symptoms that resemble osteomyelitis. A malignancy affecting connective tissue is called a *sarcoma* (literally meaning 'a swelling of the flesh'). Ewing's sarcoma affects younger children and is named after the doctor who described it, James Ewing. This malignant tumour consists of small round cells and destroys long bones. The outcome for children with these tumours has been greatly improved by the use of chemotherapy. Previously the likelihood of a child living for two years after being diagnosed with Ewing's sarcoma was poor, however, with modern treatment involving chemotherapy this has improved to between 50% and 80%.

Osteosarcomas are the second most common malignant tumour of bone in childhood. They tend to affect slightly older children (in adolescence) than Ewing's sarcomas. Bones that are affected are often those that are most rapidly growing, i.e. the proximal humerus, distal femur and proximal tibia. Chemotherapy has also greatly improved the outcome for these children recently.

These children are best treated by a team approach. Once the imaging is completed, surgery is performed to obtain a tissue specimen to confirm the diagnosis. After chemotherapy, surgery is performed to remove the tumour in addition to the chemotherapy. Some tumours occurring around the spine and pelvis cannot be removed surgically owing to the possibility of damage to the surrounding structures and radiotherapy may also be helpful in this situation.

For a malignant tumour that affects the limbs, it has been historically the practice to remove the tumour with amputation of the affected part. More recently it has been possible to remove the tumour with a sufficient zone of normal tissue that the limb can be preserved without compromising the chances of getting a recurrence of the tumour. The defect that has been left by removing the diseased bone may be filled with a metal prosthesis (such as a massive knee replacement), or with bone that has been transplanted from another part of the body or from another donor. Despite this because normal tissue also has to be removed with the tumour, this might result in that limb's function being affected and adaptive devices may be required to manage this deficit.

Trauma

Children sustain different injuries than adults, although the principles of management are the same (Chapter 9). Children are different from adults in many ways – not only are their bones growing but they are also more pliable. This means that the bones break with incomplete, greenstick fractures, rather than complete fractures (that more brittle adult bones sustain). Children may also sustain major injuries to the soft tissues without breaking bones. An example is in the spine – it is possible to have a spinal cord injury without radiological abnormality (SCIWORA) to the bones of the spinal column. There are certain patterns of injury that children sustain because of their activities and size, e.g. falling off climbing frames, or as pedestrians being hit by cars. They also have differences in the way that they respond to trauma. Children's bodies are able to compensate for a lot of blood loss with few signs of decreased blood pressure, but they can then rapidly decompensate and run into severe problems.

There are types of injury to the bones that can lead to problems with their growth, which can then lead to deformity of the bones or bone that does not grow to the length of the same bone in the opposite limb – leading to limb length difference.

Non-accidental injury

Children may sustain injuries at the hands of those who are supposed to be looking after them. Four main forms of abuse are recognised; physical, sexual, emotional abuse and neglect. Often children may have experienced more than one form of abuse. There are patterns of injury that should raise concern about a child and sometimes this can be manifested through orthopaedic injuries. Excellent advice is available through local courses and via the National Society for the Prevention of Cruelty to Children (NSPCC) website (www.nspcc.org.uk).

Certainly child abuse can be prevented, if there's the will to do something about it, however, everyone needs to be prepared to act. If there is suspicion that a child has been abused, it is any member of the team including the occupational therapist's responsibility to report this to an appropriate manager, named doctor or named nurse for child protection. In this way the child and their carers can receive the appropriate support to prevent further abuse.

The role of functional assessment

There are several orthopaedic conditions where a functional assessment of daily living activities will guide the surgical treatment. For example, in radio-ulnar synostosis, the two bones of the forearm develop fused together. This means that there can be no rotation of the forearm and often the hands are held in an over-pronated position. Surgery can be performed to rotate the forearm into a more functional position, and this is best guided by a functional assessment of the activities that are compromised (such as receiving change in a shop, which is difficult to do unless one hand can be supinated).

Summary

Children's orthopaedics is a fascinating area to work in. Children have a unique view on life, are always changing, there are interactions with the whole family and there are a wide variety of conditions that present. These can be grouped into conditions that children are born with, conditions that lead to a predisposition to a problem later in life, and problems that can affect children while they are growing up. This is a wide field and more detail can be found in the references at the end of this chapter.

Further reading

Benson, M. K. D., Fixsen, J. A., Macnicol, M. F., & Parsch, K. (Eds). (2002). *Children's Orthopaedics and Fractures* (2nd edition). London: Churchill Livingstone.

Herring, J. A. (Ed.). (2002). *Tachdjian's Pediatric Orthopaedics* (3rd edition). Philadelphia: W.B. Saunders.

Staheli, L. T. (2003). *Fundamentals of Pediatric Orthopaedics* (3rd edition). Philadelphia: Lippincott Williams & Wilkins.

Wenger, D. R., & Rang, M. (1993). *The Art and Practice of Children's Orthopaedics*. New York: Raven Press.

Useful web addresses

Great Ormond Hospital for Sick Children – www.GOSH.org

National Society for the Prevention of Cruelty to Children (NSPCC) –www.nspcc.org.uk

Online Mendelian Inheritance in Man (OMIM) – www.ncbi.nlm.nih.gov

Contact a family (for families with disabled children) – www.cafamily.org.uk

Ponseti technique – www.uihealthcare.com/topics/medicaldepartments/orthopaedics/clubfeet/index.html

Steps charity (for people with lower limb conditions) – www.steps-charity.org.uk

Chapter 8

Occupational therapy for children and young people with orthopaedic conditions

Natalie Evans

Introduction

The occupational therapist's role in working with children with orthopaedic conditions is to assist the child in optimising all areas of occupational performance and socialisation when living with their condition. This may include assisting the child to regain independence following orthopaedic surgery, perform everyday activities and to participate in their environment – at home, in school and in the community. A vital element of the role is to support parents and carers to adjust and cope with the changes relating to the condition or following surgery, which may be temporary or permanent.

Although the principles of orthopaedic management are similar to those of adults, the occupational therapist's approach to the management of a child with an orthopaedic condition or following orthopaedic surgery will be different from that of an adult. Firstly, this is because the paediatric orthopaedic condition affects the growing and developing individual; any impairment to the musculoskeletal system can influence child development and therefore must always be carefully considered during assessment and intervention. Secondly, there is usually a significant impact on the parents or primary care giver and siblings; therefore, they must be involved in the interventions. Thirdly, paediatric orthopaedic conditions often present alongside a broad range of other diagnoses and disabilities. Therefore, the occupational therapist requires a thorough knowledge and wide range of skills in order to provide the best care for these.

The ongoing management of a chronic condition or surgical intervention can have an impact on the child's development, and affects how they manage at home and school, and results in great disruption to the family. The occupational therapist plays a major role in lessening the effects on the child and their family.

Occupational therapy and children and young people with orthopaedic conditions

The occupational therapist will encounter children of all ages who require surgery, some as young as 3 months. Many of these children will have on-going treatment throughout their childhood into their adult years. Others will have only a brief intervention. The child will usually be admitted to a specialist children's hospital or orthopaedic unit for elective surgery, and will receive care from a multi-disciplinary team, including an orthopaedic surgeon and medical team, paediatrician, occupational therapist, physiotherapist, nurse, teacher, and play therapist, and sometimes a clinical psychologist and other specialist allied health professionals or nurses. The most common conditions encountered and requiring occupational therapy are:

- Developmental dysplasia of the hip
- Multi-level surgery (for children with cerebral palsy)
- Scoliosis
- Talipes equinovarus (clubfoot)
- Leg length discrepancy
- Perthes' disease.

These conditions and their medical management are described in Chapter 7. Some of these conditions may be partly due to neuromuscular disorders such as cerebral palsy, or associated with syndromes e.g. Rett's or Prader–Willi. Children with muscular dystrophy can develop major orthopaedic problems such as scoliosis due to weakened musculature; children with cerebral palsy frequently develop contractures and deformities because of spasticity.

Some children will develop only mild symptoms from diseases such as Perthes' or mild scoliosis and grow up without a disability and the complications of frequent appointments and treatments. In a specialist orthopaedic unit, the occupational therapist may also encounter children with rare conditions such as Marfan's syndrome, osteogenesis imperfecta, achondroplasia, arthrogryposis and bone tumour. In all of these children, the inability of one system, e.g. musculoskeletal or neurological, to function adequately will impact on another, and the occupational therapist will need to be mindful of this throughout treatment (Pratt and Allen 1989). The occupational therapy interventions will be carried out within the context of the family and school life, growth, age and stage of development.

In hospital, the child may have to cope with plaster casts, splints or external fixators, immobility or changed mobility and posture, pain, mobility aids and wheelchairs and a renewed dependence on their parents. This unfamiliar environment can be very daunting and frightening, so the occupational therapist needs to assist the family during this difficult time and to make the transition by providing emotional and practical support to enable them to return home as quickly and safely as possible.

Occupational therapy will be provided within an acute setting and therefore the child will only stay a relatively short time in hospital. Efficient planning and prioritisation is required to maximise rehabilitation and discharge planning arrangements. It is not the paediatric orthopaedic occupational therapist's remit to carry out a full developmental assessment and interventions during this time, but to be aware of children who may have potential developmental issues that have not been identified and to make onward referrals to other paediatric services for maintaining the continuum of care. Accurate assessment, treatment and discharge planning in conjunction with the family are essential, as is the ability to liaise effectively with hospital and community based multi-disciplinary teams. Interventions will be carried out within the context of the family and school life, growth, age and stage of development.

Summary of key roles, skills and objectives

The key roles and objectives of the paediatric orthopaedic occupational therapist working in a specialist paediatric orthopaedic unit are (Moersch 1989):

- To understand how orthopaedic conditions and surgery, treatment and postoperative management can impact on function and child development
- To liaise with the family, school and community team to facilitate smooth discharge from hospital
- To have extensive knowledge of specialist assistive equipment, including hoists, wheelchairs and minor home adaptation
- To enable children to participate in everyday activities according to developmental stage
- To train parents and carers in the use of safe manual handling techniques
- To be an advocate for child development (physical and mental health)
- To facilitate play experiences and relaxation to help children adjust
- To undertake environmental assessment (home and school visits) where required
- To be a skilled problem solver (often there are no ready made solutions available)
- To work effectively as part of the multi-disciplinary team providing specialist advice regarding appropriate activities
- To act as an expert to provide advice for other professionals who deal with children with orthopaedic conditions less frequently
- To understand the impact of and what is involved in parenting a child with a disability.

Assessment and interventions

As the child's admission date to hospital is usually known in advance, it is possible to plan the assessments of occupational performance skills: sensorimotor, cognitive, psychosocial and environmental, and occupations: self-maintenance, productivity and leisure (Hong and Howard 2002) required throughout their stay. This commences with a preoperative assessment preferably several weeks before admission. Other assessments may include standardised paediatric evaluation and assessment tools (Richardson 2005; Stewart 2005) depending on the nature of the presenting diagnosis and problems, and functional, general and risk assessments used locally.

Preoperative assessment

The hospital environment can be a fearful place, full of unknowns and events over which the child has little control (Crooks and Wavrek 2005). The child may be exposed to strange people and experiences including pain and discomfort, as well as separation from the family and normal routines. For these reasons, hospital admissions are kept to a minimum. Preoperative assessment clinics are often held, which give the child and their parents or carers an opportunity to meet the multi-disciplinary team and visit the ward environment where they will be staying after their surgery (McIlroy and Koranyi 1989). The occupational therapy assessment commences at this point and focuses on gathering background information, carrying out an initial assessment and establishing rapport. The occupational therapist should provide information (both written and verbal) to help prepare the child and the family for surgery thus alleviating emotional stress and anxiety. This may include discussing concerns regarding functional ability and how the family will manage at home when the child is discharged from hospital. Therefore, it is essential that the occupational therapist has discussed the postoperative management with the team and clearly understands any limitations and the postoperative regimen, required and for how long this will be in place. The family can often feel overwhelmed at this stage as they try to assimilate much information in a short period. It is important that the occupational therapist is able to provide time to reassure and give advice according to the family's individual needs.

The assessment comprises a verbal interview with the child and family, and will include observation of the child's behaviour and function. The following information should be gathered:

- Social situation
- Siblings
- Parental work and caring responsibilities
- Stage of the child's development
- All aspects of activities of daily living
- Physical and sensory assessment
- Likes, dislikes and family routine
- Details and contacts of any professionals involved already
- School details and contacts.

If the child is a wheelchair user, it is useful to document the model and size, any postural support or accessories used and the supplier of the wheelchair. This may be needed as the wheelchair and postural support system may require adjustment or re-provision following surgery. If a child is likely to require a wheelchair following surgery, this is an ideal opportunity to carry out a wheelchair assessment, so that advance planning and preparation can occur before admission.

Careful observation of the child playing will offer the occupational therapist an opportunity to record the child's developmental level, functional ability and mobility. Specific assessments may be required, e.g. postural, upper limb or hand, if the surgeon requires further information to decide on the surgical approach, positioning and postoperative management.

Postoperative assessment

Following the surgery, the family and child will usually welcome a familiar face. The occupational therapist will plan the postoperative assessments and interventions, having read the operation note to confirm the details of the surgery, any contraindications and the postoperative management plan. Discussion with the multi-disciplinary team will confirm the care plan and likely length of stay. Post operatively, a biomechanical approach is recommended because the disability and surgery will impact on task performance and activities (Pratt and Allen 1989). Assessment post operatively focuses on these deficit areas.

A typical assessment tool may include a checklist of daily living skills appropriate to the child's development stage. The occupational therapist will carry out a thorough functional and mobility assessment and practise with the family. Intervention will commence early while the child is recovering in bed and then to continue by assisting the transition to the normal routine by practising transfers and mobility (ambulant or wheelchair). Skills will need to be evaluated for the different environments the child needs to operate in, such as school or home, and it may be appropriate to carry out assessments in the relevant environment. Previously smooth and easy feeding regimens, nappy changing or a regular trip to school can be extremely difficult, so the occupational therapist needs to work closely with the family to find acceptable solutions and sometimes compromise in these areas, using compensatory approaches and strategies.

Parents will require emotional and practical support and be included in all decision making, as family involvement is paramount. Parents can often feel disempowered and weary of telling their story again to the many professionals involved in their family's care. The occupational therapist should ensure that they do not request information that has already been given to another team member. The occupational therapist should also be mindful in communicating and providing information without using medical terminology and jargon.

Child development

As an orthopaedic condition can impact on physical development, cognitive and psychosocial development (Pratt and Allen 1989), the child may have reduced ability to explore, play and reach independence. The occupational therapist should plan activities at the appropriate developmental level and assist other team members or parents to do so; this may include help in choosing suitable toys and activities (Case-Smith 2005). The knowledge of age-appropriate developmental tasks and understanding of purposeful and therapeutic activity can also help a child to achieve a sense of control and cope better in the strange hospital environment (Case-Smith 2005). Strategies to facilitate coping and adjustment to hospital include:

- Enabling the child to participate in their care regimen
- Encouraging independence
- Providing opportunities for play where they may otherwise be physically limited
- Using relaxation techniques with older children and young people, or working with the play therapist and teachers advising on age-appropriate developmental activities.

It is also important that parents are encouraged to develop coping strategies.

Team working and discharge planning

Communication is a pivotal role of the occupational therapist. Particularly when working with children with disabilities, this often involves liaising with a multitude of professionals within health, social and educational sectors involved in the child's care. For some children not previously seen by a community team, referral is often necessary due to the resultant support needs required for the child and family following the child's surgery. Early liaison and information sharing will help to ensure seamless care between agencies and provide advance notification of on-going care and support required, which may include:

- Arranging provision of specialist equipment, e.g. adjustable bed, hoist, toileting, bathing equipment
- Rearranging school attendance and transport arrangements
- Referrals and funding for a wheelchair and postural support systems
- Planning inter-agency visits to the school or home
- Arranging inter-agency care packages.

Inter-agency working is essential to facilitate the on-going care of the child and family. The occupational therapist working in a specialist unit will inevitably receive referrals from all over the UK and sometimes from overseas, so communication with the many different services and teams will be particularly challenging, as each service sets different access and eligibility criteria. It is essential that referrals include information about the child's condition and postoperative management, as many community teams may not be familiar with recent advances in surgery and new ways of managing post operatively.

Specialist equipment

Equipment to assist independence and mobility is often required following surgery, to manage the child while in hospital and at home. For home, equipment may be arranged through local social and community services, specialist equipment loan stores or equipment libraries, and local and specialist charities. Wheelchairs with postural adaptations, cut-away toilet seats, hair washing trays, long handled aids, and adapted car seats and buggies are all common pieces of equipment necessary after orthopaedic surgery.

Wheelchairs

Many children undergoing lower limb surgery will be immobilised in casts or braces and some may be unable to weightbear; therefore, they will require the use of a wheelchair during their postoperative recovery. Some children will only require a simple non-adapted wheelchair for longer distances which they cannot manage using walking aids. These can usually be loaned by the occupational therapy department or the local loans store. Specialised wheelchairs or those required for longer loan are generally available from the occupational therapy department, local wheelchair service or appropriate charitable organisation. If the child already has their own wheelchair or buggy, it may be possible to adapt this with elevating leg rests or reclining backrest and change in seating.

The occupational therapist should be competent in wheelchair assessment and postural management of children. Factors to consider for wheelchair assessment are:

- The environment in which the chair is to be used, e.g. indoors or outdoors, at home, school or both (including access)
- Ability of both the child and carers, e.g. self-propelling or attendant controlled wheelchair required
- Size and weight of the chair – can the chair be stored, managed and transported easily
- Physical assessment of child – size, weight, posture management, and mobility requirement. Consideration of changes to the centre of gravity because of casts and fixators should be taken into account and a risk assessment or adaptations may need to be made.

Accurate dimensions are essential to prescribe the correct size (Pratt and Allen 1989):

- Hip width – measurement of the widest part across the thighs and hips when the child is seated
- Seat depth – the back of the buttocks to behind the knee minus approximately 5 cm
- Leg length – from the heel to under the thigh
- Back height – from the seat base to axilla, or to top of shoulders or top of head depending on amount of support required.

Other considerations as part of the assessment include:

- Frame – fixed or folding
- Tilt in space (whole unit tilts rather than increasing recline angle) or recline only
- Leg rests – fixed or elevating to accommodate casts, braces or orthoses
- Armrests – correct support given, to assist transfers or working at a desk
- Push handles – height for parents (especially if chair is reclined); use of extended handles
- Brakes – does the child need to be able to operate these independently? Wherever possible the child should be given the opportunity for self-initiated mobility as opposed to being seated for safe positioning although not at the risk of compromising the surgery (Wright-Ott 2005).

Children with developmental dysplasia of the hip

The occupational therapist's primary role will be the management of the functional consequences of a child being immobilised in a plaster spica or harness with the hips maintained in flexion and either abduction or internal rotation (see Figures 7.5, p 115, and 7.6, p 116). The plaster spica can be distressing and disruptive for the child and parents, and can cause many problems with mobility and personal care (Hinde 2000). Generally, the younger child is easier to manage, as manual handling is less of a problem and the children can often be seated in their own pushchair.

At the pre-admission clinic

Preparing both the child and their parents is essential so that they know what to expect after the surgery. It is useful to liaise with the surgeon to ascertain the likely surgical procedure, e.g. open or closed reduction and the method of immobilisation and position (see Chapter 7). Parents may often present in an anxious state after their discussion with the surgeon, and have many questions regarding how they will manage.

A portfolio of pictures of children who have undergone this type of surgery and immobilisation and illustrations of practical solutions to show parents is helpful, along with written information booklets that reinforce the discussion and act as an *aide memoire* and resource for the future. It is reassuring for parents to see photographs of real children crawling, playing and having fun with their spica or brace *in situ* and to give them a realistic expectation of what their child will look like in a plaster or harness. Children can often associate with a doll with a spica in place, and parents can obtain an idea of how much their child in a plaster is likely to weigh.

During the assessment, the occupational therapist should discuss the functional implications of the application of the spica or harness. This will include:

- Seating and posture
- Manual handling and moving
- Toileting
- Bathing and personal care
- Feeding
- Clothing and dressing
- Mobility and transportation.

As well as the general initial assessment described on pages 130–31, at this stage for younger children, the occupational therapist should assess the child's pushchair or buggy to ascertain whether it may be suitable following surgery. It will also be essential to review the child's car seat, as safe seating in a car is often a difficult issue to solve post operatively and it may be necessary to advise the parents that they may need to loan or purchase a different car seat.

Post operatively

After the surgery and the application of a cast or harness, the occupational therapist should assess the child's position. The plaster will usually be reinforced 24 hours after surgery has taken place.

Moving and handling

Once the plaster is dry and the child is stable medically with any pain well controlled, the occupational therapist can instruct the parents how to move their child safely. The child may feel awkward and heavier to begin with, but practice and use of techniques in a safe environment will build confidence. Hoisting may be required for the older child, or where parents have existing medical problems. The occupational therapist will assess and recommend a hoist and suitable sling compatible with the home environment, and will lead the training of the parents and some members of the team who may not be familiar with hoisting.

Positioning

In bed

The occupational therapist and parents should problem solve together to find a position that the child is safe and comfortable in; this usually means using additional pillows or large beanbags to support extremities and to prevent pressure areas.

If the skin is not checked regularly, pressure areas and rubbing can easily occur, especially around the waist and on the heels. Parents should be instructed on how to check for redness and skin breakdown. In conjunction with the nursing team, the occupational therapist should ensure the parents are able to change nappies with the hip spica or harness in situ (if appropriate) and instruct on the importance of keeping the skin dry to maintain tissue viability. Older children may need to use a urinal and slipper pan for toileting and will require assistance from their parents or an over-bed rail.

On the floor/playing

Parents will need to understand the importance of continuing to give their child opportunities to play, explore and be involved with siblings while the hip spica is *in situ*. The occupational therapist can reinforce the importance of this by practising how to get their child positioned comfortably for floor play, and also up from the floor safely. A beanbag that moulds to the child's temporarily unusual shape, foam wedges or many pillows are all helpful. A child in a spica is often quite comfortable lying on their stomach supported by pillows, so that their arms are free to play and explore. Some learn to drag themselves around in a crawling posture and some can pull themselves to standing in the spica. It is advisable to obtain clarification from the surgeon whether weightbearing through the lower limbs is contraindicated. Although specialist or bespoke chairs and seating can be manufactured, these are not usually required.

Provision of specialist equipment

Pushchair or wheelchair

Except for very young or small children, most children will require the temporary loan of another pushchair or wheelchair to accommodate their new seating position. The young or small child may be seated safely in their own pushchair or a larger pushchair with pillows for support. Usually children over 14 months to 2.5 years require the loan of a double pushchair with a bench-type seat and variable angle of back recline, or a specialist pushchair as they are unable to sit in a standard push chair due to the extended angle at their hip joint. Children between 2.5 and 4 years often need a small junior wheelchair with a reclining backrest and a spica board to support their legs in the cast.

Older children may need to be seated in a larger or small adult wheelchair that reclines with a spica board in situ. Suitable cushions, headrests and push handles will need to be provided. A full risk assessment should be carried out to ensure that all aspects of the wheelchair prescription and provision are safe and have been covered.

The occupational therapist will provide training in the use of the wheelchair by the child, who should usually be able to self-propel unless there are any other limitations or impairments. Parents or carers should be instructed in the safe use, handling, dismantling and transportation of the wheelchair or pushchair including loading and unloading this into their car. It is useful to provide parents with a well-illustrated booklet, which explains how to safely use the wheelchair and reminds parents after their initial instruction.

Car seating

Transfers in and out of a car and the provision of a safe car seat are extremely challenging for carers who have a child in a hip spica or a brace. In all cases, it is essential that the occupational therapist is aware of the country's legislation on child restraint in a vehicle and that any recommendations made comply with this. Some younger or small children may be able to use their own car seat without modification; however, the majority will require an alternative solution temporarily. Child car safety seats are available with less built up seats and reduced lateral support, with an adjustable harness to accommodate the increased bulk of the plaster and strapping.

Local car seat safety centres and car safety advisors can provide advice to occupational therapists and their clients. In some areas in the UK, it is possible to hire or loan a suitable car seat. This will be fitted by an expert to ensure all safety requirements and legislation regarding child restraint in the individual vehicle is covered. Harnesses are available that clip to the seat belt system which allow a child to travel safely while lying across the width of the seat, however, this prevents the carrying of siblings or other passengers.

In some cases it will not be possible to achieve a safe seating position within the car and therefore special transport may be required, e.g. ambulance with stretcher to take the child home from hospital. The lack of suitable transport would impact on the family and their normal routine and activities. Therefore, early provision of accurate, relevant information regarding the loan of car seats is essential so that arrangements can be made in a timely way to facilitate discharge and to enable families to resume their normal lifestyle.

Usually the child will need to be manually handled into the car by carers.

Feeding

It may be difficult for the child to feed normally due to their position within the spica. The use of corrective seating, beanbags or additional pillows can help. Parents are often ingenious at finding solutions and these can be shared with other parents encountering similar difficulties.

Personal care

Personal hygiene can be easily compromised by the presence of the plaster or brace. The occupational therapist should work closely with the nursing staff to facilitate effective personal care and to assist parents in managing these activities at home. An adjustable bed or bed raised to a correct height to facilitate personal care and transfers may be necessary. A variable height over-bed table may be useful to enable the child to participate in some self-care. It is unlikely that the child will be able to get very near to a washbasin and will be unable to bathe or shower while they are in plaster. Special attention should be given to the plaster area following toileting. Hair washing will also be difficult and a plastic or inflatable hair-washing tray may be recommended for use with the child lying supine in bed, with surplus water draining into a bowl or bucket.

Toileting is difficult while the child is supine. A combination of slipper bedpans and urinals can be tried. Older children may be able to assist in this activity by raising themselves using an over-bed rail. For younger children, parents should be advised how to position nappies, how to prevent soiling of the plaster and how to check the skin near to the plaster edges regularly.

Loose and stretchy clothing is advisable and in some instances may need to be adapted due to the bulk of the plaster.

Cerebral palsy

To work effectively with children with cerebral palsy, the occupational therapist needs to understand the classification and severity of the condition and the specific effects on development and movement patterns along with the deprivation of experience caused by motor and sensory deficits. Usually an extensive multi-professional team is involved in the child's care.

The occupational therapist may be presented with a child requiring multi-level orthopaedic surgery due to the effects of spasticity on the growth and development of their musculoskeletal system. As a result, the child may present with scoliosis, kyphosis, hip subluxation or dislocation, hip and knee flexion contractures, heel cord shortening or foot rotation. Typically, these problems present in combination and therefore the multi-level approach is usually taken (as described in Chapter 7). The child may be immobilised in a brace for six weeks or longer and will always undergo extensive physiotherapy treatment and mobilisation. This recovery period can be very stressful for the child and family; however, if they are prepared and have appropriate equipment and resources in place, this can be alleviated.

Common postoperative issues include:

- Seating and positioning
- Mobility
- Toileting
- Transfers
- Activities of daily living and personal care
- Access – home, school
- Socialisation and play.

Preoperative assessment

The preoperative assessment will focus on the current ability of the child and identifying potential issues post operatively. The use of a preoperative assessment tool will ensure that all important areas are covered (as described above). It is likely that the child will require a wheelchair after surgery even if they do not use one beforehand, and therefore the parents and child should be introduced to this idea and a wheelchair assessment carried out if practicable, so that the wheelchair can be obtained and prepared in advance.

At this stage, it will be important to liaise with the child's usual paediatric specialist team to ensure there is continuity of care between community and secondary care services and to ensure all parties are aware of the forthcoming changes. Some children may be resident at a special school and the staff there may be used to receiving children back home after complex surgery and have the skills and resources to care for this group of children.

Transport to and from school will need to be considered. Transfers and transporting the wheelchair in the parent's car or school transport, e.g. bus, will need to be considered and whether special transport will need to be arranged when the child is able to return to school. There is extensive legislation regarding the transport of people in wheelchairs and this must be adhered to when making any temporary or permanent arrangements.

Postoperative intervention

Interventions should be planned and carried out according to the child's developmental stage and abilities. They may include:

- Assessment, modification or provision of customised postural support and seating (including 24-hour postural management)
- Wheelchair assessment and prescription
- Mobility and transfer assessment and practice
- Manual handling and instruction for parents/carers
- Facilitation of play and developmental activities
- Assessment and provision of adaptive equipment and environmental adaptation (including home or school visits)
- Facilitation of personal care and dressing (including consideration of adapted clothing) according to developmental level
- Access to transport
- Graded activity and goal setting to increase joint range of movement and muscle strength.

Perthes' disease

Generally, children with Perthes' disease have been fit and well before developing hip pain and a limp. The presentation of Perthes' disease can be mild or the child can be significantly affected by pain and reduced mobility. Usually the child and their parents will be seen in the preoperative clinic where information gathering and initial assessment can take place. At this stage, the postoperative weightbearing status may be confirmed, as well as whether the child will be required to wear a brace post operatively. If so, then a wheelchair will be required temporarily.

Following surgery, the occupational therapist's role will be to assist the child to regain independence, which may include advising on compensatory methods of achieving everyday mobility and activity, and equipment prescription. As surgery is usually performed in middle childhood, it is particularly important to discuss managing at school, including carrying items, access to toilets and facilities, and sports and activities.

Scoliosis

Corrective surgery for children and adolescents is complex with a long recovery period. The occupational therapist will be involved at all stages of the care pathway.

Adolescent idiopathic scoliosis

The occupational therapist's approach to the management of a young person will vary from that of a younger child. Independence, body image and peer issues are very important to a young person and their level of receptiveness and engagement will impact on therapy. Missing school and the loss of interaction with friends and peers can impact on the young person's development, esteem and socialisation. Therefore, their coping skills, pain management, family and peer dynamics and their ability to deal with stress can all impact on the postoperative management. For some young people, surgery is extremely frightening and can cause immense anxiety. The occupational therapist may recommend anxiety management and relaxation and sometimes refer to a clinical psychologist or counsellor for additional support. Some adolescents who have endured noticeable physical signs such as kyphoses, humps, short stature as well as chronic pain and discomfort will welcome surgical intervention and will be well motivated to proceed.

Assessment

As surgery is usually elective, preoperative assessment will usually be carried out in advance of the operation. This allows information gathering, multi-disciplinary assessment, information sharing and planning the surgical intervention and postoperative regimen and care. This is an invaluable opportunity to obtain rapport and confidence of the young person at a stage before the postoperative period, when they may experience pain and change in their functional ability.

The initial interview should establish the young person's priorities: their likes and dislikes, current functional capacity and stage of education. The occupational therapist will need to consider how the young person will cope post operatively at home, within the community and at school or college. The learning environment can create barriers, and peers and teachers will most likely be unaware of any limitations and constraints following surgery. Therefore, the occupational therapist should discuss schooling with the young person and parents. This may include mobility, i.e.: getting to school or college, and around the school campus; limitations in bending and reaching; managing everyday tasks; carrying bags and rucksacks; and classroom seating and participation in physical activity.

Postoperative precautions are likely to be in place for three months, and following major surgery, it is likely that the young person will become easily fatigued during the normal school day. The occupational therapist may liaise with the schoolteacher and carry out a school visit to ensure that all staff are aware of the assistance required and to advise on any temporary adaptation required.

It is beneficial to issue a home measurement form (to obtain furniture and fitting heights) and request the parents to bring the completed form with them on admission. This will inform the occupational therapist if there are any major concerns with furniture heights, and the dimensions of sanitaryware should toileting and bathing equipment be required.

It is likely that both the young person and their parents will have many questions and concerns about how they will manage after the surgery, and therefore the occupational therapist should allow plenty of time to for discussion. Written information can also be provided at this stage, which can be shared with other members of the family and friends.

Postoperative assessment and treatment

Post operatively, activities of daily living will be the primary focus of the occupational therapist and intervention will be planned and evaluated according to pain tolerance, energy levels, and any postoperative care advised by the surgeon. Some young people may be required to wear an external brace made of either thermoplastic materials or plaster for protection of the internal fixation. This can create further difficulties with everyday activities and may affect the young person's independence and functional ability, i.e. the restriction this brings often feels worse than their preoperative state, which can cause frustration and anxiety although it is temporary in nature. In some services, the occupational therapist will be involved in fabricating the brace or plaster cast. In any case, building confidence and stamina is an important part of the occupational therapist's role.

Personal care and dressing

Long handled equipment such as a shoehorn, sock aid or reacher may be recommended for the young person who prefers to be as independent as possible. Perching on the edge of the bed or high seat chair may make it easier to dress the lower half. Sometimes lower garments can be put on while the young person lies supine in bed and bends their knees up toward them to get their trousers or socks on, then bridges on the bed to pull the garment up to the waist. Particular attention should be made to the fitting of the brace and techniques to put on and take off a stockinet vest for comfort should be explained. Loose stretchy clothing is recommended and sometimes larger T-shirts or sweatshirts might be needed to fit over the brace or plaster.

Washing can be restricted and the young person may find a perching stool helpful to use at the washbasin in the early stages of recovery. Long handled washing aids may be recommended or parents may help to wash hard to reach areas such as feet and back.

Transfers

The minimum sitting height should be calculated and all transfers practised. The home measurement form should be reviewed to ascertain if the furniture, fittings at home, and school are suitable for safe transfers and whether any modification is required. Transfers on and off chairs and bed should be practised.

Young people without an external brace or with a removable brace are able to shower in a walk in shower or may use a bath board for an over bath shower. A shower stool may be required for confidence, to assist with fatigue or to reduce the risk of falling. Getting up and down from a low toilet can be difficult. In some cases, a raised toilet seat and freestanding rails can help. Getting in and out of a car can be difficult, but usually managed with the car seat slightly reclined and the seat pushed back to give more legroom. Long journeys are not recommended.

Therapeutic activities

Engaging the young person in therapeutic activity can be challenging, so the occupational therapist and the young person should choose activities that are meaningful and motivating. Activities should be graded and structured to increase stamina and tolerance. Group or individual work involving creative activities, games (usually computer) music or cooking can be successful ways of engaging young people. In all cases, the occupational therapist needs to apply activity analysis, and consider the likes and dislikes of the individual and any postoperative care before recommending participation in activities. Collaborative goal setting can be a method used to involve hard to engage young people.

Discharge planning and return to education

Discharge planning will be multi-disciplinary and it is likely that prescribed criteria will need to be met before the team decides that the young person can leave hospital. The occupational therapist will ensure that any modification to the home or school environment is in place and will make referrals onwards to community paediatric teams if required.

Return to education should be graded to encourage a gradual return to activities. For example:

- Having a buddy or class room assistant to assist carrying heavy bags and books
- Modifying seating and position within the classroom to avoid twisting and poor posture
- Allowing sufficient time to move between classrooms to avoid the rush between lessons
- Considering the distance walked to, from and during school or use of transport, e.g. school bus, which may jar the surgical site.

Scoliosis in children with complex needs

Spinal surgery and the postoperative management of the child with an additional significant physical disability or condition is a much more complex undertaking, and parents will often require a high degree of support within the hospital and at home after the surgery. Preoperative planning can help to ensure all processes run smoothly and facilitate a timely discharge from hospital.

A group of children commonly requiring spinal surgery are boys with Duchenne's muscular dystrophy. Scoliosis can develop after the child becomes unable to walk. The scoliosis can be marked and can lead to pelvic obliquity and deformity of the chest resulting in restriction to lung capacity (Harpin et al. 2002). It can cause pain and a tendency towards chest infections and can limit the time a child is able to sit comfortably. Surgical intervention as well as 24-hour postural management may be necessary to improve quality of life. Surgery can affect the child's function and this is discussed on page 144.

Preoperative assessment

The preoperative assessment process will be the same as for idiopathic scoliosis described above, however it is likely that the child will have a plaster jacket *in situ* following the surgery, and this will impact on the management of the child. Key issues are:

- Manual handling and transfers – these children should not be lifted following their surgery as this could compromise the procedure, and therefore a hoist is recommended.
- Seating – many children will have custom made seating and postural support in their wheelchair, which has been provided to provide correction and support for the deformity caused by the scoliosis. This postural management system will no longer be suitable and therefore early referral for an alternative to the local wheelchair service is advisable.
- Care – additional time and effort will be required by the parents or caregivers after the surgery. Early referrals to social workers and community services are advisable to plan the additional care required.
- School attendance – it is unlikely that the child will manage a full day or week at school to begin with, so the school will need to be informed and supported to make any necessary changes to the environment or routine.
- Communication – early communication with community professionals is essential to make timely referrals for any specialist equipment or modification.

Postoperative management

In children with Duchenne's muscular dystrophy, the spine is lengthened and the child is able to sit in an upright position. The fixation and rigidity of the spine may mean that the child cannot compensate for shoulder weakness by bringing their head forward; this may commonly be seen when the child attempts to eat and can no longer get their hand to their mouth. A height adjustable table is useful and mobile arm supports may be required for those with severe muscle weakness. An angled writing slope or surface is also useful to accommodate these changes. Head control may also be affected so additional head support in the wheelchair or sling may be required, and this may affect the child's ability to lower their head while getting into some wheelchair accessible vehicles (Harpin et al. 2002). A reclining wheelchair is almost always needed for support.

Postoperative assessment will follow the same domains as in idiopathic scoliosis, however; it is likely to be focused on safe transfers using a hoist with suitable sling, and wheelchair posture and mobility. Parents and carers will require instruction and guidance in the use of new and often unfamiliar equipment, and will require reassurance and practice to become competent and confident to manage within the hospital and at home where the challenges of space and obstacles will be encountered. As the postoperative function can change significantly following surgery, a home and school visit is often advised in order to realistically assess and prescribe the equipment suitable for the home or school. Feeding, writing, using a computer keyboard, playing, dressing, personal care and toileting will need to be assessed and individual solutions found to address the issues that arise. The use of further assistive electronic equipment may be required.

Leg length discrepancy

Children undergoing limb-lengthening procedures often require a significant amount of support and input from the occupational therapist during the pre-admission stage, acute postoperative hospitalisation phase, to preparing for discharge and follow up as an outpatient. This is due largely to the practical management of the external fixator (usually an Ilizarov frame), and the functional limitations this brings, as well as psychosocial issues associated with the fixator. Some children find the application and wearing of the fixator painful and traumatic while others, according to their personality and family support, adjust well to having this in place.

Management of the child with a lower limb Ilizarov frame

The occupational therapist is likely to be part of a specialist team including a specialist Ilizarov practitioner, which supports the family and child to care for the frame. The child and their family begin to learn the skills of adjusting the frame and caring for the pin sites during the hospital stay. Children are encouraged to actively weightbear through the frame, therefore assisting bone development and prevention of muscle wasting.

Pre-admission assessment

Alongside the generic pre-admission assessment for children undergoing elective surgery, it is beneficial for the child and family to see pictures of other children with external fixators *in situ* or if possible to meet children who have undergone a leg lengthening procedure, either on the ward or at an outpatient clinic,. This can help to reassure the family, allay anxiety and help to reduce the unknown. The use of a cuddly toy or doll with a fixator in place is another less intimidating way of becoming familiar with a fixator.

At this preoperative stage, the occupational therapist can ascertain the type of frame that may be used and the length of time it is likely to be *in situ*. This will assist in planning interventions and postoperative care and liaison with other services or agencies, e.g. school. Early liaison with teachers is recommended so that they have time to prepare the environment and the child's peers.

Children with large leg length discrepancies may often require the loan of a wheelchair (if they do not already have one) for longer distances due to their compromised mobility, although most will use crutches for shorter distances. It is likely that a wheelchair will require modification to support the leg with the fixator. Activities of daily living may be affected and therefore the occupational therapist should explore the home environment and the child's usual routine and preferences at this stage. If significant issues are highlighted then a preoperative home or school visit would be beneficial in order to problem solve at the earliest stage. Parents also often benefit from information on clothing adaptation at this early stage.

Postoperative assessment and intervention

The first days adjusting the fixator can be a traumatic and painful time for the child. The occupational therapist will work closely with the physiotherapist to assist the child to mobilise and transfer safely. Assessment can be made to decide which mobility aids are required, including if a wheelchair is required. Thorough assessment is needed to recommend a suitable wheelchair that can accommodate an often bulky and awkward fixator. An adjustable elevating leg rest is usually required and careful attention should be made to the sitting position and wheelchair cushion to prevent any pressure areas to skin or to the fixator. Sometimes calf pads need to be adjusted or adapted to accommodate the fixator so that the limb is supported safely. Soft, adjustable calf support slings/harness are available to purchase, which often provide a good solution. Children with a femoral fixator may require cut away wheelchair seating to accommodate the frame so that their pelvis is aligned and they are able to sit comfortably. They may not be able to sit in the usual upright position and may need to sit in a reclined position in the wheelchair or armchair.

Transfers on and off the toilet should be practised. It is not unusual for a taller child to require a raised toilet seat with a cut-away to accommodate a fixator, which is positioned high up on the limb. Problem solving for getting in and out of the bath or shower is also necessary. The loan of a bath board or shower chair may be necessary for safety and independence, especially since good hygiene is essential for the care of pin sites.

Getting dressed and undressed can be problematic due to the size and awkwardness of the fixator, which can catch on clothing. Loose stretchy clothing is recommended, although in some cases adaptation to clothing is required to accommodate the fixator. This usually involves undoing the seams of trousers and adding a material gusset and applying hook and loop fastening. Some tracksuit trousers have popper side fastenings, which are ideal. Guidance on clothing adaptations through written information, tips and hints is useful for parents and helps them to problem solve.

Building confidence in day-to-day activities is an important part of the occupational therapist's role. As the fixator will be in place for a long period, often for up to three to eight months, the parents should be encouraged to allow the child to be as independent as possible and participate in their usual activities as far as is practicable to prevent any impact on their development. A child with a fixator in place will inevitably be tired as additional energy is required for mobility and also the laying down of new bone and healing following surgery.

Management of the child with an upper limb frame

Children with an upper limb fixator *in situ* have different but no less important issues. Firstly, the preservation of hand function and strength is very important. Hand assessment and upper limb strengthening exercises may be required to maintain upper limb and grip strength. Secondly, the occupational therapist should carry out a thorough assessment of the child's functional ability with the frame *in situ*. Dressing can be particularly difficult and bilateral upper limb activities compromised. Problem solving using new techniques and assistive equipment will be required to resolve some issues. Moving the limb and positioning may be difficult and affect eating and drinking. Adapted or angled cutlery may be required and attention should be made to the positioning of the child in relation to the activity and environment, e.g. table height and ability to reach. Sometimes a pillow or foam trough can help to support the limb comfortably. Holding writing implements can be challenging and sometimes large grip pens and pencils are useful temporarily. At school, the child may require help carrying bags and equipment.

During the time when the fixator is in place, it is important that the child's family and school staff work together to ensure that all possibilities are offered to enable the child to participate in play and sporting activities. The occupational therapist can act as an advocate for the child and provide advice on the adaptation of play activities to promote the child's enjoyment, involvement and success (Pratt 1989). Weightbearing is encouraged, but knocking the frame can be painful and therefore should be avoided.

Psychosocial issues

An Ilizarov frame can be a difficult and strange thing to look at. One can see wires extending into the limb, it looks painful and can be quite frightening to other children. Children can 'feel different' and can become the centre of attention. They need to be prepared for different reactions from their peers or strangers and be able to explain why they have the frame in place to their friends. The occupational therapist can use their skills and understanding of development to provide age-appropriate advice and information to the child's peers or help the child to do so and have the right answers to those who may be inquisitive or fearful. As the child will spend much of their time at school, support for the child in this environment is key to their re-integration. Some children like to visit the school first with their family and the occupational therapist, before they return into full time education, while others adapt easily and do not wish to be made a fuss of. In any case, a visit with or without the child present will allow assessment of access, classroom positioning and seating, distances the child will have to travel, toileting arrangements, how books and equipment will be moved and how the child will cope with all areas of the curriculum. As previously mentioned a buddy system or classroom assistant may be useful. A graded return to school is most often recommended and should be negotiated with everyone involved.

Pain management

The occupational therapist has an important role in pain management. Teaching the child about pacing, deep breathing and relaxation can be very helpful for some children.

Congenital talipes equinovarus

Following surgery or manipulation, the foot or feet are placed within plaster casts to maintain the correct position. It is the plaster technicians who usually undertake casting although in some areas occupational therapists and physiotherapists will fulfil this role. The occupational therapist's main role is to assess how the parents will manage a young child with a plaster cast. This will include mobility and transfers, personal care, care of the plaster and the effect on the child's development. A buggy or wheelchair may be required if bilateral surgery has been carried out.

Juvenile idiopathic arthritis

Children with juvenile idiopathic arthritis are usually seen within specially designated services, and the occupational therapists are often part of the specialist team caring for these children, which includes a consultant rheumatologist (with a specialist interest in this condition and age group) and a paediatrician. Occupational therapy assessment and intervention are based on both rheumatological and paediatric approaches, and therefore is outside the scope of this chapter. The occupational therapist will require specialist skills, e.g. splinting, joint protection techniques including pacing and energy conservation, relaxation, anxiety management, long-term and self-management of a condition, child and young person focused activities and activity analysis (College of Occupational Therapists, Specialist Section, Rheumatology 2003).

Rare conditions

Working in a specialist unit, the occupational therapist is likely to be involved with the care of children and young people with less frequently presenting conditions. The paediatric care and approach will remain the same as described for the more common conditions, but further background reading may be required to fully understand the effects of the condition and the likely methods of intervention. Conditions encountered are as follows.

Osteogenesis imperfecta

This condition is associated with brittle fragile bones, in which even minor trauma can lead to fractures. The child may experience multiple fractures, deformity and muscle wasting due to under use, immobilisation and inactivity. The occupational therapist may be involved in the management of fractures and their sequelae, risk assessment and modification of activity and the environment to reduce the risk of fractures occurring.

Marfan's syndrome

In this syndrome, there is excessive growth at the epiphyseal plates. Children are tall for their age with long extremities, and lax and hypermobile joints. They often develop scoliosis, coxa vara and stooped shoulders. Occupational therapy intervention, therefore, will be related to these presenting problems.

Achondroplasia

Dwarfism is the characteristic associated with this condition. Lumbar lordosis and coxa vara often develop. Surgery is often required for neurological complications and to increase function. Occupational therapists will be involved in all areas of occupational performance, particularly in environmental adaptation.

Arthrogryposis

In this condition, there is incomplete fibrous ankylosis leading to contracture at the joints. This can lead to deformities including clubfoot and dislocation of the hip. Maintaining and increasing range of movement, stretching, serial splinting and maintaining independence in activities of daily living are all important aspects of occupational therapy intervention.

Bone tumour

The occupational therapist may encounter a child presenting with malignant bone tumour, which may require extensive reconstructive surgery or even limb amputation. The occupational therapist will need to be sensitive to the family and the effect of the diagnosis and prognosis, as well as potential life-changing surgery and treatment. The skills of palliative and cancer care may be required. If an amputation is indicated, close liaison and planning with the local specialist limb centre is recommended. Post-surgical management and rehabilitation should be child and family centred (see Chapter 14).

Summary

The role of the occupational therapist working with children and young people is uniquely challenging and diverse. Advanced team working, assessment and problem solving skills are essential to provide a family- and child-centred approach. Advancing orthopaedic surgical techniques and medical management require the occupational therapist to keep up to date and modify their treatment and interventions as required to embrace these changes and to link these with occupational therapy models, approaches and frames of reference.

References

Case-Smith, J. (2005). *Occupational Therapy for Children*. St Louis: Elsevier Mosby.

College of Occupational Therapists Specialist Section. (2003). Rheumatology. *Clinical Guidelines for Rheumatology*. London: College of Occupational Therapists.

Crooks, L., & Marin Wavrek, B. (2005). Hospital services. In J. Case-Smith. (Ed.). *Occupational Therapy for Children* (5th edition). St Louis: Elsevier Mosby.

Harpin, P., Robinson, T., & Tuckett, J. (2002). Children with Duchenne muscular dystrophy. In C. S. Hong and L. Howard (Eds). *Occupational Therapy in Childhood*. London: Whurr Publishers.

Hinde, S. (2000). *The provision and availability of equipment for children in hip spicas and splints: a national survey*. STEPS. Cheshire: The National Association for Children with Lower Limb Abnormalities.

Hong, C. S., & Howard, L. (2002). *Occupational Therapy in Childhood*. London: Whurr Publishers.

McIlroy, M. A., & Koranyi, K. I. (1989). General pediatric health care. In P. N. Pratt and A. S. Allen (Eds). *Occupational Therapy for Children* (5th edition). St Louis: Mosby.

Moersch, M. S. (1989). Parent and family involvement. In P. N. Pratt and A. S. Allen (Eds). *Occupational Therapy for Children* (5th edition). St Louis: Mosby.

Pratt, P. N. (1989). Play and recreational activities. In P. N. Pratt and A. S. Allen (Eds). *Occupational Therapy for Children* (5th edition). St Louis: Mosby.

Pratt, P. N., & Allen, A. S. (1989). *Occupational Therapy for Children*. St Louis: Mosby.

Richardson, P. K. (2005). Use of standardised test in pediatric practice. In J. Case-Smith (Ed.). *Occupational Therapy for Children*. St Louis: Elsevier Mosby.

Stewart, K. B. (2005). Purposes, processes and methods of evaluation. In J. Case-Smith (Ed.). *Occupational Therapy for Children*. St Louis: Elsevier Mosby.

Wright-Ott, C. (2005). Mobility. In J. Case-Smith (Ed.). In *Occupational Therapy for Children*. St Louis: Elsevier Mosby.

Further reading

Kramer, J., & Hinojosa, J. (1999). *Frames of Reference for Pediatric Therapy* (5th edition). Philadelphia: Lippincott Williams & Wilkins.

Lyons, B., Boachie-Adeji, C., Podzius, J., & Podzius, C. (1999). *Scoliosis: Ascending the Curve*. New York: M. Evans and Co.

Parker, J. (2002). *The 2002 Official Patients' Sourcebook on Scoliosis*. San Diego: Icon Health Publications.

Part II

Trauma

Chapter 9

Principles of fracture management

Chris Harris

Introduction

There is a joke about a holistic orthopaedic surgeon being one who treats the whole bone. The aim of 'fracture' management is to restore both the injured part and the individual back to 'normal', or at least back to their pre-existing state. In order to do this we need to identify those parts that are injured, the role we have to play in facilitating their recovery and to support the individual in their environment while they go through the recovery process. We also need to identify those who will not fully recover and our role in providing long-term help for them.

A fracture is a break in the continuity of a material, in our case bone. Energy transferred to the bone takes it beyond its yield strength and once broken, the bone no longer fulfils its mechanical role of support. Part of our treatment will be geared to restoring this role of the bone. Referring back to our holistic orthopaedic surgeon, we must appreciate that the injury does not just involve the bone but also the surrounding soft tissues. The energy that fractured the bone will also have been transferred to the soft tissues and injured them. The soft tissue injury is not always readily apparent; think for example how long it sometimes takes for a bruise to appear. However, it is often the resultant state of the soft tissues that determines the overall outcome of the injury. Lastly, we must realise that the local injury does not just affect the function of the limb but also that of the individual as a whole. A fractured finger means a lot to a concert pianist and limited use of an injured upper limb may leave an elderly person unable to cope with living alone at home. In the acute setting, multiple injuries may result in a systemic inflammatory response, which may lead to organ dysfunction and threaten life (see the polytrauma section below). Injuries to more than one limb will also restrict subsequent mobilisation of the individual, who may therefore require a wheelchair for a period of time.

Basic science

Like all parts of the body, the musculoskeletal system has a function – support and movement. It consists of bones, muscles and tendons, joints and ligaments, nerves and blood vessels. Each component has a specific function and together they work as a team to produce the end result, coordinated and purposeful movement. Being highly dependent on each other, injury to any one will affect the function of another and therefore the whole. For example, nerve injury results in altered muscle function, which in turn results in altered joint function. Thus, although our focus when managing fractures tends to be on the bone, our management of any injury must involve restoration of the whole.

Bone

Bone is a highly specialised living tissue. As those who treat injuries, we are most interested in its mechanical role – that of a supportive structure making up the skeleton. Bone also has metabolic functions, however, these are not discussed in this chapter. Bone provides the rigidity and leverage that bears loads and allows the muscles to function in moving the limbs.

Composed primarily of inert substances (collagen and calcium phosphate) in a layered arrangement, a little like reinforced concrete, it is all to easy to view bone as one sees it in the classroom/laboratory – as inert. However, it is a living tissue, containing cells that both regulate its composition and hence its strength and which respond to injury with healing. As a living tissue it has a blood supply and injury to that supply, which occurs to some degree with all fractures, can result in bone death. Dead bone initially tends to have the same appearance (visually and on X-ray) and mechanical properties as living bone, but it behaves in a completely different manner as evidenced with the passage of time. The blood supply to the bones has different arrangements in different parts of the body. Long bones, like the femur for example, receive their blood supply from several sources (nutrient artery, periosteum, metaphyseal/epiphyseal vessels). Other bones, typically those that are covered with cartilage for most of their surface (e.g. talus, scaphoid) have a blood supply from only a couple of sources, which means that when injured it is more likely that the bone will become devoid of supply and die. This is termed avascular necrosis. Our treatment must be as friendly to the blood supply as possible.

The skeleton needs to be both strong and lightweight. Bones have a hard outer shell, referred to as the cortex, and a softer inner part consisting of cancellous bone. In the cortex, the bone is tightly packed together; it is thus strong but also relatively heavy. The blood vessels run in bony tunnels and are therefore vulnerable to the effects of injury and infection. Cancellous bone is made up of bony trabeculae, a bit like scaffolding bars, with marrow in between. The marrow consists of fat, nerves, vessels, and in some locations haematopoietic tissue. Cortex thickness varies greatly, both within a single bone and between different bones. In long bones the cortex is thickest in the middle (the shaft) where it best resists bending. The ends of long bones are typically expanded, presumably to increase the surface of articulation at the joints. These expanded ends are predominantly made up of cancellous bone, with only a thin shell of cortex.

Apart from the articular ends and sites of musculotendinous attachment, bone is covered by periosteum. Periosteum has two important roles. Firstly, it contributes to the blood supply of the adjacent cortical bone. Secondly, its role is that of bone formation following injury. Most methods of fracture management therefore aim to preserve the periosteum. We will discuss this later in the chapter.

Joints

Joints simply represent where two or more bones meet and move relative to each other to some degree. The bone ends are covered by a specialised tissue, usually cartilage but in some cases fibrous tissue. Surrounding structures, typically ligaments, keep the ends in correct apposition. Movement is allowed to occur but only in a set pattern (direction and amount). Joints differ in their degree of stability and therefore in the likelihood of specific injuries. For example, dislocation of the shoulder is relatively common whereas dislocation of the hip is not.

In synovial joints (with hyaline articular cartilage) the surfaces are extremely smooth. This combined with the lubrication properties of the cartilage and the joint fluid results in a low frictional state. Shock absorption also occurs for those joints requiring it, e.g. the meniscal cartilages in the knee. In this state, the joints can remain healthy for the duration of the person's life.

Injuries can adversely affect joints in a number of ways. Firstly, they can increase the risk of developing arthritis as a result of:

- Chondral damage from surface impact/dislocation
- Malunion of an intra-articular fracture resulting in a prominent edge that abrades the opposite surface
- Malalignment of a weightbearing limb (e.g. genu varum) resulting in increased loading of one part of the joint surface over another.

Secondly, they can also result in reduced range of movement at the joint as a result of:

- Stiffness from capsular scarring after injury involving the joint
- Stiffness related to immobilisation
- Altered nerve/muscle function (see below).

Muscles

Their function, like that of joints, is movement, and disuse can result in atrophy. Direct injury to the muscle may result in scarring and shortening. They may also become tethered at the fracture site. Muscles can also be injured indirectly, by a surgical approach or by a period of immobilisation. All this can result in decreased movement of the joints and weakness. In addition a nerve injury can also lead to loss of muscle function.

In general, trauma results in direct injury to most of these tissues. The bony injury (fracture) tends to take centre stage, partly because it produces immediate clinical signs (i.e. deformity) and partly because bone stands out from the crowd on the X-ray film. We must not however forget the 'soft' tissues since it is these that will predominantly determine the outcome. A good example of this is in spinal injuries. Patients with injury to the spinal column alone (bone, ligaments, discs) typically fare well, whereas those who have an associated local spinal soft tissue injury (the spinal cord) frequently fare poorly. A big pitfall of fracture management is to consider only the fracture. Bones do not exist in isolation and we must not think of them so. The challenge of fracture management is therefore not focused on the fracture but on the whole.

Fractures in general

Everyday micro-fractures (fractures of an individual trabeculae or around cement lines in cortical bone) are microscopic and do not concern us clinically; they are dealt with by the normal remodelling processes of bone. Generally speaking there are three clinical fracture scenarios.

- **Acute traumatic fractures** – The injuring force is greater than the bone can withstand, like holding a pencil and bending it until it snaps in two. This is the type of injury that we will predominantly look at in this chapter.
- **Stress fractures** – Here, a single force is not sufficient to break the bone but the cumulative effect weakens and breaks it eventually. This is like taking a plastic ruler and bending it back and forth until it eventually breaks. A good example of a stress fracture is the second metatarsal neck fracture that is seen in army recruits who are subjected to an unaccustomed level of walking.
- **Pathological fractures** – Here, the bone is weaker than it should be and therefore breaks with a force smaller than expected for normal bone to break. This is analogous to breaking a rotten log in half. An example is when a femur invaded by metastatic tumour breaks simply during walking.

We are going to focus on the acute traumatic fracture. The higher the energy the more damage it does. Think of the well known nursery rhyme character Humpty Dumpty falling off the wall – the higher the wall is the more pieces poor old Humpty will end up in. When the amount of energy is low, such as with a twisting injury of the leg while playing football, the fracture tends to be a single break. When the amount of energy is high, for example after a fall from a considerable height or being hit by a fast moving vehicle, the injury to the bone is more severe. The bone tends to be fragmented with the pieces further apart (displaced) and possibly out through the skin (open fracture). When faced with a particular injury, we can try to judge the amount of damage sustained by the history (e.g. my parachute did not open) and by the pattern of the injury/injuries. This is important, since we are interested in the chance of other injuries, the associated soft tissue damage and the way in which the injured tissues will behave as regards healing and their response to surgical insult.

Classification of fractures

We try to describe fractures in a particular manner using a variety of terms. This helps us to discuss the injury with our colleagues and helps us in deciding the management of the injury.

The location of the break

Firstly, we name the bone that is broken. It may be part of the axial skeleton (spine, ribs, pelvis) or of the peripheral skeleton (limbs). Then we describe which part of the bone is broken. We use terms such as proximal, middle or distal, medial or lateral, head or neck, condyle or malleolus. For long bones we refer to the diaphysis (shaft),

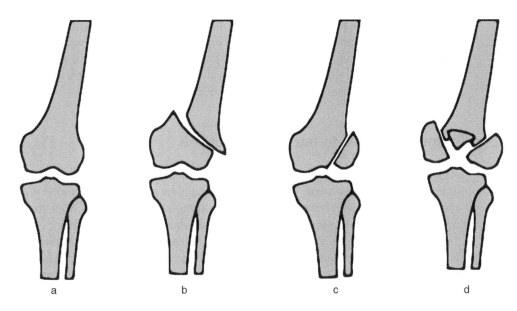

Figure 9.1 Examples of intra-articular fractures of the knee joint. (a) Normal knee joint. (b) Extra-articular fracture. (c) Partial articular. (d) Complete articular.

metaphysis or epiphysis. Fractures involving the joint surface are termed intra-articular, whereas those that do not are extra-articular.

Intra-articular fractures (Figure 9.1) are subdivided into those which separate just part of the joint surface from the main bone (partial articular) or the whole articular surface from the bone (complete articular) (Muller et al. 1990). A computed tomography (CT) scan is useful in delineating intra-articular fracture extent. Lastly, there are occasions where the fracture is extra-articular but is located within the capsule of the joint; a good example of this is the subcapital fracture of the femoral neck (see p 168–9).

The pattern of the break

Classically, fractures are described as simple (two pieces/'fragments') or comminuted (more than two pieces/fragments). Simple fracture patterns include transverse, oblique and spiral. If a third bony piece is present then it is often referred to as a butterfly fragment. Cortical bone typically breaks in this manner and so these terms are well suited to the shafts of long bones. While cancellous bone can also fracture in these patterns, it can also be impacted (squashed up), highly comminuted, (broken into lots of small pieces) or a combination of both.

Sometimes long bones are broken at two separate sites. If this results in a segment of bone being 'free' then it is termed a segmental fracture, whereas if it is more like two 'separate' fractures of the same bone then it is termed bifocal, since there are two problems to focus on.

These patterns have implications for treatment. Transverse fractures can be relatively stable under axial load so their treatment would be aimed at minimising bending or rotatory movements. Oblique and spiral fractures are much more unstable. Comminuted fractures afford no possibility of sharing the load with any implants used. Impacted fractures are the most stable but may need disimpacting in order to restore the shape of the bone. Once disimpacted, the fragments need supporting because there has been loss (squashing down) of the surrounding bone. Bone graft or bone graft substitute may be used in these situations, in addition to any fracture fixation devices.

Specific names attached to fractures – eponyms

As well as these anatomical descriptions, some fractures are so common (or notorious) as to be described by a name (eponym), either the name of the person who first described them or by a demonstrative name. A good example of this is the Colles' fracture – a fracture of the distal radius as described by Abraham Colles in 1814.

Bones tend to break at specific locations and often in one of a number of set and limited patterns. For example, fractures of the ankle fall into one of four basic categories and knowledge of the particular patterns help the treating surgeon to predict which structures are injured and which require treatment (Lauge-Hansen 1950).

Classifications specific to particular fractures

There are numerous classification systems in use. Most are called after the name of the surgeon who first described them. For example, Schatzker's classification of tibial plateau fractures (Figure 9.2), where fracture pattern I is the mildest and fracture pattern VI is the most severe (Schatzker et al. 1979). While it is not essential to know all of these classification systems, it is important to understand the basis behind them

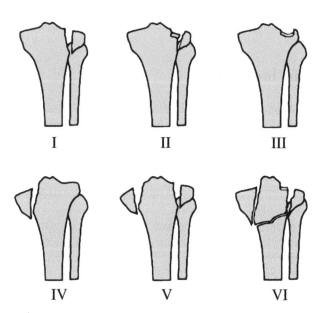

Figure 9.2 Schatzker's classification of tibial plateau fractures: I–VI.

so as to appreciate the full extent of the injury and the problems that may be encountered in treating them.

Universal (AO/Orthopaedic Trauma Association (OTA)) fracture classification system

Using this system, a fracture is represented by a five figure code, based on its location and pattern. The first figure describes which bone is involved (e.g. femur = 3, tibia = 4), the second describes the location (proximal = 1, middle = 2, distal = 3) and the third figure describes the pattern (a, b, c). The last two figures relate to the subtype. This classification system finds particular use in the research setting, where one wishes to compare injuries of similar types.

State of the overlying soft tissues

Fractures are also described as open or closed, depending on whether or not their soft tissue covering has been breached, thus exposing the bone to the contaminated outside environment.

Open fractures tend to be graded according to their severity (extent of tissue damage and risk of infection). The most commonly used classification of open fractures is that of Gustilo and Anderson where grade I is the mildest and grade III the most severe. Closed fractures have also been classified likewise, trying to estimate the extent that the local soft tissue injury will have on the outcome.

Fracture displacement

In addition to describing the fracture pattern we must include an assessment of how much the particular bony bits of the fracture are out of place. Generally speaking we use the word 'displaced' to describe fractures that overall are not in correct position.

Fractures can be (Figure 9.3):

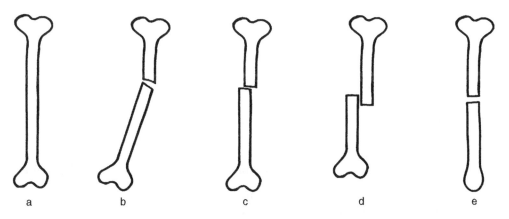

a   b   c   d   e

Figure 9.3 Examples of fracture displacement. (a) Normal bone. (b) Angulated. (c) Translated. (d) Shortened. (e) Rotated.

- Angulated (the bone is no longer straight but the pieces make an angle with each other)
- Translated (the ends have moved away from each other)
- Shortened (or distracted in some cases)
- Rotated (twisted).

How much of these displacements we can accept varies, depending on a whole number of factors. We will discuss this in more detail later.

Basic fracture healing

A famous orthopaedic surgeon, Alan Apley, often asked his students why bone heals. His reply: 'Because it was broken.' It must be remembered from the outset, that bone has a fantastic intrinsic ability to heal. As those 'treating' the patient, we are on the whole facilitating this healing process and need to ensure that our techniques do not actually prove counterproductive to this.

Exactly how a fracture heals depends on how it is treated. We will start by considering what, for want of a better word, could be considered as 'natural' fracture healing of a long bone – that which is seen with either untreated fractures or those which have been temporarily immobilised in a cast. The process is complex and not completely understood, but in general consists of a few key stages.

The broken bone bleeds and so a blood clot forms at the fracture site. This is termed the fracture haematoma. Like wound healing in general, new blood vessels invade the area, bringing in cells that together with the local cells initiate and carry out healing. The importance of local vascularity cannot be over-emphasised.

In fractures that are treated non-operatively, the challenge to the body is to restore bone, which is a relatively brittle material, in an area of abnormal movement. This is a bit like trying to super-glue two pieces of plastic together while moving the pieces about. The body manages this problem by converting the haematoma to bone via tissues of varying stiffness, until the area is stiff enough to turn to bone. So, fibrous granulation tissue is the first to form, being relatively stretchy. Then areas of cartilage, which are less stretchy, appear and merge and finally all is exchanged for bone, which is relatively rigid. At this stage the bone ends have united.

The initial type of bone is woven bone, called this because rather than being layered (lamella) its orientation is haphazard. It forms as a lump around the fractured bone ends. It is not as strong as lamellar bone but its greater amount seems to compensate for this. This new bone is called callus, which means hard. It will not be seen on X-ray for at least a few weeks. Then, over the following weeks, months, and years, the woven bone is replaced by lamellar bone and the overall amount of bone at the fracture site decreases, trying to restore the bone to its original form if possible. This process is called consolidation and remodelling.

Important factors in fracture healing can be considered in the following manner:

- Biology – the integrity of the local vascularity
- Contact – how close the bone ends are to each other
- Stability – the mechanical environment
- Stimulation – the use of the limb during healing.

There is overlap between these factors: stimulation acts via biology and in part depends on stability, bone contact affects stability, etc. Each factor plays its part in the healing process and the treating orthopaedic surgeon has control, to some degree, over each of them. A surgical approach to the fracture site, for example, will alter the biology, which may or may not be important. The amount of weightbearing permitted for a lower limb fracture balances concerns about stability with the desire for stimulation.

Too much movement of the fracture can delay or even stop the transition of the fibrous tissue and cartilage into bone, while too little movement (or stimulation) of the fracture site can make the healing process stop midway through. The result of both of these is delayed union or non-union of the fracture. Sometimes fractures fail to heal because of a large fracture gap whereas at other times fractures heal despite one. Thus fracture healing is a little like making a cake; not only are the correct ingredients required but they are also needed in the correct amounts.

The aim of fracture treatment is to restore the bone back to one solid piece, since its function of being a rigid skeletal structure depends on this. We can use either surgical or non-surgical means to obtain this. In addition to this our overall (holistic) aim, where possible, is to restore the individual back to their normal functioning lifestyle.

Non-surgical fracture treatment

Traditional non-surgical fracture management consists of a number of steps:

- Reduction
- Immobilisation until union
- Protection until consolidation.

Not all of these steps however may be necessary for a particular fracture.

Reduction

Reducing the fracture means putting the bone back into position/alignment. The fracture is reduced by closed manipulation – the surgeon grips the limb and pulls, pushes, and moves the broken bone into a better position. Fractures are initially painful, so manipulation typically requires some form of analgesia/anaesthesia. This can range from simple measures such as Entonox (gas and air) and local anaesthetic blocks through to general anaesthesia. The surgeon does not have a direct hold on the bone but rather manipulates it via their grip on the skin/soft tissues. Closed reduction of some fractures can therefore be a challenge and some amount of residual fracture displacement is often accepted.

An undisplaced fracture clearly does not require reduction. How accurate a reduction is necessary depends on a whole number of factors, relating to both the fracture itself (such as its location) and to each particular patient. Fractures that involve the joint surface (intra-articular) generally require as accurate (anatomic) a reduction as possible, to restore the smoothness of the articular surface. Some fractures simply cannot be reduced closed; there may be soft tissue interposition between the fragments or a displaced fragment may not have any soft tissue attachment whereby to pull it into place (e.g. depressed articular fragment as seen in fractures of the distal tibia).

Immobilisation until union

Using some form of external splintage, the reduced fracture is kept relatively still (immobilised) until the natural healing process (described under basic fracture healing) has caused the fragments to stick back together again or 'unite'. This takes time, typically weeks to months.

Over the ages, numerous materials have been used for external splintage. The Egyptians bound leaves around the fractured part, whereas the Anglo-Saxons used copper plates. Plaster of Paris, introduced in the 1800s has become the mainstay material for casting fractures, although synthetic materials (e.g. fibreglass casting tape) introduced in the late 1900s are becoming increasingly used.

The degree of splintage (by which we mean both the amount of the limb immobilised and the rigidity of the splint) is determined by a whole host of factors, including the location and fracture configuration. The rigidity of the splinting material itself and the rigidity conferred by its shape are also important. Sometimes a less rigid external splint is sufficient, in which case a crepe bandage or Elastoplast tends to be used. Some upper limb injuries may only require a sling for immobilisation. Undisplaced or impacted fractures of small bones (e.g. fingers) may not require any further splintage than the local surrounding soft tissues afford. Splints may be static or dynamic.

As external methods only hold the bone indirectly, via the skin and soft tissues, several issues arise. Firstly, it was traditionally felt that in order for casts to provide adequate immobilisation of the bone, they should include the joint above and the joint below the fracture. Therein lays the major drawback of such methods – relative immobilisation of joints and muscles. An illustration of the adverse effect of immobilisation is found in what used to be called 'fracture disease'. Here, individuals would come out of a cast (typically after a long period of immobilisation) with a healed fracture but there would be persistent joint stiffness, weak atrophied muscles and osteoporosis. It should have been termed 'immobilization disease' or 'plaster disease', but the fact it was not highlights how strong the belief was then in 'rest' of the injured part. For certain fractures it is not always easy to immobilize the joint above. For example, a femoral shaft fracture would require the cast to include the pelvis, rendering not only the fracture but also the individual immobile for months.

The second issue relating to the indirect holding of bone via the soft tissues is that of poor fracture control. A cast may not be able to hold the reduced position well for a number of reasons. Firstly, the cast may be too loose. It may have been applied poorly or may have become loose as the associated soft tissue swelling resolved. Moulding of the cast, so that it grips the limb in the correct areas, is one way to try to overcome this. The efficacy of cast treatment depends in part on the stability of the reduced fracture. In a Colles' fracture, for example, the intact dorsal periosteum allows us to use three point fixation to maintain the reduced position (Figure 9.4).

Some fractures are less amenable to cast treatment than others simply by their pattern or location. For example, fractures that are unstable longitudinally (comminuted, long spiral) have a tendency to shorten, something that is difficult to control using external

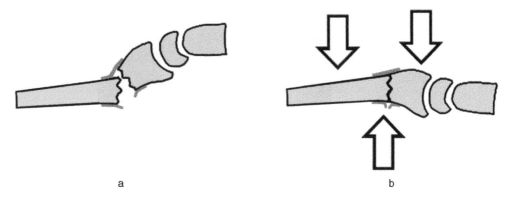

a   b

Figure 9.4 Three point fixation. (a) The fracture has an intact periosteal/soft tissue connection (hinge) on the concave side. (b) Once reduced, the forces indicated by the arrows act together with the periosteal hinge to maintain the reduction. Pressure is applied to these points by a moulded cast.

splintage. Fractures of the femur would need a cast that included the trunk and so are used in small children (who are easily portable) but not in adults who would be confined to bed if they were in such a cast. Lastly, associated injury to the soft tissues such as open wounds and skin grafts/tissue flaps may make the use of external splintage impractical or even hazardous.

Protection until consolidation

Union implies that the bone will now move as one piece. However, it may take some weeks or even months before it is strong enough for all of life's various activities. Thus the bone requires protecting from undue stresses. Such protection often equates to leaving the cast on for a little longer or changing to a removable splint. For lower limb fractures it may mean limiting the amount of weightbearing (crutches/walking stick). It may simply mean avoiding sporting activities for a time. Often the individual goes through a graduated series of such limitations while the fracture site consolidates its strength.

Functional bracing

Aware of the relative advantages of non-surgical treatment, some surgeons developed methods of external splintage that maintain joint range of movement and function. Sarmiento and colleagues have been a major force behind such treatment for fractures of the humeral and tibial diaphysis (shaft) (Sarmiento and Latta 2006). Their work was based on the philosophy that movement at the fracture site during functional activities promotes osteogenesis (bone formation). The initial cast, which immobilises the joint above and the joint below the fracture, is soon exchanged for a prefabricated adjustable plastic brace. This wraps firmly around the limb segment (arm or calf), controlling angular alignment, but does not immobilise the adjacent joints, leaving them free for functional activities. In the case of the tibia, control over shortening relies on the tether-

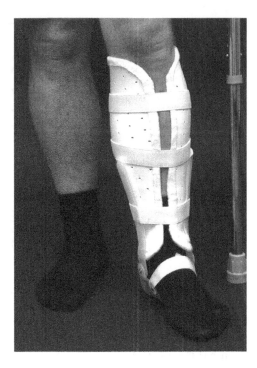

Figure 9.5 A custom made tibial brace.

ing effect of any remaining soft tissues, such as the interosseous membrane. Injury to these, resulting in an unacceptable initial amount of fracture shortening, is one of the exclusions for functional bracing for tibial fractures (Figure 9.5).

While on the subject of non-operative fracture management we must mention the role of traction. A longitudinal force is applied constantly to the broken limb, which helps to stabilise the fracture. The surrounding muscles relax and act like an external splint, which assists control of the fracture site. This decreased movement results in decreased pain.

Traction can be used for certain fractures to both reduce and maintain the fracture position. The longitudinal pull is applied either via the skin (skin traction – either directly stuck to the skin or using the frictional force) or via a bone (skeletal traction – pin or wire through either the end of the fractured bone or through a bone distal to the fractured one). Traction, like external splintage in general, has the disadvantage that it immobilises both the local joints and the individual as a whole. Femoral fractures for example may require three months of bed rest if treated in this manner. Traction finds its main use nowadays in short-term fracture stabilisation prior to formal operative fixation.

Non-surgical management on the whole is safe. One must of course not forget that an over-tight, encircling cast can result in compartment syndrome (Volkmann's ischaemic contracture) although this complication is fortunately rare nowadays. The main drawback of non-surgical management relates to the period of immobilization (and therefore its effects on the individual both locally and in general) and the limitations on the accuracy of obtaining and maintaining fracture reduction.

Operative fracture management

The disadvantages of non-operative management led surgeons to explore operative alternatives. Initial techniques, such as the use of ivory pegs seem primitive today but serve to indicate to us the desire to better the outcome for the management of certain fracture types, something that continues to this day. Using an internal 'splint' (screw, plate, nail etc) to hold the bone directly, the mechanical integrity of the bone is 'immediately' restored. This allows the limb to be moved early, aiding rehabilitation of the joints and muscles (soft tissues) and of the individual as a whole. The latter is especially important in those patient with multiple injuries, where early fracture stabilisation and movement may be critical at preventing the life-threatening complications of immobility. The phrase 'life is movement, movement is life' perhaps encapsulates the philosophy behind the huge shift from non-operative to operative management of fractures that was seen in the latter half of the twentieth century (Helfet et al. 2003).

The basic steps of surgical fracture management are essentially the same as for non-surgical:

- Reduction
- Immobilisation until union
- Protection until consolidation.

Reduction

Generally speaking the fracture can be reduced open or closed. In open reduction a surgical approach is made to the bone and the fractured ends are brought back together under direct visualisation. The main indication for open reduction is in conjunction with plate internal fixation, where the same surgical approach is used for both. However, in some cases the surgical approach to the fracture may purely be for the reduction, the bone being fixed in some other way (e.g. with an intramedullary nail – see p 166). Some approaches to the bone pass between individual muscles whereas others may divide or detach muscles. Some approaches are said to be extensile, where the exposure can safely be extended proximally/distally as required to give more access, while some are limited in extent because neurovascular structures cross the path of any proposed extension. There are a number of means of obtaining a closed reduction and examples of these will be given as we look at the various means of surgical fixation.

Immobilisation until union

While this is a useful concept (see non-operative management above), it must be realised that surgical fixation both immobilises the fracture and produces a functional union at the same time. Even before the bone has united, the fracture is held together as if united. The bone will then unite over a period of time after which the fixation becomes redundant. It can be removed at this stage (e.g. removing K-wires from a wrist fracture in clinic at three weeks post operatively) or left *in situ*. Should bony union fail to occur then eventually the fixation device would fatigue and fail itself. We must also remember that the use of the term immobilisation here relates to the fracture and not necessarily to the limb.

There are broadly speaking three categories of surgical 'fixation': internal, percutaneous and external. Fixation is performed using metallic devices – plates, screws, wires, pins and nails. Stainless steel predominates with titanium as an alternative option in many cases. There is also much interest in the development of bio-absorbable implants, which are absorbed by the body over time, obviating the need for a further operation for removal. While bio-absorbable screws are commonly used in operations such as cruciate ligament reconstruction, they have yet to realise their full potential in fracture management.

Plates are applied to the surface of the bone using screws (Figure 9.6). These typically hold well in cortical bone but can pull out of cancellous metaphyseal bone, especially in older patients with osteoporosis. This problem led to the development of locking plates – in addition to screwing into the bone the screws also screw into the plate enhancing their fixation of the fracture. In addition early plates tended to be 'one type for all locations' – the surgeon would select the appropriate length and bend the plate by hand as required to fit the bone. More recently pre-contoured plates have become available – these are location specific (e.g. clavicle) and are contoured to fit the average sized/shaped person. Such fixation allows for early mobilisation of the limb.

Nails are placed inside the medullary canal, their presence limiting movement of the surrounding bony tube. While early nails relied solely on fitting tightly into the bone to keep them in place, nowadays, nails have holes at each end allowing them to be screwed into the bone for better fixation (Figure 9.7).

Another operative option is the external fixator, where pins or wires grip the bone fragments but the bulk of the holding metalwork is on the outside of the limb (Figure 9.8). This has advantages of minimising any surgical soft tissue injury and avoiding implanted metalwork at sites at risk of infection (e.g. open fractures).

Percutaneous fixation mainly relates to K-wire fixation. The wires transfix the bony fragments, keeping them in place while they unite. The wires are left protruding from the skin, which allows their relatively simple removal in clinic a number of weeks later. Usually the individual then continues in a cast for another few weeks while the union strengthens.

With closed reduction, the internal fixation is typically performed from a surgical site away from the fracture, as seen typically with the use of intra-medullary nails. In some situations, especially for comminuted fractures, it may be better to accept a less

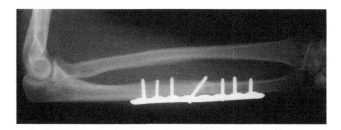

Figure 9.6 Plate fixation of an ulnar shaft fracture. The oblique screw (in the middle) was placed across the fracture site. A simple straight plate such as this can be used in many fracture locations.

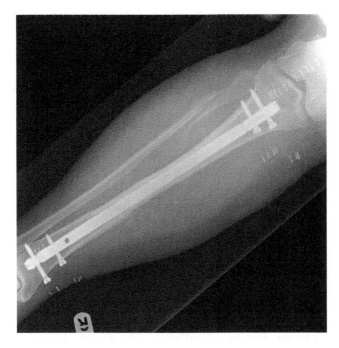

Figure 9.7 Tibial nail – the nail occupies the intramedullary canal and has screws at each end, which help lock the nail to the bone.

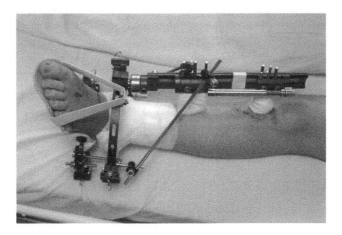

Figure 9.8 An example of external fixation using half pins in the tibial section and wires in the ankle and foot.

accurate reduction because an accurate reduction of all pieces may only be possible if the soft tissue attachments are detached from them. A good example is a comminuted intra-articular fracture of the end of a long bone, e.g. tibial plateau and pilon fractures (as described on pp 171–2) where anatomical reduction of the articular fragments is desirable but the reduction of the metaphyseal fragments does not need to be so accurate, provided that the overall alignment of the joint on the shaft is good.

Protection until consolidation

Most surgically fixed fractures will initially be protected to some degree, while we wait for the bone to unite and consolidate, otherwise excessive stresses on the fixation may cause it to fail (e.g. pull out of screws from the bone). Protection on the whole follows similar lines to that described above for non-surgical management (e.g. partial weightbearing after a lower limb fracture). Most internal fixation devices remain *in situ* long after union has occurred, thus affording some protection while the fracture consolidates.

There are, of course, disadvantages of surgical management. Openly reducing a fracture in itself creates a soft tissue injury. The biological environment of the fracture site is detrimentally altered both by the exposure of the bone ends and by any fixation attachment; local factors that ordinarily promote healing tend to be cleared from the fracture site and local vascularity is to some degree damaged. This, together with the altered mechanical environment (stability) alters the method of fracture healing. As mentioned previously, fracture healing requires the right ingredients in the right amounts. Sometimes altered healing is beneficial, sometimes detrimental. Opening the fracture to the external environment significantly increase the risk of infection, which if it occurs will be compounded by both the presence of the metallic foreign body (e.g. plate) and by the decreased local vascularity. Despite best intentions, the fracture stabilisation is not always sufficient to permit that all-important early mobilisation and in this case one may have the worst of both worlds, local soft tissues that are further damaged by the surgery and then immobilised.

External splintage is sometimes used in addition to internal fixation. Here the external splint is often used to support the soft tissues while they heal (a hinged knee brace to supplement an internally fixed tibial plateau fracture) or to protect the internal fixation from undue forces (e.g. a below knee cast after ankle fracture fixation).

Regional injuries

Femoral fractures

Proximal femoral fractures – 'hip' fractures

Fractures of the proximal femur are among the commonest injuries that we treat. Nearly all occur in older people, the effect of low energy trauma on weak bone. The individual may have a 'simple' fall, although there is nothing simple about either the factors that contributed to the fall (balance, vision, stiffness, weakness) nor its after effects on such a vulnerable group.

Bone strength decreases with age, in particular in women following the menopause. The World Health Organization defines osteoporosis as a bone mineral density 2.5 standard deviations or more below peak bone mass (measured by bone density scan). However, the diagnosis of osteoporosis can also be made in the presence of fragility fractures (fractures that occur as a result of a fall from a standing height).

Timely operative treatment is the standard for proximal femoral fractures. It allows the patient to be sat out of bed and mobilised early, thus decreasing the risks associ-

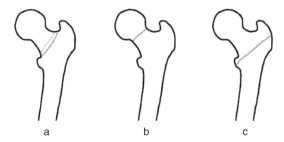

Figure 9.9 Femoral neck fractures. (a) Capsule attachment. (b) Intracapsular fracture (subcapital level). (c) Extracapsular (intertrochanteric level) fracture.

ated with prolonged bed rest (chest infection, pressure sores, venous thromboembolism, etc.). The simplest, and most useful, classification of proximal femoral fractures (Figure 9.9) is into two types – extracapsular and intracapsular.

- **Extracapsular fractures** – These are treated by internal fixation. The fracture is reduced closed (on a traction table) and fixed internally. The dynamic hip screw (DHS) has been the mainstay of treatment for several decades but cephalomedullary nails, where the proximal locking screw of the nail is into the femoral head, are also becoming a popular choice. All of these devices are designed to share the load (patient weight) with the broken bone, in order to decrease the risk of fixation failure. They do this by allowing the fracture site to collapse a little until the bone ends are in firm contact. Good bone contact together with good local vascularity means that healing does not tend to be an issue with these fractures.
- **Intracapsular fractures** – These may be complicated by damage to the blood supply to the femoral head. The risk of avascular necrosis (AVN) is proportional to the amount of fracture displacement, and since most intracapsular fractures present with some degree of displacement, we find that around a third are associated with AVN. This has significant implications for the way we treat these fractures. In 1961 Garden classified intracapsular fractures according to the amount of displacement. Garden grades I and II are termed undisplaced while grades III and IV are termed displaced.

Traditionally, younger people (those under 65 years of age and active) have been treated by fixation of the femoral head (using several screws or a dynamic hip screw (DHS)) whereas older people are treated by prosthetic replacement of the proximal femur (hemiarthroplasty). It was advocated that in younger people one should try to keep the femoral head in the belief that this gives the best long-term outcome, provided that the head survives. The fracture is therefore reduced and fixed. The individual is kept minimal/non-weightbearing initially, to protect the fixation. With this management, up to a third of fixations will fail and subsequently need revising to a total hip replacement (THR). Recent studies, however, suggest that a primary THR may be a better option.

In older patients, hemiarthroplasty was seen as best practice, a relatively simple operation with only a small reoperation risk. Hemiarthroplasty was felt to provide the simplest way back to mobility. Again, more recent studies suggest that for all but the infirm, total hip replacement gives the best outcome scores. However, it remains to be seen whether or not such recommendations will make their way into widespread clinical practice. Postoperative mortality is high in this group; around 5–10% die within the first 30 days and 25% by six months (Goldacre et al. 2002). Chest infection, venous thromboembolism and cardiovascular events (myocardial infarct, stroke) are prevalent. Many of these older patients were on the edge of coping even before the fall. They are slow to mobilise post operatively and tend to be in some form of hospital care for several weeks. Their post-injury mobility is often reduced. Some will subsequently be placed in long-term care while others will return home but with significant input from both health care and social workers. Identified osteoporosis needs to be treated to try to reduce the risk of subsequent fragility fracture (the other hip, vertebral).

Femoral shaft fractures

The femur is a very strong bone, and tends therefore to break in only one of two situations. Firstly, there is the younger person who undergoes a significant force, such as a motorbike accident. The femoral fracture may be an isolated injury or be one of multiple injuries. Polytrauma will be discussed later. Secondly there is the elderly person in whom the bone is relatively weak, typically from osteoporosis but occasionally from a bony metastasis.

Femoral fractures heal well, but being subject to large forces the femur requires adequate fixation. Intramedullary nailing is the mainstay treatment for nearly all femoral shaft fractures. A metal rod is passed either antegrade (entering proximally through the piriformis fossa or greater trochanter and passing down the medullary canal) or retrograde (entering distally through the knee joint). Treatment is the same in older people. In this group, however, it must be noted that a fractured femur is a significant insult to the body as a whole.

Fractures that have been nailed are often able to take a large amount of weight early on. For cases where it is not possible to insert a nail (presence of other metalwork such as a THR, or fracture too near the end of the bone) then internal fixation with locking plates tends to be used. Postoperative weightbearing status will be less than for intramedullary nailed fractures.

Distal femoral fractures

Like other fractures affecting the ends of the long bones these fall into two main types – intra-articular and extra-articular (see Figure 9.1). An extra-articular fracture in essence separates the shaft from the femoral condyles. Here, as with shaft fractures, an intramedullary nail can be used in most cases. Since the amount of bone 'gripped' by the nail is less, the amount of initial postoperative weightbearing may be less, to protect the fixation.

Intra-articular fractures can be partial or complete. Partial articular fractures have the advantage of an intact bone to fix the separated condyle back onto. In complete articular fractures the condyles are separated from themselves as well as from the shaft. Treatment consists in anatomical reduction of the joint (by screwing the condyles together) and connecting the restored condyles to the shaft using an intramedullary nail or plate. If chosen, a nail is typically passed into the bone through the knee joint whereas a plate sits on the lateral aspect of the bone. Strength of fixation is significantly less than for shaft fractures and so weightbearing is often limited to none for the first six weeks and then partial for the next six weeks. Hinged braces may be used during this time to give added protection.

Patella fractures

The patella is part of the extensor mechanism of the knee. Most fractures are transverse and include the soft tissue envelope (retinaculum) so that the continuity of the extensor mechanism is lost. The fracture gap is significant and those affected are unable to straight leg raise. Sometimes the retinaculum remains intact, so that the fracture gap is small and the extensor mechanism continues to function, albeit precariously. Occasionally the patella fracture can be more comminuted (stellate). The treatment of patella fractures is aimed at bringing the bone ends into contact and keeping them so while the fracture heals. At the same time, the joint needs to be mobilised to limit the amount of post-injury stiffness that ensues. Most fractures are therefore treated operatively, using wires in what is known as a 'tension band' construct to maintain the fracture reduction in association with the joint forces that occur during mobilisation. The knee is braced in extension during weightbearing (until the extensor mechanism control is regained) but mobilised soon after the operation. If the retinaculum is intact (fracture gap minimal) then non-operative treatment may be possible with the knee braced in a similar manner to protect it during weightbearing.

Tibial fractures

Proximal tibial fractures

As we discussed for distal femoral fractures, these fall into two main types – intra-articular and extra-articular. Most are intra-articular and are referred to as fractures of the 'tibial plateau'. Some are relatively simple (a few large pieces) while others can be incredibly complex (smashed to pieces). The commonest classification is that of Schatzker's: types I–VI (see Figure 9.2). Schatzker's types I–III constitute fractures of the lateral plateau of increasing severity. Schatzker's IV is a fracture of the medial plateau while V and VI describe fractures where the articular surfaces are completely separated from the shaft.

Accurate (anatomical) reduction of the joint surface is the aim, in order to minimise the risk of subsequent degenerative joint disease, while keeping the surgical approach(s) as soft tissue friendly as possible. The current choice for types I–IV is internal fixation using a periarticular plate (locking plates precontoured for that particular location). In types V and VI, where the associated soft tissues injury is more significant, many surgeons initially use an external fixator that crosses the knee ('bridging') for a week or two to allow the soft tissues to recover prior to internal plate fixation. Other surgeons prefer external fixation using a circular fine wire frame for types V and VI, after concern about the risks of wound breakdown, which was historically associated with internal fixation of these more severe injuries.

Post operatively the knee will be mobilised early but weightbearing will be minimal for the first six weeks to three months. If the fixation is felt to be tenuous (perceived poor fixation due either to bone quality in general or because of multiple small bone fragments) then a hinged brace will be used during this time. In older patients, fixation of poor quality bone is an issue. In the young, the associated soft tissue injury is the issue.

Tibial shaft fractures

As with femoral shaft fractures the 'gold standard' for some time has been intramedullary nailing, with the fixation usually being good enough for immediate weightbearing. A postoperative backslab or splint is often used at first to keep the ankle from adopting an equinus posture (and subsequent potential contracture). Since the nail is inserted proximally, either through or to the side of the patella tendon, the patient will have a scar over the front of the knee. There is a significant incidence of anterior knee pain together with some limitation of kneeling after tibial nailing and this must be taken into consideration for those patients whose lifestyle involves frequent kneeling.

Some tibial fractures are suitable for non-operative management, using functional bracing as described earlier (Sarmiento and Latta 2006; Sarmiento et al. 1989). An initial above knee cast is used, followed several weeks later by a functional brace. These allow knee range of movement while supporting the bone adequately to maintain fracture alignment. Many surgeons, however, still follow Sarmiento's earlier method, following the initial above knee cast with a patella-tendon-bearing (PTB) cast until union and only using the brace during the early consolidation period.

External fixators are also highly effective in the treatment of tibial fractures, but are nowhere near as popular a choice as intramedullary nailing. For many their role remains reserved for the more severe open fractures. It is important that the ankle joint is splinted initially, to prevent an equinus contracture developing. Once the individual is walking and performing effective stretching exercises the splint can be discontinued.

Unlike femoral shaft fractures, tibial healing is less certain. The state of the soft tissue envelope is crucial. Any surgical procedure must respect the fracture site vascularity while providing bone surfaces in contact, plus enough support to allow early weightbearing. Cigarette smoking has a clear adverse effect on bone healing (Schmitz et al. 1999) which in certain cases may be sufficient to tip the balance against bone healing. Tibial fractures are also notorious for their association with compartment syndrome, especially in young males (see p 178).

Distal tibial fractures

Again, these fall into two main types – intra-articular and extra-articular. Like the distal femur, most extra-articular fractures are amenable to intra-medullary fixation. Those fractures that are very distal tend to be fixed with a periarticular locking plate, although fine wire circular fixation is another option.

Intra-articular fractures tend to be associated with a considerable soft tissue injury component. In younger people they require a significant amount of force. They typically occur after a fall from a height, landing on the heel. The talus is driven up through the distal tibia (hence the name pilon fracture), splitting it into either a few large fragments or multiple small ones. The soft tissue envelope must be respected if one is to avoid major complications. The limb is elevated and rested for a week or more, while the local oedema decreases. Many surgeons favour a temporary external fixator placed across the ankle, which aids swelling reduction (by supporting the limb) and allows easy inspection of the soft tissue state (unlike a plaster slab). Once the soft tissues are stable, the fracture is fixed. Most surgeons prefer internal fixation with plates although some recommend external fixation as a safer option.

Ankle fractures

The talus sits beneath the tibia, nestled between the two malleoli, to which it is connected by ligaments. (This arrangement is referred to as the ankle mortise. The distal tibia and fibula are also bound together by strong ligaments.) Ankle injuries result in disruption of ligaments or bones or both; the more structures that are disrupted the more unstable the joint is. The talus may displace (sublux or dislocate), moving with whichever malleolus it remains attached to (usually the lateral one).

Treatment is aimed at maintaining the talus accurately in the ankle mortise while these structures heal. Some fracture patterns are stable enough to be treated in a cast whereas others require internal fixation (plate, screws) to maintain the reduction while healing occurs. Whatever treatment option is used, the person is kept non-weightbearing for the first six weeks. During this time they may be in a cast or some may have a brace (boot).

Foot fractures

Although any bone in the foot can be broken, a few bones deserve special mention here. In addition to the specifics for each fracture, there are some basic principles for managing foot injuries. Swelling reduction is important, using gravity (keeping the foot elevated) with or without the use of foot pumps. The foot and ankle are supported/protected using backslabs, casts or orthotics (e.g. surgical sandal, CAM walker boot). Most foot fractures require the person to be non-weightbearing initially, with subsequent progression to protected weightbearing. People with diabetes (with neuropathy and arteriopathy) are at particular risk of complications, even from minor injuries.

Fractures of the calcaneum

These typically occur after a fall from a height. They are primarily classified as extra- or intra-articular, depending on the involvement of the subtalar joint. Extra-articular fractures have a better long-term outcome but are still important to treat well since the Achilles tendon attachment is typically attached to the fractured off part. A number of authors have described the fracture pattern of intra-articular injuries (Sanders 2000). What is termed the primary fracture line passes across the posterior articular facet. This is best appreciated on a CT scan. Upward displacement of the calcaneum and secondary fracture lines account for the typical plain film appearances as described by Bohler, Gissane and Essex Lopresti (Sanders 2000). In common with intra-articular fractures elsewhere, anatomical reduction of the joint surface is the aim. Use of the extended lateral approach together with specific calcaneal plates has significantly decreased the incidence of operative morbidity. However, people with peripheral vascular impairment (diabetes, smoking) are still at considerable risk of wound complications and are often declined surgical treatment. There continues to be controversy about what is the optimum treatment for displaced intra-articular fractures of the calcaneum. While some surgeons are strongly in favour of operative treatment, some long-term studies have suggested that the clinical outcomes of non-operative treatment may not be dissimilar to operative treatment.

Post operatively the individual is kept non-weightbearing for the first six weeks and then partial weightbearing for the next six. Shock absorbing heel cups are useful initially. Physiotherapy is used for rehabilitation of ankle and subtalar joint movement. Late issues include persistent pain and subtalar degenerative change.

Talar fractures

These are potentially disabling injuries. The talus is predominantly covered with articular cartilage and has little in the way of soft tissue attachments. Its blood supply is therefore easily damaged by fractures, with the incidence of AVN being related to the amount of fracture displacement. Talar fractures fall into two main types: those of the neck and those of the body (dome). Hawkins (1970) classified talar neck fractures by the degree of displacement, which includes dislocation of the fragments. For the more severe Hawkins' types, the AVN rate is close to 100%. All but undisplaced fractures are fixed operatively. The surgical approach may require osteotomy of the medial malleolus. The fixation is typically protected with a below-knee cast and the individual kept non-weightbearing for at least the first six weeks and partial weightbearing for at least a further six. This results in stiffness and local osteoporosis. If AVN occurs, the fracture may not unite, the fixation may fail, and the talar body (dome) may collapse. All these have a significant effect on the ankle joint. Many of the more severe types culminate in a salvage ankle arthrodesis. Talar dome fractures have a similar poor outcome. Surgical access for fixation is limited and AVN rates are high.

Lisfranc injuries

Jacques Lisfranc, a surgeon in Napoleon's army in the 1800s, described an amputation technique through the tarsometatarsal joints. This part of the foot became known as the Lisfranc joint, with injuries to it bearing his eponym. Lisfranc injuries vary in severity, from simple ligament sprains to complete disruption of the joint. They are important injuries because they can result in chronic instability, pain and arthritis. Historically, Lisfranc injuries were seen in horse riders who fell from the horse with the foot stuck in the stirrup. Nowadays they tend to occur in motor vehicle accidents, unexpectedly stepping into a hole, or are sports related. They are characterised by significant swelling to the foot and pain across the tarsometatarsal joints. Undisplaced fractures tend to be treated by initial non-weightbearing in a moulded cast/orthosis, while displaced or unstable injuries require internal fixation (screws/wires). Full weightbearing tends to be resumed after three months with a return to sporting activities even later. These injuries can result in painful tarsometatarsal osteoarthritis (degenerative joint disease), which may require surgical fusion.

Pelvic and acetabular fractures

These are discussed elsewhere (pp 195–210). Forces involved are often great and result in both associated local soft tissue injuries (pelvic and abdominal organs/viscera) and other musculoskeletal injuries. Polytrauma is discussed on page 179.

Shoulder injuries

Soft tissue injuries include dislocations of the acromioclavicular (AC) and glenohumeral joints. Rockwood classified injuries to the AC joint as types I–VI, with the degree of joint displacement depending on the severity of injury to the ligaments (AC and coracoclavicular (CC)) and the supporting muscles of the shoulder (trapezius, deltoid) (Williams et al. 1989).

- **Types I and II** – Injury to the AC ligaments causes no significant displacement of the AC joint and these are treated non-operatively.
- **Type III** – Rupture of the CC ligaments results in the shoulder drooping and the lateral end of the clavicle sticking up as a visible bump under the skin. For many years type three injuries have also been treated non-operatively. This left the individual with a prominent lateral clavicle but function was deemed to be acceptable. More recently there has been a trend towards operative stabilisation of the joint, using a hook plate with or without repair of the torn CC ligament.
- **Types IV–VI** – Displacement of the AC joint is even greater. These are rarer and are treated operatively.

The initial management of glenohumeral dislocation is manipulative reduction, typically in the emergency department but occasionally in theatre. The shoulder is then immobilised for a short time in a sling. In the young, subsequent shoulder instability is often a problem and is managed by an arthroscopic stabilisation procedure, whereas in older patients shoulder stiffness is the issue. Dislocations may be associated with either fracture of the greater tuberosity or tear of the rotator cuff, each of which is treated on its own merits once the dislocation has been reduced acutely.

Bony injuries of the shoulder are predominantly fractures of the clavicle and of the proximal humerus (discussed below). For a long time, the vast majority of clavicle fractures have been treated non-operatively (sling/figure of eight bandage). The subsequent small number of resulting non-unions were treated by bone grafting and internal fixation. There is an increasing trend for the operative management of clavicle fractures, particularly those that are more displaced or comminuted. It is claimed that both the union rate is higher and the functional outcome better with operative fixation.

Humeral fractures

Proximal humeral fractures

Fractures of the proximal humerus are another group of injuries where the trend is increasingly towards operative treatment. Like intra-capsular hip fractures, the outcome is determined to a large degree by the vascularity. Neer (1970) classified proximal humeral fractures according to the displacement of the various potential fragments (head, shaft, tuberosities) and whether or not there is an associated dislocation. Subsequent joint stiffness is a major issue for all of these injuries, especially in older patients. Internal fixation using periarticular locking plates or locking nails affords reasonable fracture stability and allows early mobilisation. Hemiarthroplasty is favoured when the fracture displacement suggests that the humeral head will be avascular. Problems with hemiarthroplasty relate to reattachment of the tuberosities and soft tissue balance. Some surgeons feel that the outcome with operative treatment is no better than with non-operative treatment in older patients.

Humeral shaft fractures

Sarmiento and associates have championed the non-operative management of these fractures (Sarmiento and Latta 2006; Sarmiento et al. 2000). This consists of immobilisation of the fracture while keeping joint immobilisation (shoulder and elbow) to a minimum. Fractures are initially splinted using a plaster of Paris slab, from the shoulder to the elbow. Then, within a few weeks, a functional brace is used. This wraps tightly around the arm but leaves the shoulder and elbow relatively free to move. Operative fixation is gaining in popularity, having the advantage of restoring upper limb function rapidly (at the risk of operative complications). There is an increasing trend in modern society for patients to opt for the less safe but more 'convenient' option, allowing them to return to work/play more rapidly. Operative treatment of humeral shaft fractures involves the use of either an intramedullary nail or a plate. While nails have the advantage of relative percutaneous insertion, they have a couple of disadvantages. Firstly, for those nails that are introduced antegrade (proximal insertion and distal passage) the insertion point may cause some damage to the rotator cuff area with concerns about subsequent shoulder issues. Secondly, unlike femoral and tibial fractures, there is a not insignificant incidence of non-union after humeral fractures are nailed. Plate fixation remains the popular choice, having the disadvantage of extensive exposure but good union rates.

The radial nerve winds around the humerus (formerly known as the musculospiral nerve) in close proximity to the bone, and can therefore be injured in fractures of the shaft. While most such injuries recover on their own, typically by about eight weeks, not all do. A nerve injury in itself does not mean that the fracture needs operative intervention unless the injury followed the reduction or is associated with an open fracture. The nerve is also vulnerable to injury during a surgical approach and fixation. Radial nerve palsy leads to a wrist drop and loss of sensation over a small part of the dorsum of the hand. The wrist and hand is dynamically splinted (lively splint) until the nerve recovers.

Distal humeral fractures

These can be either extra- or intra-articular. In older people, where bone quality is poor, these can be some of the most unrewarding fractures to treat. Since these fractures are too close to the elbow to permit functional bracing, non-operative treatment involves immobilisation of the elbow joint until fracture union occurs. An above elbow cast/ sling is used for four to six weeks or more, accepting that the elbow will become stiff. It may not even be possible to hold the fragments well reduced by closed methods. In selected older patients some surgeons advocated early joint mobilisation ('bag of bones' treatment), feeling that subsequent fracture non-union at least preserves some 'elbow' movement. Because of these difficulties many surgeons attempted internal fixation but historically the rates of failure were high in older patients due to pull out of the metal ware. The fractures are so close to the elbow that only a few screws can be inserted. Surgeons were therefore reluctant to allow early joint mobilisation. The extensive surgical dissection only contributed to the postoperative stiffness. It was therefore for good reason that the elbow was viewed as the surgical graveyard! Like other metaphyseal fractures in older people, locked precontoured plates have gone some way to addressing these issues. Typically two plates are applied, one to each side of the distal humerus. The elbow is immobilised initially and then moved when the surgeon feels confident enough in the fixation. More recently some surgeons have been treating selected distal injuries by elbow replacement.

In young patients with good bone quality, open reduction and internal fixation is the norm. With articular fractures, where the distal humeral joint surface is split into two or more pieces, the operative approach may include osteotomy of the olecranon to allow adequate visualisation for the reduction. Post operatively the elbow is mobilised early in an attempt to minimise stiffness.

Elbow injuries

These constitute dislocations and fracture dislocations. Dislocations occur as the joint is forced to extend beyond its limits. The stabilising ligaments are torn. Simple dislocations are reduced usually in the emergency department. The elbow is initially immobilised in a flexed position (backslab and sling) since it may re-dislocate if extended early on. Most dislocations are treated non-operatively. The elbow is mobilised in a hinged brace, which is initially locked to prevent terminal extension. The brace is discontinued after six to eight weeks. However, some elbows are particularly unstable and for these repair of the ligaments is performed to facilitate early mobilisation. Long-term outlook is good, although some elbows go on to dislocate again with more minor trauma and some people complain of instability.

With fracture dislocations, not only is there ligamentous disruption, but there is also loss of some of the bony stabilisers. They usually involve one or more of the following;

- Radial head
- Olecranon
- Coronoid.

The reduced elbow is usually not stable enough to mobilise early, therefore operative treatment is performed to restore the integrity of these bony stabilisers and allow early mobilisation. Postoperative management is then similar to that of dislocations as described above.

Olecranon fractures

Olecranon fractures share some similarities to patella fractures. Not only are they intra-articular but the triceps inserts via the olecranon and any fracture gap represents a change in the length (and therefore function) of the extensor mechanism. Like patella fractures they are typically fixed using a tension band construct, thus allowing early elbow mobilisation. More comminuted olecranon fractures are treated by plate fixation, typically one of the newer precontoured plates.

Radial head fractures

These are intra-articular injuries and so accurate reduction is important. Mason (1954) classified radial head fractures according to the degree of comminution and displacement. Where possible, displaced fractures are internally fixed. When the radial head is too fragmented to fix it is replaced. Radial head excision should be avoided since it can lead to instability issues for the elbow and wrist. Post operatively the elbow is mobilised early and a hinged brace is used if there are associated ligamentous injuries compromising elbow stability.

Forearm fractures

The radius and ulna function together, to allow rotation of the wrist/hand. This occurs via the proximal and distal radioulnar joints. The forearm complex as a whole should therefore be viewed as a joint, and so anatomical reduction is the order of the day for these injuries. Fractures of the forearm occur in one of three general patterns. The commonest injury is when both bones fracture. Open reduction and internal fixation (ORIF) using plates, followed by early mobilisation, is the typical treatment. We also sometimes see a fracture of one of the bones with dislocation of the other. Monteggia described fracture of the ulna with dislocation of the proximal radius while Galeazzi described fracture of the radius with dislocation of the distal ulna. Lastly, sometimes there is an isolated fracture of only one bone. These usually result from a direct blow. Fracture of the ulna (nightstick fracture) is more common than fracture of the radius. After internal fixation these injuries are usually mobilised early although it will be a number of months before the individual can return to forceful use of the arm.

Distal radial fractures

These, together with fractures of the wrist and hand, are discussed in Chapter 12 (p 211).

Compartment syndrome

Compartment syndrome is a condition in which raised pressure in an enclosed fascial space decreases tissue perfusion leading to ischaemia. Tissues receive their oxygen from the blood, which flows through them down a pressure gradient. If the tissues themselves are under high pressure (for whatever reason) then the blood cannot flow properly. Starved of oxygen, the ischaemic tissues swell, increasing the pressure further in a vicious cycle.

Ischaemia is very painful and continued will lead to tissue death. Nerve and muscle are particularly sensitive to ischaemia. Pressure is typically raised because bleeding and oedema at the site of injury occupies space at the expense of the muscles. Ischaemic nerves fail to work, so paraesthesiae followed by numbness is the early sign of compartment syndrome. Likewise, ischaemic muscle is painful, especially to stretch and likewise fails to work (paralysis). Urgent decompression of the fascial space is necessary to save the tissues from necrosis. Failure to do this results in necrotic muscles being replaced by contracted fibrous tissue (Volkmann's ischaemic contracture) with permanent loss of function. Compartment syndrome can complicate any injury, but is most commonly seen with fractures of the calf and forearm bones. Young males seem particularly at risk. It is an acute complication, occurring within the first 72 hours after injury.

Polytrauma

In the multiply injured person, there is a massive challenge to haemostasis, with potential for metabolic derangements and organ failure. The initial trauma and any subsequent surgeries are seen as 'hits' to the immune system. Hyperstimulation of the immune response, either by single or multiple hits, can result in acute respiratory distress syndrome or multiple organ failure. Thus, the management of this group of people involves controlling both the local injuries and the systemic injury. Damage control surgery involves stabilisation of the individual while minimising the second hit. From the orthopaedic perspective this typically involves the initial application of external fixators, which may later be exchanged for definitive internal fixation once the person is surgically more stable. Once the systemic injury has passed, these individuals with multiple injuries (limb and visceral) pose a particular challenge for rehabilitation.

Summary

The challenge is to manage the individual injury within the context of the individual person, aiming not just for healing of the bone but also for restoration of the whole. For many fractures there are various treatment options, each having its own advantages and disadvantages. These have to be weighed up in each specific case, applying the basic principles described at the beginning of this chapter.

References

Goldacre, M. J., Roberts, S. E., & Yeates, D. (2002). Mortality after admission to hospital with fractured neck of femur: database study. *British Medical Journal, 325,* 868–869.

Hawkins, L. G. (1970). Fractures of the neck of the talus. *Journal of Bone and Joint Surgery, American Volume, 52*(5), 991–1002.

Helfet, D. L., Haas, N. P., Schatzker, J., Matter, P., Moser, R., & Hanson, B. (2003). AO philosophy and principles of fracture management – its evolution and evaluation. *Journal of Bone and Joint Surgery, American Volume, 85,* 1156–1160.

Lauge-Hansen, N. (1950). Fractures of the ankle II, combined experimental-surgical and experimental roentgenologic investigations. *Archives of Surgery, 60*(5), 957–985.

Mason, M. L. (1954). Some observations on fractures of the head of the radius with a review of 100 cases. *British Journal of Surgery*, *42*, 123–132.

Muller, M. E., Nazarian, S., Koch, P., & Schatzker, J. (1990). *The Comprehensive Classification of Fractures of the Long Bones*. Berlin: Springer-Verlag.

Neer, C. S. (1970). Displaced proximal humeral fractures. Part I. Classification and evaluation. *Journal of Bone and Joint Surgery, American Volume*, *52*(6), 1077–1089.

Sanders, R. (2000). Current concepts review – displaced intra-articular fractures of the calcaneus. *Journal of Bone and Joint Surgery, American Volume*, *82*(2), 225–250.

Sarmiento, A., & Latta, L. (2006). The evolution of functional bracing of fractures. *Journal of Bone and Joint Surgery, British Volume*, *88*(2), 141–148.

Sarmiento, A., Gersten, L. M., Sobol, P. A., Shankwiler, J. A., & Vangness, C. T. (1989). Tibial shaft fractures treated with functional braces – Experience with 780 fractures. *Journal of Bone and Joint Surgery, British Volume*, *71*(4), 602–609.

Sarmiento, A., Zagorski, J. B., Zych, G. A., Latta, L., & Capps, C. A. (2000). Functional bracing for the treatment of fractures of the humeral diaphysis. *Journal of Bone and Joint Surgery, American Volume*, *82*, 478–486.

Schatzker, J., McBroom, R., & Bruce, D. (1979). The tibial plateau fracture. The Toronto experience, 1968–1975. *Clinical Orthopaedics and Related Research*, *138*, 94–104.

Schmitz, M. A., Finnegan, M., Natarajan, R., & Champine, J. (1999). Effect of smoking on tibial shaft fracture healing. *Clinical Orthopaedics and Related Research*, *365*, 184–200.

Williams, G. R., Nguyen, V. D., & Rockwood, C. A. (1989). Classification and radiographic analysis of acromioclavicular dislocations. *Applied Radiology*, 29–34.

Further reading

Charnley, J. (1999). *The Closed Treatment of Common Fractures*. Cambridge: Colt Books Limited.

Pynsent, P. B., Fairbank, J. C. T., & Carr, A. J. (1999). *Classification of Musculoskeletal Trauma*. Oxford: Butterworth-Heinemann.

Chapter 10

Occupational therapy within orthopaedic trauma

Madeleine Mooney

Introduction

Working in an orthopaedic trauma unit can be a uniquely challenging experience for the occupational therapist. The majority of people referred for assessment and treatment present with one or more fractures and possibly soft tissue damage usually acquired as the result of a traumatic event. Accidents can happen to anyone at any time and as they do not respect age, social position or ethnic origin, the resulting caseload on an orthopaedic trauma ward will often reflect this, consisting of people of all ages and from a range of backgrounds. In addition to this they will present with a wide variety of injuries acquired as a result of many different types of accident. For the occupational therapist the end result of this is a caseload that is as varied and diverse as it is challenging. With this in mind, the occupational therapist, as part of the multi-disciplinary team, is responsible for ensuring that each person achieves their maximum level of functional independence throughout the different stages of the healing process.

This chapter hopes to address some of the issues and challenges faced by the occupational therapist in the management of a person with traumatic orthopaedic injuries. With the help of case studies it will look at the role of the occupational therapist through the different stages of the occupational therapy process and in the different areas they might find themselves working. Other more specific injuries, which present on an orthopaedic trauma ward, such as pelvic and acetabular fractures, hand injuries and traumatic amputation are dealt with in separate chapters.

Guidance for intervention

In common with other areas the occupational therapist in the orthopaedic trauma setting works very much as part of the multi-disciplinary team. The end result for all the team members is to help each person to achieve maximum function of the injured part and, where possible, to return them to their pre-injury level of independence and where this is not possible to their optimum level of function. For this to be achieved the person will require guidance from all team members from the time of their injury through to full recovery. The acute nature of a fracture/traumatic injury means that the healing process will follow a natural course with the individual slowly returning to full independence as the healing process progresses.

In many instances developments in orthopaedic surgery have decreased the need for lengthy hospital inpatient rehabilitation. As a result of this occupational therapists may find themselves assessing and treating fracture and trauma patients in a variety of settings. This may include the emergency department, acute orthopaedic ward or the person's own home, as part of an early supported discharge scheme. Despite the location the core concepts and beliefs of the profession remain the same.

Frames of reference

Although it is outside the scope of this book to discuss the many frames of reference, approaches and models of practice that might lend themselves to the practice of occupational therapy within orthopaedic trauma, it would not be complete without some mention. Given the proximity with which the team members work together and the fact that their overall aims and objectives are similar it is not surprising that they find themselves working with reference to common approaches as opposed to profession specific ones. It follows, therefore, that individuals may feel that professional boundaries are becoming blurred and that they are losing their professional identity (Atkinson 1995; Feaver and Creek 1993 and Joice and Coia 1989 (cited in Atkinson 1995)). It is, however, important that occupational therapists can draw on the theory underpinning the profession so that their practice is informed.

The biomechanical approach, which is based on biomechanical and physiological principles related to movement, might be viewed as a '*Primary Frame of Reference*' as it includes information, which originates from sources external to occupational therapy and can be used by the multi-disciplinary team. It can also, however, be viewed as an '*Applied Frame of Reference*', having been adapted by occupational therapists for intervention within orthopaedic trauma. Treatment plans are formulated to address such issues as limitations in range of movement, decreased strength and lack of stamina in completing tasks.

Hagedorn also identifies several approaches within this frame of reference, which may be used separately or at different stages in the treatment programme. These include the graded activities approach, the activities of daily living approach and the compensatory approach (Hagedorn 2001).

Models of practice

If occupational therapists are to work effectively within a multi-disciplinary team without surrendering their professional identity it is important to work with reference to an occupational therapy model. This will provide the therapist with definition and focus within the area of clinical concern. For the experienced therapist much of the theory, which guides our everyday practice, is used unconsciously. It is important that this theory is brought to the fore, particularly with novice practitioners, in order that we might validate and guide our practice appropriately (Atkinson 1995).

In more recent years the Canadian Model of Occupational Performance has provided a clearer account of the core concepts and values of occupational therapy together with a process for person-centred service delivery. Central to this model is the belief that the person must undertake the process of determining need and planning action – the therapist's role is to enable the process. Adopting this, however, may result in problems if the person is unable to determine their own goals or the person determines goals meaningful to them but not necessarily considered practical or desirable by the occupational therapist (Hagedorn 2001).

Assessment and treatment within orthopaedic trauma

Background information

In common with all other areas of intervention the occupational therapist must obtain all relevant background information before commencing intervention. Of particular importance is the nature of the injury and surgical intervention undertaken, as the mechanism of the injury and force of the impact may be significant in determining the course of treatment. Two different people may be referred, both diagnosed with a fractured tibia. The first may have tripped over a loose paving flag and fallen heavily resulting in a closed, undisplaced midshaft fracture which might easily be treated in a plaster of Paris cast and the person discharged home fully weightbearing on elbow crutches. A car, travelling at speed, may have hit the second person, resulting in an open, comminuted tibial fracture with significant soft tissue damage. This will require debridement, surgical fixation and possibly skin grafting. The course of rehabilitation both in terms of intervention and length of time will be significantly different for these two people although the diagnosis of 'tibial fracture' on the referral may be the same.

It is important to have an understanding of the orthopaedic management of the fracture in particular the nature of the injury, surgical intervention and likely course of fracture healing. In addition a careful note should be made of the postoperative precautions prescribed by the surgeon with regard to movement at or near the fracture site. Postoperative instructions will generally indicate a person's weightbearing status. The surgeon will have determined this having taken into account the severity and location of the fracture, the person's weight, the integrity of their bone quality, the ability of the fixation device to withstand stress, and the person's cognitive state (Goldstein 1999). While orthopaedic surgeons will advise of this close liaison with the physiotherapist is also important to establish the person's current level of mobility, choice of walking aid, exercise regimen and expected progression to ensure that this is reinforced by the occupational therapist in their treatment programme and not contradicted.

It may be that the surgeon wishes to restrict or control the movement within a given range. In this instance the occupational therapist may be required to fabricate a splint to allow the person to adhere to this regimen while pursuing functional independence. In addition to their current orthopaedic problems, the occupational therapist needs to take note of the individual's past medical history as this may significantly affect the rehabilitation process. Where the injury was the result of an accident involving other people, or may have resulted in the death of other individuals, then the occupational therapist should be aware of the possible psychological effects this may have had on the person and how this might influence their progress.

Similarly, where the injury is a direct result of someone else's negligence then the person may not be as motivated to progress quickly because the thought of compensation is uppermost in their mind. Only when all the background information is available should the occupational therapist proceed to assessment of the patient.

Assessment

In theory there is very little difference in the assessment of a person with an orthopaedic trauma problem to that of a person with any other medical condition. Generally speaking a person is referred to the occupational therapist because they are experiencing some degree of limitation in their occupational performance. This has been defined by the College of Occupational Therapists as the 'interaction of the individual with the environment through the selection, planning and carrying out of activities that contribute to occupations and roles' (College of Occupational Therapists 2005). With this in mind, the occupational therapist, having gained the person's consent, needs to obtain information from them regarding their level of occupational performance prior to the orthopaedic injury. In addition to this it is necessary to ascertain how able the person is to engage in activities of importance at the present time and what their expectations are for the future.

The assessment process usually begins with an initial interview where the person provides the information regarding their usual routine, home circumstances, work circumstances and activities of importance. This will give the therapist a clearer idea of what the person is aiming for and whether it is realistic or not. Establishing what activities a person engages in and the degree of importance to them will assist the occupational therapist in determining what functional tasks are of relevance when completing a baseline assessment. This can be better understood by comparing the following case studies.

Case study 10.1

Diagnosis – Fractured neck of femur

Hannah – female, aged 77 years

Hannah underwent a hemiarthroplasty for a fractured neck of femur. She had tripped over a raised threshold in her flat. Prior to admission she lived alone in a ground floor flat. She was independently mobile around her flat and was able to get in/out of bed, up from her chair and the toilet without difficulty. There was a shower over the bath but she had been unable to climb into the bath for some time and found it difficult reaching her lower half to wash and dress. She was able to make herself a hot drink and snacks but found meal preparation more difficult. A carer attended twice daily to assist her with personal care and to prepare a meal. Her sister undertook her shopping. She spent her day watching television, reading and looking out of the window.

Hannah wished to return to her pre-admission level of function, which was not considered unrealistic. Tasks considered relevant to her rehabilitation were aimed at improving mobility and transfers, independence in personal care and domestic skills. On discharge she was mobile with a walking frame around her flat. The occupational therapist had arranged for the raised thresholds to be removed and made good for safety reasons. She was able to get herself in and out of bed, up from her chair with provision of chair raising unit and up from the toilet following provision of a raised toilet seat.

A shower board was provided for use over the bath but a carer was still required to assist. She was also able to dress her lower half independently using long handled equipment. She was able to stand for long enough to prepare hot drinks and snacks and was provided with a trolley to transport the items through to her living room. It was arranged that the carer would resume daily visits to prepare a hot meal and assist with personal care. Her sister would continue to do her shopping.

Case study 10.2

Diagnosis – Fractured neck of femur

Tom – male, aged 74 years

Tom is a farmer who, despite his age, had shown no sign of retiring from work. He sustained a fractured neck of femur when he was knocked over by one of his sheep while rounding up his flock up in the hills. He also underwent a hemiarthroplasty fixation.

Prior to admission, Tom was fully mobile and independent and had spent his entire working life as a sheep farmer in the rural community where he lived. He had two sons and a wife who assisted him with the running of the farm. His wife also undertook all the domestic tasks. Tom had one goal and that was to be back to work on his farm within the week. Although it was anticipated that, given his previous level of physical fitness, he would make a speedy recovery and return home, returning to heavy manual work so soon was considered to be unrealistic. The occupational therapist had to spend time educating him with regard to postoperative precautions and determining a course of rehabilitation which would initially get him home and eventually back to work should he choose to continue along this route.

Tom returned home within ten days of admission. He was mobile with elbow crutches, independent up and down stairs and independent in all transfers. He was provided with a toilet raise and toilet frame, chair raisers and long handled dressing equipment to assist him with compliance of postoperative precautions. Arrangements were also made for a grab rail to be fitted in the shower to make it safer when he stepped in.

He was advised, and reluctantly agreed, to let his sons undertake all heavy manual farm duties for the foreseeable future. Due to the isolated location of the farm and his determination to get around his land Tom was taught how to transfer in and out of the passenger side of the car without compromising the need to follow postoperative precautions.

Given the pressure on acute hospital beds and the fact that fracture/orthopaedic trauma patients are not ill in the true sense of the word it might appear easier and quicker to ask the person to describe their own ability in a given task. However, should the patient be anxious to please and more importantly anxious to be home, the response given may provide inaccurate information as to their true ability. Observation of a person is, therefore, the easiest and most reliable way to determine a person's current ability in a given activity and from this form an appropriate plan with them.

Although the occupational therapist is assessing function in daily living tasks it may be necessary to break down the assessment to look at more specific impairments in order to better explain each individual person's limitations in occupational performance. Assessments should therefore progress, where applicable, to look at more specific components such as range of movement, strength, endurance or cognitive impairment to name but a few. It is beyond the scope of the book to go into detail on component assessments but further information can be found in many standard occupational therapy texts.

It is important for the occupational therapist to be aware that occupational performance is personal to each individual and will be strongly influenced by who they are, what they do, where they live and work and their life experiences. As a result of this the occupational therapist must recognise the importance of a client-centred approach and involve the person in decisions around goal setting, treatment planning and the desired outcome of intervention.

It is this person uniqueness which can make the use of standardised assessment more difficult as the assessment cannot cover all aspects of an individual's occupational performance. However, it can provide us, in some instances, with a more accurate assessment and evaluation of problems allowing the occupational therapist to determine the success/outcome of the intervention.

The 'Functional Independence Measure' (FIM) is one such assessment, which can be of use to the occupational therapist with a person following an orthopaedic injury. It includes 18 items, which are divided into 13 motor domains and five cognitive domains. Each domain is scored from 1 to 7, representing a measure of overall performance in activities of daily living. Each level of scoring is defined from 1, which equals total assistance, to 7, which equals complete independence. The person would be assessed on admission, on discharge and at follow up enabling the occupational therapist to monitor progress and evaluate the outcome (Ottenbacher 1997).

The Barthel Index can also be of use in orthopaedic trauma, as it is designed to measure improvement in daily living activities during the rehabilitation of older people with physical dysfunction. It does, however, only cover the daily living skills of feeding, personal toilet, transfers, bathing, mobility, dressing and controlling bowel and bladder, but unlike the FIM, it does not assess function in the areas of communication and cognition (Murdock 1992).

Completion of a functional assessment might show that a person needs a more specific assessment, for example for a wheelchair. Alternatively, the person might have been referred for a wheelchair or a specific splint, and on assessment for these it becomes apparent that a more detailed assessment of occupational performance is going to be required. The occupational therapist's holistic approach to treatment necessitates that all appropriate assessments are completed and treatment provided accordingly.

Where the assessment takes place is also of importance. Many different settings can be used such as the hospital ward, the therapy assessment flat or a community setting. This may affect the person's performance and the occupational therapist should be careful not to take the results of an assessment in one setting and assume that the person will perform the same in another setting (Law 2002).

Due to the acute nature of the injury and the predicted outcome, people with orthopaedic injuries can often be discharged immediately after assessment. It is not uncommon for only temporary modification to the home environment being all that is required for the duration of the fracture healing. There are others, however, who due to the nature and complexity of their injury will require much intervention from the occupational therapist to restore them back to their pre-admission level.

Intervention

It would be impossible within the scope of this book to cover in detail every aspect of occupational therapy intervention for all the many different types and combinations of fracture and soft tissue injury, and the degrees of disability resulting from them.

During the assessment process it will have become apparent to both the person and the occupational therapist what areas of intervention are required to ensure that the person reaches their optimal level of function on discharge. The nature and degree of intervention will be dependent on the type of injury and degree of temporary or permanent disability resulting from it. It is likely to cover one or more or all of the following areas.

- **Practice of daily living skills** – This includes mobility, transfers, personal care and domestic rehabilitation.
- **Modification of the home environment** – This may include provision of equipment either short term or long term, minor adaptations or in some instances advice on major adaptations or re-housing.
- **Assessment and provision of a wheelchair** – This may be for short-term or long-term use and involve the occupational therapist linking in with the specialist wheelchair therapist. It will also require the occupational therapist to teach the person mobility and transfer techniques in the wheelchair.
- **Orthotics** – The manufacture and provision of thermoplastic splints and fracture braces. Alternatively, custom-made splints may be required. The occupational therapist who issues a splint is responsible for ensuring that the splint fits correctly, is appropriate for need and that the person and/or their carer is educated in the wearing regimen and care of the splint. The occupational therapist involved in the manufacture of splints should have appropriate training and experience to perform this task.
- **Upper limb activities** – This includes remedial activities to increase range of movement, strength and endurance and thus to ultimately improve the person's functional ability (see Chapters 5 and 13).
- **Work/leisure rehabilitation** – It is important to bear these in mind from early in the assessment process. The person may need referral for benefits advice and it may be necessary for the person to notify their employers as to when or if they will be able to return to work. Later in the rehabilitation process it may be necessary for the occupational therapist to undertake a job analysis in order to advise the person and employer on returning to work especially if a change in work role is required or a graded return to their existing job.

Settings for intervention

As identified earlier the occupational therapist may be asked to assess and advise on a person with a traumatic injury in a variety of settings. It is proposed to illustrate this intervention by means of a number of case studies.

Case study 10.3

Emergency department – rehabilitation unit – community setting

Annie – female, aged 79 years

History

Annie was brought to the emergency department by ambulance following a fall at home. She had slipped on the back step injuring her left ankle. X-rays revealed an undisplaced bimalleolar fracture without talar shift, which it was agreed to treat conservatively in plaster of Paris. She was to be allowed up non-weightbearing on her left leg. She was referred to the occupational therapist to see whether or not she would manage if discharged home from the emergency department as she was experiencing difficulty with the non-weightbearing aspect of mobility.

Social situation

Annie reported that she lived alone in a house. Her bedroom, bathroom and toilet were all located upstairs. There was a banister rail on the left side of the stairs (ascending). Prior to admission she had managed at home being able to undertake all necessary daily living activities. She had one son, who lived 25 miles away and visited her from time to time.

Annie enjoyed reading and regularly visited her local library, where she was an active member of a retired persons' social group.

Assessment

- **Mobility** – Managed short distances with a walking frame and non-weightbearing on her left leg. Tired easily. Unable to manage stairs.
- **Transfers** – Bed transfers assessed on a hospital bed, able to go from lying to sitting, sitting to standing and vice versa. She reported that her bed at home was quite low.
- **Chair** – Independent from sitting to standing and vice versa.
- **Toilet** – Unable to manage without using grab rails on both sides.
- **Personal care** – Able to reach lower limbs for washing and dressing purposes while seated at wash bowl.
- **Domestic** – Unable to mobilise sufficiently well to undertake tasks in the kitchen. Unable to carry items about kitchen while using her walking frame.

Conclusion

Annie would be unable to manage at home due to her reduced mobility, which affected her ability to function safely. She did not, however, require admission to an acute orthopaedic trauma bed.

Plan

Annie would transfer to a nurse led elderly rehabilitation unit to work on improving her mobility and overall functional level and so that arrangements could be made for adequate support at home on discharge. From an orthopaedic point of view she would be followed up as an outpatient in the fracture clinic.

Elderly rehabilitation unit

Annie was able to work on her mobility with the physiotherapist firstly increasing her stamina and independence with the walking frame until eventually after a week she was able to progress to elbow crutches. She still had difficulty though managing the stairs.

Annie was able to walk to the bathroom and back to wash herself. She was independent washing both upper and lower body while seated at the wash hand-basin. Standing tolerance was poor but after working in the kitchen with the occupational therapist she was able to make herself hot drinks and light snacks while seated on a perching stool.

Following a home visit and discussion with Annie it was decided that she would return home with her bed downstairs and a commode initially. Her bed was to be raised by the occupational therapist for easier transfers. A perching stool would also be provided for her to use in her kitchen. A carer would visit each day to empty the commode and bring a bowl of water through so that she could wash and dress. The carer would also leave out the necessary items for meal preparation and drinks each day. Annie's son had agreed to visit weekly and undertake her shopping and exchange library books for her. Several friends were also regular visitors.

Community rehabilitation team

On discharge Annie received on-going therapy at home. As fracture healing progressed and Annie was able to fully weightbear she was soon able to manage the stairs. The occupational therapist provided a second banister rail and a grab rail by the toilet to assist independence. Her bed was replaced upstairs and the bed raisers were no longer required. As Annie was now accessing her bathroom the carer was no longer required and with her increasing confidence she was soon visiting the library and shops again.

Case study 10.4

Intensive care unit – acute setting – out-patient

Ben – male, 34 years, involved in a road traffic accident

History

Ben was employed as a police officer and was returning home from work when his motorcycle was hit by another vehicle. He was admitted to the emergency department where his injuries were identified and from there he was transferred to the intensive care unit via the operating theatre.

Table 10.1 details the injuries received and the surgical intervention for each.

Table 10.1 Injuries received and the surgical intervention for these

Injury	Surgical intervention
Open fracture right tibia; severe soft tissue damage; large area of skin defect	Debridement and application of monolateral external fixator; fasciotomy
Comminuted fracture right femur; 10 cm – 10 cm skin defect	Debridement of right thigh and retrograde nail; Skin defect for review by plastic surgeons and grafting
Fractured right neck of femur	Cannulated screw fixation
Comminuted fracture left femur	Retrograde nail and patellectomy
Segmental fracture right ulna; 20 cm – 10 cm skin defect	Debridement, plate on radius and long Recon. Plate to the ulna; plastic surgeons to review skin defect
Fracture left distal radius	Manipulation under anaesthesia and K-wiring

Intensive care unit

Initial assessment and intervention:

- **Problem** – Ben's right foot was resting in plantar flexion and he was unable to actively dorsiflex to plantigrade.
- **Solution** – Resting foot drop splint was manufactured to position foot/ankle at plantigrade to preserve soft tissue length and alignment.

After two days Ben was transferred to the acute orthopaedic trauma ward where he remained as an inpatient for a period of four months.

Acute orthopaedic trauma ward

Once on the ward the occupational therapist was able to reassess him and in conjunction with Ben come up with a treatment plan. Table 10.2 details the problems and the aims of treatment.

Over the next two months Ben received intervention from all members of the multidisciplinary team including daily physiotherapy, advice from the dietician, medical and surgical intervention and nursing care. Occupational therapy intervention included:

- Provision and monitoring of foot drop splint.
- Provision and monitoring of right and left wrist extension splints for day time use. These supported the wrist and enabled combined finger flexion and extension and active range of movement of the thumb. They were serialised at regular intervals to increase wrist extension.
- Right and left night resting splints to maintain fingers in extension at night-time.
- Provision of attendant propelled wheelchair with right extended leg rest as unable to fully flex knee. Initially Ben was hoisted in/out of wheelchair.

Table 10.2 Problems identified and the treatment plan for these

Problems identified by the occupational therapist	Aims of treatment
Decreased active range of movement left ankle, leg length discrepancy	To maintain range of movement and prevent residual deformity
Left wrist resting in flexion, patient unable to actively extend	To encourage left wrist extension and position to prevent deformity
Decreased activity right wrist extension and finger extension (ulnar graft subsequently completed)	To encourage right wrist and finger extension and position to prevent deformity
Decreased functioning and strength in both upper limbs	Increase function and strength in bilateral upper limbs
Decreased independence in mobility	To encourage functional mobility
Decreased independence in transfers	To encourage independence in transfers
Decreased independence in personal care	To encourage independence in personal care and dressing
Decreased independence in ability to perform domestic activities of daily living	To encourage independence in domestic tasks in preparation for return home
Unable to fulfil work role	To encourage return to some form of employment as appropriate in the future

- Upper limb rehabilitation commenced with light hand activities to encourage range of movement and increase grip strength.

Initial interview completed

Environmental visit completed to Ben's home to give the occupational therapist an idea of the minimum function Ben would need to be able to manage at home, what equipment might be needed and whether it would fit.

At approximately two months post accident Ben was able to mobilise short distances with the aid of two gutter crutches and one other person. He required assistance of one to get in/out of bed and on/off a chair and he still required assistance with personal care and toileting.

Two months after his accident, Ben returned to the operating theatre for further surgery. He underwent bone grafting to his fractured right ulna and application of a six ring Ilizarov frame with tibial and fibula osteotomies for lengthening of his right leg by means of bone transport. The lengthening process was to begin at seven days post operatively.

Immediately post operatively Ben was seen by the occupational therapist and provided with a night resting splint for his right arm and encouraged to use the arm as pain allowed during the day. He was also fitted with a dynamic foot drop splint. This consisted of a thermoplastic foot piece attached to his Ilizarov frame with resistance exercise band. The aim was to prevent the formation of contractures around the ankle joint, anticipated as a result of the resistance of the soft tissues to the distraction process (Mooney and Gilbody 2006). Ben was also able to plantar and dorsiflex his foot in the splint to encourage maintenance of range of movement.

Occupational therapy intervention continued as an inpatient for a further two months and included:

- **Wheelchair mobility** – Ben had now progressed to a self-propelling wheelchair and could transfer in/out of the wheelchair using a sliding board.
- **Light hand activities** – and use of the BTE work simulator (see Figure 5.7, p 82) to increase upper limb strength.
- **Monitoring** – and adjusting of splints accordingly.
- **Provision of temporary raised shoe** – which was adjusted as required at regular intervals to accommodate the lengthening of his right limb.
- **Personal care** assessment and practice.
- **Domestic activities**.
- **Home assessment** – with Ben to determine what equipment if any would be required for discharge home.

After four months in hospital Ben returned home. He was mobile around the ground floor of his home with two gutter crutches. He was able to mobilise around his kitchen using one gutter crutch and the work surface for support – he was provided with a perching stool for use in the kitchen and was able to prepare hot drinks and snacks, this was important as Ben's girlfriend was at work during the day.

The occupational therapist also provided the following equipment to assist independent transfers:

- Toilet frame and raised toilet seat
- Adjustable height commode with detachable arms
- Armchair raisers
- Bed raisers
- Shower board

Despite initial reluctance on Ben's part he finally agreed on discharge to be referred to counselling to help him address the psychological issues he had following his accident. He was also referred to the outpatient therapy department for ongoing occupational therapy and physiotherapy.

Outpatient department

Ben attended twice weekly for treatment continuing with his upper limb rehabilitation where he showed a slow but steady improvement in strength and range of movement. He continued to attended outpatient physiotherapy to improve mobility and stamina. Nine months later the Ilizarov frame was removed but unfortunately Ben had a re-fracture through the regenerate bone, requiring a plaster of Paris cast for a further nine weeks. After this was removed he returned to occupational therapy for provision of a custom made tibial brace (see Figure 9.5, p 164). With this he was able to continue weightbearing while mobilising with elbow crutches. Fifteen months after the accident Ben returned to work on light duties and within four months of this he was back undertaking most of his previous duties at work.

Needs of the older fracture patient

Vellas et al. (cited in McIntyre 1999), stated 'falls in elderly persons are a typical example of new diseases directly linked with aging which have appeared with the increase in longevity.' This rise in the older population and the incidence of falls has resulted in a number of initiatives designed to improve the care of this particular group of people. In the UK, the National Institute for Health and Clinical Excellence (NICE) recommends that all older persons coming into contact with a health care professional should be questioned on whether or not they have had a fall in the past year and if so the nature and characteristics of the fall. For those people who are considered at risk of falling or who have had a fall, a multi-factorial falls risk assessment should be completed. Intervention from the multi-disciplinary team should include a review of the following (NICE 2004):

- Strength and balance training
- Home hazard assessment and intervention
- Vision assessment and referral
- Medication review/withdrawal.

This increase in the older population and the increase in the number of falls has resulted in many older persons presenting with fractures, the management and rehabilitation of which is a large and ever expanding area of orthopaedic trauma.

Any fracture is likely to prove distressing and disruptive to an older person but a fractured neck of femur is particularly so. Hip fractures occur most commonly in the older population, and in particular with those who are frail, more dependent and often exhibiting a host of pre-existing medical problems. Persons with a fractured neck of femur make up a large percentage of any orthopaedic trauma unit and their treatment has become almost routine, with many hospitals having set up care pathways. However, hip fractures like any other fracture vary in both their severity and outcome. The aforementioned assessment and intervention needs to be followed but, for people who have undergone a hemiarthroplasty procedure, it might be necessary for them to follow precautions as for a total hip replacement for up to six weeks post operatively. Individual therapists should check with the operating surgeon as to the length of time/

necessity for precautions as these are known to differ from hospital to hospital. With the older person, rehabilitation can often take longer, due in part to their frailty, which leads us to question whether or not an acute orthopaedic trauma ward is the best place to rehabilitate these people.

Problems in rehabilitating this group are experienced all around the world so it is not surprising that many different approaches, which reflect local resources and health care systems, have been described. The one thing that they have in common is an emphasis on the collaboration between the specialist services for older people and orthopaedics, early and efficient discharge planning and increased community support (Stewart and McMillan 1998).

In Scotland the development of the SIGN (Scottish Intercollegiate Guideline Network) guideline for fractured neck of femur emphasised the importance of early assessment by the multi-disciplinary team. This was so a decision could be made as to the person's rehabilitation potential and their destination for this. Indicators as to an individual's success in rehabilitation include the person's pre-admission mental state, motivation and co-operation. These should be considered alongside the type of fracture, surgical intervention and mechanical stability (Eldar et al. 1995).

An older person admitted from home who was previously managing independently might reasonably be expected to recover quite well and may either be discharged from the acute unit with support after a short period of rehabilitation or discharged into an early supported discharge scheme. Frailer, more dependent persons, who may have been considered precarious at home, may benefit from transfer to an orthopaedic rehabilitation unit or nurse led intermediate care setting. These are multi-disciplinary inpatient units where a consultant specialist in older persons medicine or a general practitioner oversees the medical care and rehabilitation. Orthopaedic input still needs to be maintained and the rehabilitation staff should have an understanding of the orthopaedic condition (SIGN 2002).

Summary

This chapter has provided an overview of the intervention required from the occupational therapist for an individual with an orthopaedic injury. The principles of occupational therapy intervention remain the same as for all other groups of people but the occupational therapist must have an understanding of the nature of fracture management and the healing process in order that the intervention is appropriate to the particular stage of healing.

The nature of the acute orthopaedic trauma setting requires the occupational therapist to work efficiently and effectively to ensure that each person is discharged to the most appropriate setting in a timely fashion in order that bed occupancy is maximised. In doing so it is important not to compromise on care and to ensure that the person's needs remain the focus of their intervention.

References

Atkinson, K. (1995). Do we need to use models in occupational therapy practice. *British Journal of Therapy and Rehabilitation*, 2(7), 370–374.

College of Occupational Therapists. (2005). *Occupational Therapy Standard Terminology Project Report*. London: College of Occupational Therapists.

Eldar, R., Tamir, A., & Susak, Z. (1995). Determinants of rehabilitation following fracture of the hip in elderly patients. *Clinical Rehabilitation*, 9, 184–189.

Goldstein, T. S. (1999). *Geriatric Orthopaedics Rehabilitative Management of Common Problems* (2nd edition). Maryland, Gaithersburg: Aspen Publishers.

Hagedorn, R. (2001). *Foundations for Practice in Occupational Therapy* (3rd edition). London: Churchill Livingstone.

Law, M. (2002). Assessing roles and competence. In M. Trombly & R. M. Vining (Eds). *Occupational Therapy for Physical Dysfunction* (5th edition). USA: Lippincott Williams & Wilkins.

McIntyre, A. (1999). Elderly fallers: a baseline audit of admissions to a day hospital for elderly people. *British Journal of Occupational Therapy*, 62(6), 244–248.

Mooney, M., & Gilbody, J. (2006). Techniques in splintage and support during reconstruction of the tibia. *Strategies in Trauma and Limb Reconstruction*, 1(1), 58–65.

Murdock, C. A. (1992). Critical evaluation of the Barthel index, part 1. *British Journal of Occupational Therapy*, 55(3), 109–111.

National Institute for Clinical Excellence. (2004). *Falls: The Assessment and Prevention of Falls in Older People*. Online. Available at: www.nice.org.uk/cg021 (accessed 9 April 2009).

Ottenbacher, K. J. (1997). Methodological issues in measurement of functional status in rehabilitation outcomes. In S. S. Dittmar and G. E. Gresham (Eds). *Functional Assessment and Outcome Measures for the Rehabilitation Health Professional*. Maryland, Gaithersburg: Aspen Publishers.

Scottish Intercollegiate Guidelines Network. (2002). *Prevention and Management of Hip Fracture in Older People*. Edinburgh: SIGN Executive, Royal College of Physicians. Online. Available at: www.sign.ac.uk (accessed 9 April 2009).

Stewart, L. S. P., & McMillan, I. R. (1998). Rehabilitation schemes for elderly patients with a hip fracture. *British Journal of Occupational Therapy*, 61(8), 367–371.

Chapter 11

Pelvic and acetabular fractures: management and occupational therapy

Dawn Miller

Introduction

Fractures to the pelvis and acetabulum are primarily the result of a traumatic event, although in some instances it may be due to bone disease. This chapter outlines the types of injury that may occur to the pelvis and acetabulum, their orthopaedic and surgical management, and includes an overview of the role of the specialist occupational therapist.

Intervention from the occupational therapist is essential for individuals in this group and should begin within the hospital environment. The severity of the injury will determine the length of time the person remains in hospital but the length of stay could vary from a few days to many months. The occupational therapist's input will involve helping the person to overcome the physical and psychological challenges they are likely to face. From a psychological point of view they may require expert help in coming to terms with any long-term disability issues or in dealing with the effects of post-traumatic stress. Physically these individuals will experience difficulty in all aspects of daily living and the occupational therapist will need to assist each of them to achieve their maximum functional ability in order for them to return home. Once home occupational therapy should continue in the community until the person has achieved all their functional goals and overcome any psychological issues related to long-term disability.

Types of trauma resulting in pelvic and acetabular fractures

In the main pelvic and acetabular fractures result from high impact injuries. These include:

- Road traffic accidents
- Falls from a height
- Crush injuries.

They are particularly critical, as they are often associated with significant soft tissue injuries, severe blood loss and shock. As they usually involve high speed or heavy weights they are commonly associated with other significant injuries:

- Head injury
- Fractures to other bones
- Peripheral nerve injury
- Skin lacerations, burns or foreign bodies
- Thoracic injury
- Abdominal trauma, often affecting the bladder, spleen, liver or kidneys
- Blood vessel damage.

Less commonly, however, a simple fall may result in a pelvic or acetabular fracture, this would usually be seen in frail older people or those people with osteoporotic bone.

Incidence

Fractures of the pelvis and acetabulum account for between 1% and 3% of all skeletal injuries (Patient UK 2005). As they are uncommon the occupational therapist is unlikely to see many unless working in a specialist unit. Injuries may vary from minor, which will heal without intervention, to complex requiring surgical repair and many months of rehabilitation for the person to regain functional independence.

Anatomy of the pelvis and acetabulum

The pelvic girdle consists of the two coxal bones, which are united anteriorly at the symphysis pubis and posteriorly to the sacrum. The pelvis is the bowl created by the two hip bones, the sacrum and the coccyx (Figure 11.1). The acetabulum is a deep lateral fossa, which receives the head of the femur. This sits solidly in the acetabulum balancing the weight of the body (Figure 11.2) (Tortora and Anagnostakos 1990).

The pelvis has several functions:

- It supports and protects the pelvic viscera
- It supports and transmits the weight of the body from the vertebral column to the lower limbs in standing and the ischial tuberosities in sitting
- The swing of the pelvis enables a person to walk reasonably well
- It provides attachments for muscles
- In the female it provides bony support for the birth canal (Palastanga et al. 1994).

Pelvic ring stability is provided by ligaments that attach bone to bone, providing strength and stability and restricting excessive movement (Kapit and Elson 1977). The pelvis also has a rich supply of blood vessels, which are frequently damaged as a result of pelvic trauma (McRea and Esser 2002).

Classification of pelvic injury

Pelvic injuries can be simply divided into two groups, stable and unstable. In order to further understand and classify pelvic injury it is necessary to look at the mechanism of injury. Solomon et al. (2001) describes three major forces involved in injuries to the pelvis. These are:

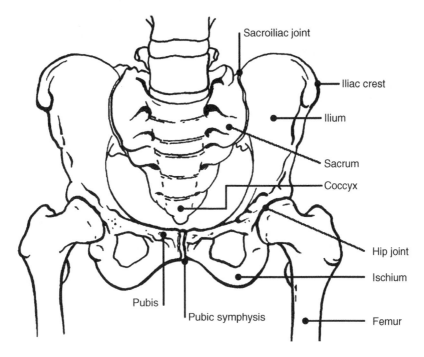

Figure 11.1 The pelvic bones. Reproduced by kind permission of EMIS and PiP, 2005.

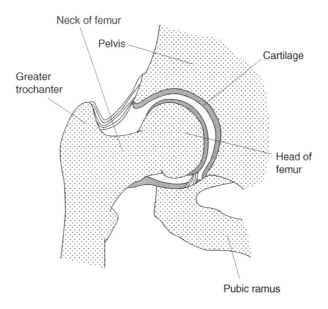

Figure 11.2 The hip joint showing the head of the femur sitting within the acetabular socket. Reproduced by kind permission of EMIS and PiP, 2005.

- Antero-posterior compression – usually caused by an impact at the front of the pelvis (resulting in direct trauma to the posterior iliac spines or forceful external rotation of the lower limb). If the pubic rami are fractured and there is disruption of the symphysis the innominate bones will externally rotate, leading to the so called 'open book' injury.
- Lateral compression – results from a side on blow to either the iliac crest or femoral head. The result is a fracture of the pubic rami on one or both sides; together with a severe sacroiliac strain or a fracture of the sacrum or ilium either on the same or opposite side of the pubic rami fracture.
- Vertical shear – usually the result of a fall from a great height where the person lands on one leg. The innominate bone on one side is displaced posterosuperiorly fracturing the pubic rami and disrupting the sacroiliac region on the same side. It is associated with massive skeletal and soft tissue damage and a high mortality rate.

Where a person presents with a combination of the above injuries, it would be classified as a severe pelvic injury.

There are several classifications in use to further define pelvic injury. These include Tile's classification (1984) and Young and Burgess (1986) (Pynsent et al. (1999). Tile classified fractures to the pelvis into three groups (Table 11.1); this can be better understood by reference to Figure 11.3.

It is beyond the scope of the book to go into further details but further reading is recommended for the occupational therapist working within a specialist unit in order to more fully understand the nature of these injuries.

Acetabular fractures are also associated with high-energy injuries and despite the increase in road traffic accidents the incidence remains low.

Acetabular fractures like pelvic fractures are extremely complex but also involve joint disruption. The numerous variations make classification difficult. The most widely accepted classification is by Judet and Letournel who suggest two major types, elementary fractures and associated fractures with five sub-groups in each (Pynsent et al.

Table 11.1 Classification of Tile (1984)

	Direction of injurious force	**State of posterior sacroiliac complex**
Stable	Anteroposterior compression *Type I:* Open book (stages I–III) *Type II:* Four rami fracture	Intact
Stable	Lateral compression *Type I:* Ipsilateral anterior and posterior *Type II:* Bucket handle *Type III:* Four rami type	Impacted
Unstable	Vertical shear	Disrupted – unilateral, bilateral

Miscellaneous	Complex
	Bilateral sacroiliac joint disruption with
	  an intact anterior arch
	Acetabular fracture associated with
	  pelvic ring disruption	

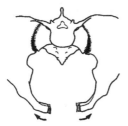

a. Anteroposterior compression (Type I): open book pelvic fracture.

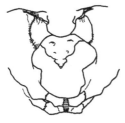

b. Anteroposterior compression (Type II): four rami fracture.

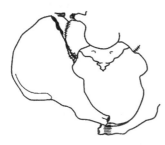

c. Lateral compression (Type I): ipsilateral anterior and posterior injury.

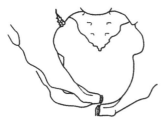

d. I. Lateral compression (Type I): locked symphysis (variation in anterior injury pattern).

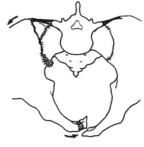

e. Lateral compression (Type II): contralateral anterior and posterior injury (bucket handle).

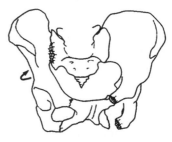

f. Lateral compression (Type III): four rami type (Straddle or butterfly fracture).

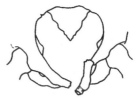

g. Lateral compression (Type III variation): superior pubic rami fracture involving the anterior column of the acetabulum.

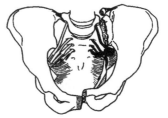

h. Unstable pelvic fracture: vertical shear (Malgaigne fracture).

Figure 11.3 Tile's classification (1984). Source: *Classification of Musculoskeletal Trauma*, Pynsent PB, Fairbank JCT, & Carr AJ. 1999: 95, Elsevier.

1999). Again, it is beyond the scope of the book to go into further detail but further reading is recommended.

Medical management

Early intervention

Following pelvic trauma the single most life threatening complication for the individual is haemorrhaging to the abdominal area (Unwin and Jones 1995). As with any major trauma the paramedic should first check that the individual's airway is clear and that breathing is not impaired, immediate attention to blood loss is then required. Their lower body can then be securely strapped to a stretcher in such a way as to restore anatomical alignment as well as assisting in the reduction of blood loss. Once stabilisation has been achieved the individual can then be moved to the nearest hospital emergency department for stabilisation.

Correct diagnosis and knowledge of the extent of the injury is essential in order to formulate the most appropriate treatment plan. There are several methods of determining this. Observation, clinical examination and communication with the individual may give an indication of the extent of the injury and provisional diagnosis. Imaging such as X-ray, magnetic resonance imaging (MRI) or computed tomography (CT) will be required to confirm this. Where intra-abdominal injuries are suspected, referral to the appropriate speciality is required.

Surgical management

Reconstruction of the fractured pelvis or acetabulum is considered a specialist area of orthopaedic trauma in the UK. Therefore transfer to an appropriate specialist reconstruction unit might best serve the interests of the person with a significant pelvic or acetabular fracture.

There are two clear stages involved in the management of any major fracture of the pelvis. The first stage will include reducing internal haemorrhaging and stabilising the person sufficiently to allow further investigations and intervention for other injuries. This may include application of an external fixator and perhaps a pelvic clamp for pelvic fractures and application of traction for acetabular fractures. The second stage is the definitive treatment that will follow and may take different forms depending on the severity of the fracture.

Pelvic fractures

- Bed rest/possibly combined with traction – for minimally displaced fractures, open book fractures, where the anterior gap is less than two centimetres and there are no posterior injuries, and iliac blade fractures.
- External fixation – for more severe open book fractures.
- Internal fixation – fractures of the iliac blade with marked displacement, associated ring fractures or separation of the symphysis pubis.
- Skeletal traction, combined with external fixation and bed rest – for very severe and vertical sheer injuries (Solomon et al. 2001).

Acetabular fractures

- Non-operative treatment – for minimally displaced, those that do not involve the weightbearing aspect of the acetabulum, older persons and those persons with medical contraindications for surgery.
- Operative treatment – indicated for unstable hips and where a femoral head fracture is also involved (Solomon et al. 2001).

Postoperative management

It is not unusual following pelvic or acetabular reconstructive surgery for the surgeon to recommend that the person follow a postoperative regimen that places restrictions on movement and weightbearing. This is to protect the injured area from further damage until the bone, muscles and ligaments around the injured area have healed and strengthened. These precautions will relate to the area and severity of the injury and the stability of the fixation. As different surgeons use a range of operative techniques, it is important to adhere to local protocols relating to postoperative advice. Currently there is no national or internationally agreed regimen. These precautions are usually recommended for a prescribed length of time, commonly 12 weeks following surgery.

Common postoperative precautions

- Non-weightbearing – this may be unilateral or bilateral. As the person is advised not to put weight through the leg for the instructed length of time they cannot stand or push through their legs when in the sitting or lying position. A wheelchair will be required for a person who is non-weightbearing bilaterally.
- Avoiding excessive hip flexion – common in patients who have a fracture of the posterior wall of the acetabulum. The surgeon may recommend that the person sit in a reclined position to prevent the head of the femur pushing against the posterior wall of the acetabulum (Figure 11.4). This will not affect the person's ability to straighten their leg to stand or to lie flat.

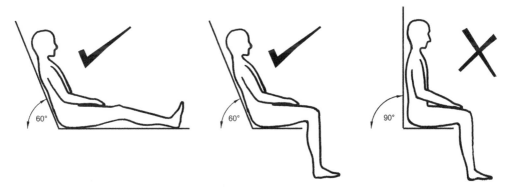

Figure 11.4 Postoperative sitting precautions to prevent the head of the femur pushing against the posterior wall of the acetabulum.

The occupational therapist will need to take into account any other postoperative care instructions resulting for other associated injuries.

Complications of pelvic injury

The following complications are associated with injury to the pelvis:

- Early:
  - Blood loss/uncontrolled haemorrhaging
  - Infection
  - Thrombo-embolic disease.
- Late:
  - Malunion
  - Non-union
  - Leg length discrepancy
  - Gait abnormality
  - Erectile dysfunction in some males as a result of disruption to the urethra
  - Nerve injury.

Team work and the person-centred approach

It is essential that effective collaboration and communication occur between the multi-disciplinary team and the individual to ensure a consistent, unified approach to treatment. As with any injured person all members of the team should be clear about the goals of treatment and be working together to assist them to achieve the optimum level of functional independence that they can.

Dependent on the nature and extent of the pelvic injury there may be additional members of the multi-disciplinary team working with the person to advise on such aspects as pressure care, wound care and pin site care where an external fixator is in situ. A clinical psychologist/trauma counsellor is also considered to be an essential part of the team. Where the extent of the injury results in a dramatic change in the person's circumstances or was the result of such a traumatic event as to cause the person psychological issues then the trauma counsellor can help to address these. They can also offer support to the person's family, friends and carers.

Occupational therapy intervention

Any fracture to the lower extremities is likely to disrupt normal mobility resulting in impairment to many areas of occupational performance. Occupational therapy intervention for the person with a pelvic or acetabular injury is likely to follow a similar care pathway from the acute phase through to their eventual return to the community.

All departments will have protocols around timing and prioritisation of referrals but occupational therapy can commence when:

- The person's medical condition is stable
- There is no further plan for major surgery (the person may still have numerous minor surgical interventions planned such as wound debridement)
- The person is able to commence functional activities within the limits of pain tolerance.

As with any person with an orthopaedic injury the occupational therapist should first review the person's history from the multi-disciplinary team and the case notes. Having established this then an initial interview and baseline assessment is required in order to establish with the individual the goals of treatment.

With pelvic and acetabular injuries particular consideration should be given to:

- The events leading to the trauma – This may be obtained from the medical notes and ambulance report which may include details of the accident, how it happened and other people involved. If the accident resulted in fatalities then it may have an impact on the person's state of mind. Where there is concern as to the emotional and psychological state of the individual then referral to a trauma counsellor is indicated. As a result of their experience the person may present with anger, decreased motivation, sadness or anxiety.
- Postoperative protocols/regimens – These may restrict range of movement or weight-bearing dependent on the nature of the injury and type of fixation. Internal fixation will not be visible but may restrict movement; soreness and the extent of the wound may also be a factor to consider. External fixation will protrude from the body and will therefore obstruct normal activity. Both will need to be considered in relation to activities of daily living.
- Patient goals – Sumison (1999) states that the essence of occupational therapy is the collaboration or partnership between the client and the therapist, working together to achieve the client's goals. Therefore the person is the most important component in any intervention.
- Associated injuries – As previously discussed there are likely to be other injuries, which must be taken into consideration. The occupational therapist may need to consult with other specialist therapists and other health professionals in order to ensure appropriate care is given.
- Psychological trauma – The person may suffer psychological trauma following their injury, resulting in post-traumatic stress disorder. It is important that all persons are offered the appropriate support and counselling in order to address their psychological needs.

Initial interview

This intervention is aimed at establishing the individual's previous level of function, support network, environment, expectations and any plans they may have already made. With a pelvic injury the following specific points should be discussed alongside a general initial assessment:

- Pre-morbid functional ability – The person's functional ability prior to injury is important to ascertain in order to ensure an appropriate level of function can be achieved.

- Age – A younger person who was previously fit and well may have the capacity to heal at a faster rate than an older person. These people may have increased potential for successful rehabilitation.
- Occupation – A person who is in employment will have natural concerns about time off work, loss of income and whether or not they will be able to resume their job. This will need to be considered in treatment planning and referral to appropriate employment advisors/back to work schemes should be considered.
- Locality – If the person is in a specialist hospital for treatment this may be some distance from their home. Administrative time will be required to liaise with local services for the provision of temporary assistive equipment, wheelchair services provision and minor home adaptations or care packages.

Following the initial assessment the occupational therapist should discuss with the person the aims of treatment and set goals that will focus on optimal functional independence and safety. Short- and long-term goals will be dependent on the complexity of the injury.

Treatment planning

Goals are a method of setting realistic, achievable and measureable aims for therapy intervention. Short-term goals will reflect the initial needs of the individual in order to return home or to a rehabilitative setting. Long-term goals, whilst dependent on the extent of the injuries, should be given some consideration so that the individual has a realistic idea of what they are aiming for. It is possible that an individual will return to their previous level of function. However, in more complex situations they may need to consider major changes in their lifestyle such as moving to ground floor accommodation or a new work role.

Following the initial goal planning session the occupational therapist may need to assess the person in specific areas of function such as personal care or ability to transfer to determine a baseline from which to commence intervention.

Mobility and transfers

The person's mobility will be dependent as much on the nature and extent of the pelvic injury as on other injuries that may have been sustained. They may be allowed to fully weightbear bilaterally, partial or non-weightbear unilaterally or bilaterally within the limits of pain and precautions. It is for the physiotherapist to determine the most appropriate walking aid and instruct the person in correct use and appropriate gait pattern. It is important though for the occupational therapist to be aware of the techniques adopted and to reinforce the advice during assessment and treatment sessions.

Where a person is non-weightbearing bilaterally then a wheelchair will be required for mobility until the restrictions are lifted. A wheelchair may also be indicated where the person has upper limb injuries preventing them from using an appropriate walking aid such as a frame or elbow crutches. Local protocols should be followed for the assessment and provision of an appropriate wheelchair.

The type of wheelchair and accessories prescribed will be dependent on the person's overall medical condition and other injuries sustained. Should the person have upper limb injuries then an attendant propelled chair may need to be considered. If the pelvic surgery has resulted in the person having restrictions placed on the range of movement at the hip joint then a wheelchair with an adjustable reclining backrest may be indicated.

In issuing the wheelchair the occupational therapist must ensure that the person is aware of all the relevant health and safety requirements pertinent to the wheelchair issued, that they can mobilise safely in the wheelchair and can safely transfer in and out of the wheelchair (see Chapter 8, p 134).

Transfer techniques

It is important to assess all individuals transferring in and out of bed, getting up and down to a chair and toilet and in/out of the bath or shower in order to ensure that their technique is safe and that any required equipment is available on discharge home. It is particularly important where a person is non-weightbearing either unilaterally or bilaterally.

Unilateral non-weightbearing

Technique

This person should be able to hop on their good leg using an appropriate walking aid such as elbow crutches or a frame for support. A standing pivot transfer allows them to stand on one leg and pivot around to the next surface. It is important that the surfaces, such as the bed and the wheelchair, are next to one another, preferably at a 90° angle, and of a similar height.

Possible problems

- Difficulty lifting their legs up when getting into bed
- Difficulty getting up and down from low surfaces such as a toilet or low chair
- Pain and postoperative precautions may restrict movement
- Inability to step into bath or shower.

Potential solutions

- Provision and instruction in use of a leg lifter
- Appropriate raising equipment for chair or toilet. Grab rails or frame to assist balance when rising from sitting
- Appropriate bathing equipment such as a bath board or shower chair.

It is important that a person with pelvic or acetabular injuries does not attempt to get down into the bottom of the bath initially. Also a person with pin-sites and covered wounds should not soak them in the bath.

Bilateral non-weightbearing

Technique

This person will be required to slide for all transfers, sideways, backwards or forwards. They will need to be careful of any postoperative requests that require them to sit slightly reclined, as they will have to maintain this position when transferring. As the person is non-weightbearing they will need to push through their upper limbs and avoid at all costs pushing through their lower limbs.

Possible problems

- Lack of upper limb strength in order to transfer
- Inability to lift legs to position them when seated
- Lack of confidence to transfer self
- Unequal height of surfaces
- Lack of space, especially within the person's home.

Potential solutions

- The person may require assistance of one or two people
- Provision of and instruction in the correct use of specialist manual handling equipment such as sliding sheet and transfer board
- Chair with removable arms for sideways transfers
- Specialist equipment to raise other surfaces such as bed raisers, chair raisers and toilet raise
- Environmental assessment to ensure that there is adequate space for correct use of equipment.

If a person is unable to transfer with appropriate equipment and assistance, it may be necessary to consider the use of a hoist to transfer. Consideration must be given to postoperative precautions and the position of the person in the sling. There may well be occasions where it is safer to nurse the person in bed rather than to compromise the fixation in an attempt to sit them out.

Personal care

A personal care assessment should be undertaken early on in the person's intervention. Where possible they should be encouraged to undertake as many tasks for themselves as is possible. The individual who is non-weightbearing bilaterally may find it easiest to wash and dress while lying on the bed. Those who can, should be encouraged to mobilise to the bathroom where they may need to sit on a perching stool to wash or use a shower chair or bath board as appropriate and a long handled sponge or toe washer to reach their lower limbs.

Anyone who is unable to bend as a result of pain or the postoperative regimen, will have difficult reaching their lower limbs for dressing. Long handled equipment such as a helping hand, long handled shoe horn or sock aid will assist them towards independent dressing. It may be necessary for some people to have assistance from a carer for some or all aspects of personal care.

Home environment

Consideration needs to be given to the person's home environment early on in treatment so that intervention can be focussed towards returning them there as soon as is practicably possible. Ideally a home visit from the hospital setting would be most appropriate but this is not always possible if the person is in hospital some distance from the locality in which they live.

If unable to carry out a home visit, the occupational therapist needs to establish as much information as is possible from the person and their family about their home circumstances. The information required includes:

- Type of accommodation – In particular the type of house or flat, whether there are steps or stairs to negotiate, approximate size of rooms and if there is room for a bed and other equipment downstairs.
- Access – Whether or not this needs to be suitable for a wheelchair.
- Furniture heights for appropriate transfers – The family can be requested to assist by providing the measurements of the height of the bed, chair, toilet and width of the bath. They will also need to give a description of the type of furniture it is so that the most appropriate raising equipment can be ordered.
- Level of support available from family and friends – The occupational therapist will need to establish if anyone is available to assist with personal and domestic tasks and for how long. It should be remembered that caring for relatives is not easy and that family members will often have other commitments and should not be made to feel that they are responsible. It may be more appropriate to have an employed carer from an outside agency, which it may be possible to arrange through the social worker.

With the information to hand the occupational therapist will need to liaise with the appropriate agencies for the provision of all essential assistive equipment in readiness for discharge.

Long-term goals

These will usually be addressed by the occupational therapist in the community. The individual may attend a rehabilitation centre or receive visits from a community occupational therapist dependent on the resources available in their area. Once home they should continue to work towards independence in mobility and activities of daily living. As they improve their dependence on assistive equipment may lessen until it is no longer required.

The occupational therapist should also address with each individual the need to return to work or education. This may involve working with the person's employer on what aspects of the job they can and cannot do and working out a timescale for a graded return. Where an individual is unable to return to their previous job then referral to appropriate agencies may be required to look at alternatives and the possibility of incapacity benefits.

Case study 1

Diagnosis

John – male, 40 years old

John was admitted to hospital following a road traffic accident in which his motorcycle collided with a lorry. Prior to admission John was fit and healthy with no significant past medical history. He was employed as a motorcycle courier and the accident happened while he was in work.

Injuries sustained:

- Bilateral pelvic fractures
- Urethral rupture
- Sacral nerve injury
- Lacerations and bruises, vulnerability of skin on all bony prominences.

Having been stabilised at the scene of the accident, John was transferred to the emergency department and then to a specialist centre for further treatment.

Surgery included:

- Application of external fixation to his pelvis
- Laparotomy
- Colostomy
- Debridement and dressing of all wounds.

Postoperative precautions:

- Non-weightbearing both legs for 12 weeks
- Only to sit up 60° for 12 weeks

Occupational therapy intervention

Initially John was not considered medically well enough for occupational therapy but the occupational therapist was involved in close liaison with the multi-disciplinary team about the patient's progress and the most appropriate time to commence intervention. An initial interview was completed and it was established that prior to the accident John was fit and well and independent in all activities of daily living.

John was employed full time as a motorcycle courier and had been in the area working when the accident happened. He lived alone in a first floor flat, accessed by a staircase. He had an active social live with a good network of supportive family and friends. Of immediate concern to John was how he was going to manage alone in the flat, accessing the flat and financial concerns due to loss of income. It was established that he was entitled to sick pay and his family undertook to liaise with his employers.

Initial goals agreed with him:

- To be able to get out of bed
- To have greater independence mobilising
- To be independent washing and dressing his top half.

John was assessed for and provided with a recliner wheelchair with a pressure relief cushion. The type of cushion had been determined by using a standardised tissue viability scoring system. Joint occupational therapy and physiotherapy sessions were set up daily to initially assess and then practise transfers from the bed to the wheelchair. Initially, on the ward, John was hoisted out of bed by the nursing staff and allowed to sit for short periods in order to increase his tolerance in sitting.

He was taught to transfer from the bed to the wheelchair using the backwards forwards technique. Once in the sitting position he used a sliding sheet, his upper limb strength and three therapists assisting to lift himself back into the wheelchair. The therapists were positioned one on either side holding onto the sliding sheet to aid the movement backwards and the third supporting his lower legs to prevent them from taking any weight.

Once in the wheelchair he was taught how to manoeuvre it safely and awareness of space and the environment. Transfer and mobility practice continued for a number of weeks and during this time the occupational therapist also saw John for washing and dressing practice. John was able to manage washing and dressing his top half while sitting supported in bed, assistance was required for his lower half.

Further goals were discussed and set:

- To increase sitting tolerance on a daily basis
- To reduce the number of people required to assist with transfers
- To reduce the assistance required for personal care
- To involve the family in assisting with transfers and personal care
- To plan for discharge back to his family home.

At this stage John agreed to be referred to the trauma counsellor as he was suffering from flashbacks and nightmares related to the accident. He felt that he required some psychological support to assist him to cope with this.

Over the next few weeks the hoist was withdrawn as John's ability to transfer improved. With increased practice his strength and stamina improved until he only required one person, to assist with positioning his lower limbs, when transferring into the wheelchair. He was able to tolerate sitting in the wheelchair for up to an hour at a time and was showing signs of further improving on this. He continued to improve in personal care skills but still required assistance with his lower half.

A multi-disciplinary case conference was held with John and his family and it was decided that arrangements would be made to discharge him back to his family home, as this was more suitable. A room could be made available on the ground floor to accommodate a bed and wheelchair and his family were willing to assist in whatever way they could. Although the family were available it was agreed that an outside carer would attend daily to assist him with his personal care so that the family had some respite.

In anticipation of discharge the occupational therapist discussed with the family the exact nature of the accommodation available and obtained a measurement for the height of the bed. As this was very low and could not be raised it was considered unsuitable and it was agreed that a hospital bed would be required. The occupational therapist liaised closely with the local equipment store to ensure that all items were in place in readiness for discharge. These included:

- Hospital bed – an electric profile bed was arranged as John would benefit from the height adjustable feature and the backrest
- Sliding sheet
- Commode
- Urine bottle.

John's local wheelchair service also delivered a recliner chair with a pressure relieving cushion to his family home and reported that they would provide an ongoing review of his wheelchair needs once he was home. In order to meet John's ongoing rehabilitation needs he was referred on discharge to a local therapy rehabilitation team, which would provided regular input initially at home and as he improved at his local hospital.

Six months after discharge from hospital John is able to mobilise around his home with elbow crutches. He still uses a wheelchair for longer distances outdoors but no longer has the backrest in the reclined position. He transfers independently but has chair raisers and a toilet frame to assist him. He is independent washing and dressing himself and is able to shower over the bath using a bath board. He continues to attend outpatient physiotherapy, hydrotherapy and regular occupational therapy reviews and the long-term functional outcome is looking very positive.

Summary

This chapter has provided a brief overview of the nature of the problems resulting from a pelvic or acetabular injury. As with all fractures this is traumatic for the person and requires the combined efforts of the multi-disciplinary team to help them to adjust and recover to their maximum potential. The occupational therapist is better equipped to assist the person to achieve their goal of maximum functional independence if he or she has an understanding of the underlying injury and the course of healing for that pelvic injury.

References

Kapit, W., & Elson, L. (1977). *Anatomy Colouring Book*. New York: Harpur and Collins.

McRea, R., & Esser, M. (2002). *Practical Fracture Management* (2nd edition). Edinburgh: Churchill Livingstone.

Palastanga, N., Field, D., & Soames, R. (1994). *Anatomy and Human Movement, Structure and Function* (2nd edition). Oxford: Butterworth Heinemann.

Patient U. K. (2005). Pelvic fractures. Online. Available at: www.patient.co.uk (accessed 10 April 2009).

Pynsent, P. B., Fairbank, J. C. T., & Carr, A. J. (1999). *Classification of Musculoskeletal Trauma*. Oxford: Butterworth Heinemann.

Solomon, L., Warwick, D. J., & Nayagam, S. (2001). *Apley's System of Orthopaedics and Fractures* (8th edition). London: Arnold.

Sumison, T. (1999). *Client Centred Practice in Occupational Therapy. A Guide to Implementation*. London: Churchill Livingstone.

Tortora, G. J., & Anagnostakos, N. P. (1990). *Principles of Anatomy and Physiology*. New York: Harpur Collins.

Unwin, A., & Jones, K. (1995). *Emergency Orthopaedics and Trauma*. Oxford: Butterworth Heinemann.

Chapter 12
Hand injuries

Neil Davidson and Daniel Brown

Introduction

Hand injuries of varying degrees of severity are very common and the surgical and therapeutic treatment of these is extremely important due to the part the hand plays in a person's functional ability. Much has been written about the best way to manage these injuries and all authors agree that the best results are achieved by a team approach with the hand surgeon and therapists working together with the individual person to achieve their goals.

In this chapter we will deal with some of the more important aspects relating to the surgical management of hand trauma. To assist the reader the chapter has been divided into sections to cover all the main areas but it is important to remember that the hand-injured person may present with a combination of injuries, which may complicate their treatment.

Bone injuries (fractures)

Fractures of the wrist and hand are extremely common and a comprehensive account of the treatment of these injuries is outside the remit of this book. The following section will outline the basis of treatment for some of the more frequently presented injuries. Readers wanting further information are directed to standard orthopaedic texts as outlined in the Further reading section at the end of this chapter.

Distal radius fractures

These are more often referred to as 'wrist' or 'Colles' fractures and are the most frequently presented injury in the fracture clinic. They represent a broad range of injuries from the insufficiency fracture in elderly osteoporotic bone to complicated intra-articular injuries resulting from high energy trauma. Fractures of the distal radius make up one-sixth of all long bone fractures and have three distinct peaks of distribution.

- **Fractures in childhood (5–14 years of age)** – These tend to be low energy injuries and are often incomplete. Torus (or buckle) fractures (Figure 12.1) are the commonest fractures; they are incomplete fractures, are stable and can be considered as a 'bone bruise' requiring no more than simple splinting. Greenstick fractures are also incomplete but are relatively unstable. They are usually treated in plaster of Paris (POP) cast, following manipulation under anaesthesia (MUA) if the fracture is significantly displaced. Complete fractures (usually situated more proximally than their adult counterparts) are unstable again and often require K-wire fixation.
- **Fractures in young adulthood** – These tend to be higher energy injuries, e.g. sports injuries or road traffic accidents (RTA). They are injuries of normal bone. These fractures are often displaced and usually unstable (Figure 12.2). Treatment depends upon the fracture pattern, amount of displacement and instability of the fracture pattern. Simple fractures are again treated in POP with more complex fractures traditionally being treated with K-wires (Figure 12.3) or external fixation and more recently with locking plates (Figure 12.4).
- **Fractures of old age** – These tend to be low energy injuries, e.g. simple falls, in osteoporotic bone. They again tend to be displaced and can be unstable. Treatment options are as above, however, the indications for more 'aggressive', operative,

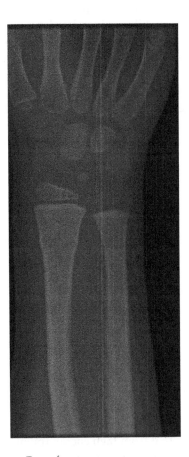

Figure 12.1 Anteroposterior view – Torus fracture.

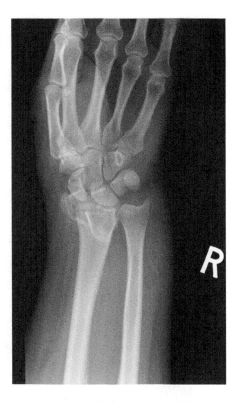

Figure 12.2 Anteroposterior view – young adult fracture.

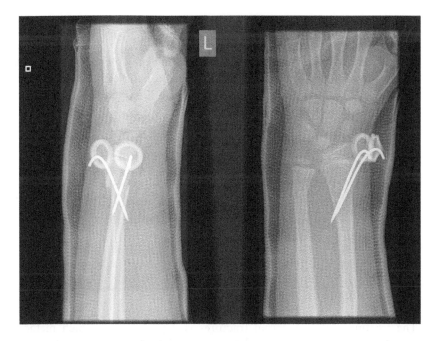

Figure 12.3 Fracture post K-wire fixation.

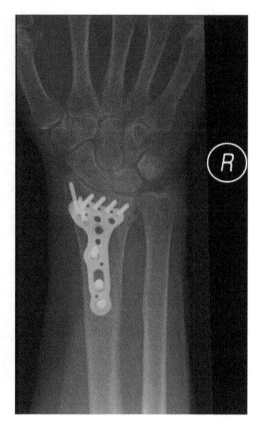

Figure 12.4 Anteroposterior view of a wrist fracture post ORIF.

treatment in this group, however, depend not only on the fracture configuration but, more importantly, on the age, general medical status and functional demands of the person. What appears a terrible fracture on X-ray does not always correlate with a poor result in these individuals.

Hand fractures

Fractures to the bones of the hand are common, particularly in the young male working population. Most fractures are stable and have a good outcome with conservative management.

Metacarpal fractures

The treatment of metacarpal fractures is dependent on which metacarpal is injured and the area of the metacarpal affected. Fractures affect base, shaft, neck, or head of

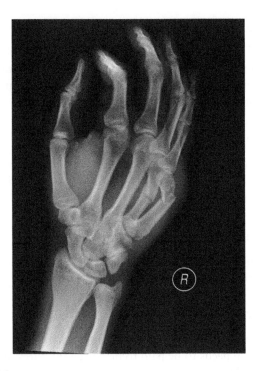

Figure 12.5 Metacarpal fracture.

the metacarpal (Figure 12.5). Fractures to the head of the metacarpal are uncommon. If the fracture enters the joint treatment is aimed towards anatomical restoration. Displacement of the articular surface or malrotation deformity should be corrected and stabilised. Stable fracture patterns may only require immobilisation in cast or splintage. The unstable injuries will usually require surgical stabilisation.

Fractures of the neck are often the result of an axial load to the clenched fist (boxer's fracture) and commonly affect the fourth and fifth metacarpals. Fractures to the metacarpal shaft often result in a flexion deformity. In general angular deformities, in the plane of movement, are tolerated better than other deformities. This is especially the case in the ring and little finger because of the greater degree of mobility at the carpometacarpal (CMC) joints in the fourth and fifth rays. Rotational deformity is tolerated poorly, and results in finger overlap when making a fist.

More commonly seen fractures are now described.

Thumb metacarpal base

The injury is caused by axial load to the flexed thumb with the fracture being either intra- or extra-articular (the commonest fracture being the intra-articular Bennett's fracture). Stable fractures that are outside the joint are usually treated conservatively in a cast with thumb extension. Displaced or unstable fractures usually require internal stabilisation, with wire or screw fixation. Poor results after this injury can affect pinch grip and the motion of opposition to the fingers.

Fifth metacarpal base

Often referred to as a reverse Bennett's fracture. The fracture often displaces dorsally. Usually manipulation under anaesthesia and K-wire fixation is required. More complicated, comminuted fractures will require open reduction and internal fixation. These are commonly associated with fractures of the hamate bone.

Fifth metacarpal neck (Boxer's fracture)

The boxer's fracture is the result of a direct blow to the metacarpal head of the little and ring fingers. The common result is a fracture displaced into flexion. A relatively high degree of this angulation is acceptable.

Fifth metacarpal shaft

Only fractures with marked angulation or any rotation will require manipulation to improve the position. Stabilisation is then usually provided by K-wires or plate fixation.

Other metacarpal fractures

Fractures of the index, middle and ring metacarpals are less tolerant of displacement. Careful attention needs to be paid to displaced fractures of the index finger metacarpal. As a general rule, single fractures tend to be stable while multiple fractures are not; third and fourth metacarpal fractures are similarly more stable than those of the index or little fingers.

Phalangeal fractures

These are very common injuries in the hand. The anatomical descriptions include base, shaft, neck, intercondylar and epiphyseal fractures. Evaluation of the fracture will also include deformity and associated injury to nerve, artery or tendon. Tuft or crush fractures are also included with these (see crush injury below).

The aim of management of these fractures is for accurate reduction of the fracture if required and early mobilisation as fracture stability allows.

Proximal and middle phalanges

Fractures of the proximal and middle phalanges when undisplaced usually cause no problems. Neighbour strapping to the adjacent finger for three to four weeks is commonly used to treat them (Figure 12.6). Displaced or angulated fractures may require manipulation under anaesthetic with suitable stabilisation. When the fracture is unstable and cannot be reduced or fails closed means of stabilisation, then K-wires, screws and plates or dynamic external fixation may be indicated.

Mallet fractures

This injury has a classic drooping finger appearance with the distal phalanx in a flexed position. The injury is caused by forced flexion of an extended finger. The insertion of

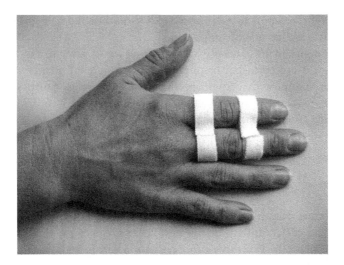

Figure 12.6 Neighbour strapping.

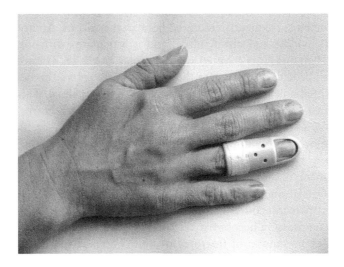

Figure 12.7 Mallet splint.

the extensor tendon is pulled from its anchor point, with or without a piece of bone. Unless a large part of the joint is affected by the fracture fragment treatment involves using a mallet splint (Figure 12.7). Large fractures into the joint often result in joint subluxations, which may require surgical reconstruction.

Tuft fractures (crush injuries)

Fractures to the terminal phalanx, result from blunt injury to the distal finger. Fracture configuration varies, but generally is regarded as a soft tissue injury with an underlying fracture. If the skin is broken, treatment should include a thorough clean, prophylactic antibiotics, analgesia and support.

It is important to carefully assess a fracture of any part of the ray for a rotational deformity. If a metacarpal or phalanx heals in a small degree of rotation, it can cause major problems with grip from fingers overlapping. Stiffness and swelling can be problems resistant to treatment. A displaced fracture into a joint has a higher risk of developing osteoarthritis in the long term.

Carpal injuries

Carpal bones each have six surfaces. These are the proximal, distal, medial and lateral articulating surfaces, with dorsal and volar surfaces for the ligament attachments (see Figure 4.4, p 50). Fractures can occur in isolation but should herald a search for an associated fracture or dislocation of adjacent structures.

Scaphoid

This is the most frequently fractured bone in the carpus. Anatomically it is divided into proximal, middle and distal thirds, and it articulates with four carpal bones and the radius. Therefore, it is covered with articular cartilage. The waist (middle third) has a small non-articular area where the blood supply enters the bone; the blood supply to the proximal pole therefore travels from distal to proximal. This is an important feature when considering management of the fracture. Waist fractures will result in decreased blood flow to the proximal pole and occasionally frank avascular necrosis of the proximal pole occurs. Non-union is common for the same reason. Seventy per cent of all fractures are middle, 20% are proximal and 10% distal third.

Treatment of non-displaced fractures requires cast immobilisation for six to 12 weeks. Displacement greater than 2 mm requires fixation. Techniques used include open and percutaneous fixation. The method of fixation is generally a screw, which creates compression across the fracture site and is buried completely within the bone. Delayed or non-union of fractures treated conservatively may require curettage, bone graft and fixation. Inadequately treated scaphoid fractures can lead to later degenerative osteoarthritis.

Lunate

Fractures in isolation are rare. Volar pole fractures require fixation if displaced, but the more common chip fractures are treated non-operatively.

Triquetrum

These most commonly involve impaction of the proximal pole. If the injury results from forced ulnar deviation with dorsiflexion, the ulna styloid can shear off a fragment. Displaced fractures require fixation. Undisplaced fractures are treatment non-operatively.

Capitate

Capitate fractures are often associated with scaphoid fractures as a combined injury resulting from extreme dorsiflexion. The diagnosis is easily missed when the proximal pole flips through 180° and presents an X-ray which can look remarkably normal. The clinical picture should alert the examiner to a more severe injury. Avascular necrosis may occur as a result of a disturbed blood supply. Undisplaced fractures can be treated conservatively.

Hamate

These can be either hook or body fractures and result from a direct blow to the hand. If missed, chronic symptoms of pain from a non-union should be treated by excision of the fragment. Body fractures are commonly associated with fractures of the fourth and fifth metacarpal bases. These often require open reduction and internal fixation.

Trapezium

Non-displaced fractures are treated conservatively. A displaced body fracture should be fixed internally, and any painful non-union (usually of the ridge) should be treated by excision of the painful part.

Trapezoid

These are rare fractures in isolation. This should be suspected as an associated injury if dislocation of the index carpometacarpal joint occurs. Again, non-operative management is required for undisplaced fractures, and internal fixation for the fracture dislocation.

Joint injuries

These can present as either a dislocation, where the joint surfaces are completely displaced and no longer in contact, or a subluxation, where the joint surfaces are partly displaced but still opposed to some degree. In the acute setting they are usually secondary to trauma whereas in the chronic and recurrent setting they are secondary to ligament laxity or joint incongruity.

Wrist dislocations

This is more correctly termed dislocation of the carpus, and is a relatively uncommon injury. The mechanism of injury is usually a fall onto the outstretched hand. There are several types, however, two are common:

- **Perilunate dislocation** (or trans-scaphoid peri-lunate) – Here the lunate (possibly with part of the scaphoid) remains attached to the radius and the rest of the carpus dislocates from them (usually dorsally)
- **True dislocation** – Here both carpal rows remain aligned with the distal radius and one or two bones (usually the lunate) dislocate dorsally.

Treatment of wrist dislocations

Usually fracture dislocations are reduced by closed reduction manipulation and it is rare for open reduction to be required. Once the dislocation is corrected cast immobilisation is commenced for six weeks. Any associated scaphoid fracture will be treated on its merits and may require internal fixation. The scapho-lunate ligament must, by definition be ruptured in these injuries (see p 221).

Finger dislocations

Dislocations of the distal interphalangeal, proximal interphalangeal and metacarpophalangeal joints are common hand injuries. They are usually the result of a forced hyperextension injury to the joint. Most finger dislocations are posterior and are treated by closed reduction (simple traction being applied with pressure over the base of the affected phalanx). Treatment involves early immediate mobilisation of the joint. If the joint is unstable this may indicate an associated fracture or a more severe soft tissue problem. Further assessment and perhaps immobilisation will be required. Dislocation of the metacarpophalangeal joint of the thumb may be difficult to reduce due to the presence of sesamoid bones at this joint.

Ligament injuries

Injuries to any joint can result in either an incomplete tear (sprain) or a complete tearing (rupture) of the joint ligaments.

Distal radioulnar joint (DRUJ) instability

This may complicate fractures of the radius, ulna or both. Eponyms are given to two specific fractures that affect the DRUJ. Galeazzi fracture-dislocations (fracture to the shaft of radius with associated disruption of the DRUJ) by definition generate instability, and the Essex Lopresti injury (comminuted radial head fracture, with disruption of the interosseous membrane and injury to the DRUJ as a result of a longitudinal compression force). Injury to the triangular fibrocartilage complex (TFCC) often forms part of this injury. Instability and dislocation as a result of these injuries can be either dorsal or volar.

Treatment is dependent on the associated injuries but should include early reduction and stabilisation with percutaneous wire fixation and immobilisation in an above elbow cast. Chronic instability can be treated conservatively with specialist bespoke splints, or surgical stabilisation using tendon grafts may be required.

Carpal instability

The stability of the bones in the wrist depends upon the shape of the bones and the ligaments to keep them in position. This means that instability can arise from either a change in the shape of the bones or a problem with the restraining ligaments. Instability of the carpus describes the presence of an abnormal position of the carpal bones and descriptions relate to the proximal carpal row. The abnormal position may be present all the time ('fixed') or, more commonly, the abnormal position may only be present intermittently with certain movements of the wrist ('dynamic'). Clinically instability presents as pain with clicking and clunking with different movements.

Carpal instability is a difficult concept to understand and the classification and terminology are complicated; however, the distal carpal row is fixed to the metacarpals, while the proximal row 'floats free' (as an intercalated segment) between the mid-carpal and radiocarpal joints. The intrinsic ligament arrangement (that is scapho-lunate and luno-triquetral ligaments) creates movement in all three bones of the proximal row. Normally flexion and extension occur simultaneously at both the mid-carpal and radiocarpal joints. Lack of the intrinsic constraints may cause the radiocarpal joint (or part of it) to flex while the mid-carpal joint extends (or vice-versa). With an intrinsic tear, the bones ulnar to the tear do not move with the scaphoid. Therefore:

- In a scapho-lunate tear the scaphoid flexes while lunate and triquetrum extend (causing a dorsal intercalated segment instability – DISI).
- In a luno-triquetral ligament tear the scaphoid and lunate flex while triquetrum extends (causing a volar intercalated segment instability – VISI).

It should be noted that instability detected at examination or X-ray may not be the cause of the symptoms.

Ulnar collateral ligament injuries of the thumb (gamekeeper's thumb)

A tear of the ulnar collateral ligament (UCL) of the thumb metacarpophalangeal joint is caused by forced abduction of the thumb. The original description of gamekeeper's thumb was applied to a chronically lax UCL but is now often applied to injury in the acute setting (an injury probably better described as a 'skier's thumb'). The result is instability at the metacarpophalangeal joint to abduction (i.e. in lateral pinch). The ligament injury may include an avulsion fracture of the bony insertion at the base of the proximal phalanx (Figure 12.8). The adductor aponeurosis can interfere with ligament healing if it interposes between ligament and bone (Stener lesion).

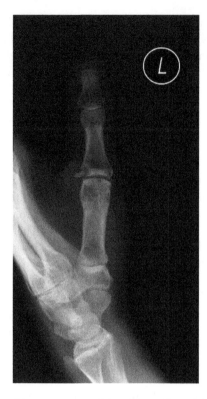

Figure 12.8 Avulsion fracture of bony insertion of the ulnar collateral ligament.

Tendon injuries

Tendon injuries are usually associated with a penetrating injury, lacerations or deep abrasive injuries. Associated injuries to nerves and vessels are common. Repair is desirable in the acute setting, as delayed or staged repair is complex and complications more common.

The number of injuries and their location largely dictates the approach to tendon injuries. The surgical repair of tendons is probably not as important as the postoperative rehabilitation. The principles of tendon repair and rehabilitation are based around the stages of tendon healing.

Tendon healing

Tendon healing occurs in three phases:

- **The initial inflammatory phase** – The initial injury generates bleeding and inflammation. Neutrophils predominate and the injured dead tissue is removed by macrophage activity. These in turn release chemical factors, which stimulate a cascade of new blood vessel proliferation and activity of tendon repair cells. These tenocytes synthesise type III collagen, which lasts for around five days, during which time the strength of the tendon is that of the sutured repair.

- **The regenerative phase, fibroblastic (collagen producing phase)** – This begins at five days and continues for three weeks. Synthesis of type III collagen peaks during this stage. Water content and glycosaminoglycan concentrations remain high during this stage. The strength of the repair increases rapidly with granulation tissue bridging the defect. Passive mobilisation in a controlled manner is recommended at this stage in order to encourage collagen fibre alignment, encourage excursion and reduce adhesions.
- **The remodelling stage** – This commences after six weeks and the tissue is consolidated and matured. In the first part of the remodelling stage the repaired tissue consolidates from a cellular repair structure and becomes fibrous, the collagen fibres become aligned in the direction of stress. In the second part of the remodelling, the maturation stage, the fibrous tissue changes to a tendon like scar tissue. The maturation occurs for 12 months.

Anatomy of tendons

Extensor tendons

The extensor tendons lie superficially and are easily palpable. Their anatomy is simpler than the flexors. The long extensors are the only tendons on the dorsal aspect of the hand. They pass through the wrist area in six separate dorsal extensor compartments.

Just proximal to the metacarpophalangeal joint the tendons are joined to each other by three variable oblique bands. The deep portion of each tendon has an attachment to the capsule of the metacarpophalangeal joint. It divides into three slips. The central slip inserts into the base of the middle phalanx, the lateral slips take attachment from interossei and lumbricals, together they form a broad structure, which covers the proximal part of the proximal phalanx, the hood. The extensor tendon has multiple attachments to the intrinsic muscles of the hand. On its own the extensor tendon provides extension of the metacarpophalangeal joint whereas the intrinsic muscles flex the metacarpophalangeal joint. However, working together with the extensor expansion the extensor tendon assist the intrinsic muscles to extend the proximal and distal interphalangeal joints.

The lateral slips pass back toward the midline as they become more distal until they join to insert into the base of the distal phalanx. In general terms therefore, injury to the lateral slips will affect distal interphalangeal joint extension, injury to the central slip will mainly affect proximal interphalangeal joint extension. Tendon injury proximal to the division will affect extension of both joints. Careful examination should exclude extensor tendon injury even if metacarpophalangeal joint extension is possible.

- Partial laceration of the extensor tendons proximal to the metacarpophalangeal joint may or may not require repair.
- Partial lacerations of the extensor tendons at or distal to metacarpophalangeal joint level must be repaired.

Flexor tendons

The digital flexor sheath is a closed synovial system consisting of both membranous and retinacular portions. The membranous portion invests both the flexor digitorum profundus (FDP) and flexor digitorum superficialis (FDS) tendons in the distal aspect of the hand. The flexor sheath has three main functions:

- It facilitates smooth gliding of the tendon
- The retinacular component acts as a fulcrum, adding a mechanical advantage to flexion
- It is a contained system with synovial fluid bathing the tendons and aiding their nutrition.

The retinacular component consists of tissue condensations arranged in cruciform, annular and transverse patterns that overlie the membranous or synovial lining aiding their nutrition. There are five annular pulleys and three cruciate pulleys.

Tendon zones

Injuries to tendons around the hand are classified according to zones. This descriptive method allows principles of surgical repair and methods of rehabilitation to be standardised and monitored to give predictable results. There are major differences in the approach to extensor tendon injuries and flexor tendon injuries.

Extensor tendon zone classification and injuries (Figure 12.9)

Zone I	distal interphalangeal joint
Zone II	middle phalanx. Usually tendon injuries in this location are partial, since the extensor tendon extends over the dorsal half of the digit
Zone III	proximal interphalangeal joint
Zone IV	proximal phalanx – at this level there is only two or three millimetres of tendon excursion between flexion and extension, so even minor adhesion can result in significant functional loss
Zone V	metacarpophalangeal joint
Zone VI	the area overlying the metacarpals of the fingers
Zone VII	the area of the wrist under the extensor retinaculum (dorsal carpal ligament)
Zone VIII	the area of the distal forearm, proximal to the extensor retinaculum

Hand therapy is a vital adjunct to operative repair.

Flexor tendon zone classification and injuries (Figure 12.10)

Zone I	distal to FDS insertion, FDP is the only tendon affected. Repair is attached using a pullout button,
Zone II	both FDS and FDP travel in the tight fibro osseous tunnel. This is a demanding repair and often has the worst outcomes. Often referred to as 'no man's land'.

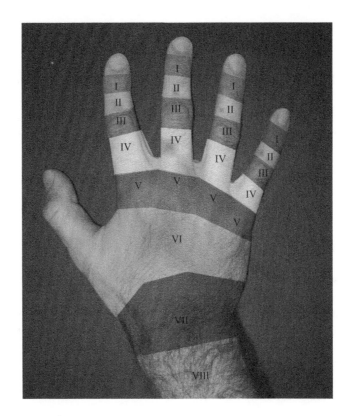

Figure 12.9 Extensor tendon zones.

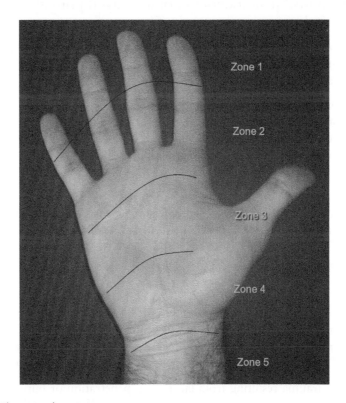

Figure 12.10 Flexor tendon zones.

Zone III	injury in the palm of the hand. Both tendons are affected, but there is no tight pulley or tunnel so good results are achieved. Vascular injury can complicate surgery in this zone
Zone IV	at the level of the wrist and carpal ligament. Can be complicated by injuries to ulnar and medial nerve.
Zone V	proximal to the carpal ligament. No sheaths with plentiful space. But multiple tendon lacerations are characteristic and have a good prognosis for repair in this zone.

Tendon repair

Primary repair is recommended for most lacerations to the flexor tendons, regardless of zone. In general terms, the flexor tendon sheath is preserved, the A2 and A4 pulleys, which are broad and sited between the joints, need to be preserved to avoid the bow-stringing of the tendon. The A1 (lying over the metacarpophalangeal joint) and the A3 (lying over the proximal interphalangeal joint) pulleys are less important in terms of function. Repair is usually by a combination of a strong 'core' suture for strength and a weaker 'peripheral' suture to improve tendon gliding. The aim is for the repair to be strong enough for early mobilisation.

Delayed treatment (definition of a delayed primary repair is after three weeks)

A tendon graft is often required to bridge the defect, because of contracture within the muscle-tendon unit.

The approach to treatment is:

- Delayed primary direct repair, if possible
- If not, proceed to single stage tendon graft
- If not, proceed to two-stage graft
- Failure or unsuitable for reconstruction, then consider arthrodesis, tendon transfer or amputation.

An experienced surgeon, with the support of an experienced hand therapist and a compliant and well-informed patient, should carry out all tendon reconstruction of this nature.

Peripheral nerve injuries

Nerve injury is commonly seen with associated soft tissue or bony injury around the hand or in isolation (e.g. penetrating injury). Examination of the injured extremity should always include a thorough documented neurological assessment of sensory and motor function, and a regular review. Acute injury is as a result of:

- Direct trauma resulting from laceration, penetration or burns
- Indirect injury from traction on the nerve or the effects of displaced fracture fragments.

Chronic or delayed manifestations may present later because of fracture callus formation or malunited fracture resulting in chronic nerve stretch and irritation.

Classification

As discussed in Chapter 1, injury to the nerve is classified into three types. For revision these are:

- **Neuropraxia** – blunt trauma causes compression and a local reaction. The axons and sheath remain intact. Wallerian degeneration (axonal loss) does not occur. Injury is manifest as a temporary physiological conduction delay. Recovery is usually spontaneous in less than six weeks. The least severe of nerve injury types which may only last a few hours.
- **Axonotmesis** – blunt trauma or stretch injury, which causes discontinuity of axons but the sheath remains intact. Wallerian degeneration does occur. Axons recover and regenerate in an antegrade direction through the original intact sheaths. Stretch injury has a poorer prognosis than blunt injury. Recovery can take months depending on the nerve injury site distance from the end organ. Average regeneration is 1 mm a day.
- **Neurotmesis** – injury results in a discontinuity of all nerve structures over part of its length. The proximal axons die back while the distal axons and sheath undergo degenerative change. The nerve recovery is limited and re-establishing connections to the end organ is patchy. If nerve ends are apposed and surgical repair undertaken better results are achieved. In general the more peripheral injuries fare better.

Common nerve injuries around the hand

- **Median** – At the wrist, the median nerve enters the hand through a confined space – the **carpal tunnel**. It is at risk in fractures of the distal radius and carpal injuries. Sensory loss is in the lateral three and a half fingers (i.e. thumb, index, middle and the radial half of the ring finger) and it is the most important deficit at this level. The expected motor loss from an injury at the wrist is of all the thenar muscles except adductor pollicis (ulnar nerve). In reality this is not always seen due to a cross-over from the ulnar nerve supply. More proximal injuries to the median nerve in the forearm will produce 'pointing sign', caused by paralysis of the flexor digitorum profundus to the index finger.
- **Ulnar** – At the wrist, the main deficit is motor. Sensation over the little finger and ulnar side of the ring finger is lost. The ulnar nerve supplies the intrinsic hand muscles (which flex the metacarpophalangeal joints and extend the interphalangeal joints). Loss of power creates the classic ulnar claw position, (i.e. no opposition to extend the metacarpophalangeal and flex the interphalangeal joints). The index finger is less affected because the lateral lumbricals are supplied by the median nerve. Adductor pollicis function is lost, giving rise to Froment's sign. The test is positive if the thumb interphalangeal joint flexes while asking the person to resist the pull of paper from between the thumb and the index finger, i.e. loss of adductor pollicis

function is compensated for by the flexor pollicis longus. Beware of the anatomical oddity of the ulnar paradox – higher ulnar nerve lesions will create *less* of a claw because the long flexors to the ring and little fingers (which create the claw) are paralysed. Injuries to the nerve at the wrist level will result in loss of some function after repair and patients in dextrous professions should be aware of the expected deficit.

- **Radial** – the radial nerve is primarily a motor nerve. Higher injuries to the radial nerve will manifest as motor deficit in the wrist and hand. Injury around the wrist and hand would only manifest as minor sensory deficit. Distally it provides sensation to the dorsum of the thumb; the superficial branch innervates the dorsal aspect of the first web space and hand. This sensory loss is not a problem to most people whereas the motor deficit creates a wrist drop, the paralysis affecting the extensors to wrist, fingers and thumb.

Digital

Digital nerve repair is only indicated when proximal to the distal interphalangeal joint. Recovery is usually only partial and full normal sensation is uncommon. The aim of repair is to provide protective sensation to the injured finger.

Treatment options

- Primary repair – Should be undertaken in all nerve divisions if there is no contamination. The aim is to realign the nerve sheath usually done by simply repairing the nerve's outer sheath (epineural repair). The final repair should be tension free and protected by plaster immobilisation for two weeks. A sensory and motor rehabilitation programme is required.
- Secondary repair – Is only used for contaminated wound problems. For better functional results the repair should be carried out at around the six week mark (but before three months). The aim is the same as for primary repair, but resecting the scar tissue at the injury site may mean tension of the repair and need for a nerve graft.
- Nerve graft – Indicated in secondary repairs and failed primary repair. The choice of the graft donor nerve is made from either the sural nerve, intercostobrachial nerve or the medial cutaneous nerve of the forearm. The donor is sutured to span the defect. Due to size difference the sural nerve is laid in parallel bundles. More recently artificial neural tubes have been used with good effect.
- Tendon transfers – Failed nerve repair or grafting means the loss of muscle function of that nerve can be accommodated by using a functioning muscle tendon unit and redirecting its function by a re-routing surgical procedure. The tendon being used should have synergistic muscles to accommodate the loss of its function. An example is the transfer of flexor carpi ulnaris (FCU) to provide extensor function in radial nerve injury. The FCU functional loss is provided by the flexor carpi radialis (FCR) and palmaris, and so active flexion is preserved.

General considerations

The patient's age gives the best indication of success in the nerve repair.

Skin and other soft tissue injuries

Thermal burns

This refers to the destruction of tissue by heat. First degree burns are superficial and present with erythema, occasional blisters, and some pain. Second degree burns are deeper, a partial thickness skin injury. They present as erythema, large numbers of blisters and with extreme pain. Third degree burns involve loss of the whole skin layer. Sensation to the area is lost and therefore pain is not a major feature. Treatment will depend upon the degree of the burn. Generally speaking second and third degree burns will require careful attention to prevent infection. Splinting and early mobilisation is important to minimise contractures across the joints.

Frostbite

This results from tissue freezing after prolonged periods of exposure to sub-zero temperatures. It is caused by the extracellular formation of ice crystals, subsequent cell dehydration, the failure of local microcirculation and ultimately cell death. Treatment is rapid re-warming of the affected part in circulating water at 40 °C. Revascularisation during this phase is extremely painful. Debridement or amputation is left until a clear level of tissue demarcation has occurred.

Electrical injuries

Electrical injuries to the periphery should not be considered in isolation and examination and investigation will need to exclude other electrical injuries. Specifically relating to the hand there are three elements causing injury:

- Ignition – a burn at the site of direct contact
- Conductant – injury along the path of conduction in the neurovascular structures
- Arc – high voltage current propagates along the flexor aspect of the joints.

These injuries result in contractures.

Ring avulsion injuries

These are injuries caused when a ring (jewellery) gets caught and is forcibly removed from the finger. This causes varying degrees of de-gloving. The Urbanaik classification dictates both treatment and prognosis:

- Class I – circulation is adequate. Standard bone and soft tissue management is indicated
- Class II – circulation is inadequate, bone, tendon and nerves are intact. Vessels are repaired to preserve viability
- Class III – complete de-gloving or amputation occurs. Poor prognosis with 30–70% complicated by cold intolerance. The best outcomes are with amputation, especially if the proximal interphalangeal joint is damaged or proximal phalanx is fractured.

Amputations

Elective amputations of the hand and wrist are rarely performed; indications include chronic osteomyelitis, malignant tumour, congenital deformity and Dupuytren's disease (see Chapter 4). This section will only consider traumatic amputations. Finger tip injuries are discussed below.

Following traumatic amputation of any digit and certainly of the hand and wrist, consideration must be towards replantation or revascularisation of the injured part. Crush and avulsion injuries generate more soft tissue problems and result in a reduced chance of a viable extremity. In general most digit amputations can be reattached and vascularity returned. This, however, is not the only measure of a positive outcome and functional capacity is the major factor when considering the possibility of such a procedure.

General rules apply. Favourable indications are:

- All injuries in a child. Good recovery and adaptation give good function.
- Multiple digit amputation. Replantation of all is not always possible, priority in order of importance is: thumb, middle, ring, little, index.
- Thumb. In thumb amputation focus is on maintaining length, which is vital for function. Replantation is considered as far distal as the nail base, although good sensation remains the most important factor of function.
- Entire hand (especially of the tendinous rather than the muscular part of the forearm).
- Replantation. As soon as possible (ASAP). Maximum warm ischaemic time for digits is 12 hours.

Unfavourable conditions are:

- Finger amputations proximal to FDS insertion
- Severe crush
- Multiple level amputation
- Severe vessel injury or pre-existing vascular problem

Joint stiffness, sensory problems and cold intolerance are the cause of poor outcomes in these situations.

Finger tip injuries

These are defined as injuries occurring distal to insertion of both deep flexors and the extensor tendon. The aim is to provide a finger with normal sensory function, a cushioned pulp and no pain. Preservation is desirable but not always possible. These injuries can be considered generally in two groups. Those with soft tissue loss and bone exposed and those with soft tissue loss and bone not exposed.

In the absence of bone exposure and in minimal tissue loss treatment is with cleaning and regular dressing. Healing of the amputated fingertip will occur within four weeks by wound contracture and epithelialisation, with little affect on sensory perception, range of motion or cosmetic appearance.

When bone is exposed, if injuries are treated the same as the above, healing and cover is often by poor-quality scar tissue that may result in chronic ulceration. Treatment is directed towards creating a smooth bone and ample soft tissue cover. Shortening, or terminalisation, of the bone end to achieve this may not be an ideal treatment if significant shortening will result. Skin grafting for a small local defect with intact pulp can be performed. Many varieties of local and advancement flaps are in use. The aim is to achieve finger cover with similar skin from the same or adjacent digits. Kulter and V-Y advancement flaps are the more commonly used types.

Miscellaneous

Compartment syndrome

In this condition the pressure within an enclosed anatomical compartment rises sufficiently to obstruct the micro-vascular circulation causing tissue ischemia, and, if left untreated, necrosis. Compartment syndrome is less common in the upper limb than the lower limb but does occur in the forearm and less commonly in the hand.

Compartment syndromes are usually associated with fractures, dislocations or crush injuries. The most reliable clinical findings are of pain on passive stretch of the muscles within the compartment involved and uncontrollable pain beyond that expected with the injury. Nerve symptoms and particularly circulation symptoms are very late signs. Treatment is to surgically decompress the compartment.

Pressure injection injuries

High pressure injection injuries of the hand can cause significant soft tissue trauma. On superficial examination it can appear to be a minor injury, but they represent a surgical emergency because of the rapid destruction of soft tissue. Fluid (air, water, oil, paint) is injected under pressure through the skin. The degree of injury depends on numerous factors: the pressure of the device, the fluid viscosity, the toxicity of the fluid and the length of time toxic fluid is in contact with tissue.

The treatment aims are extensive, exploration of the whole zone of injury, evacuation of all injected material, debridement of all dead tissue and antibiotic prophylaxis. Postoperative hand therapy is essential to regain maximum potential of hand and finger movement. These injuries are reported to cause significant functional problems in the hand.

Infections

Hand infections are caused by multiple organisms and affect any tissue. Most infections are related to *Staphylococcus aureus*, but 30% will grow anaerobic organisms. Early diagnosis and treatment followed by intensive hand therapy are paramount. If pus is present, surgical drainage is mandatory.

Specific infections in the hand include:

- **Paronychia** – This is infection of the nail fold (usually *S. aureus*). Treatment is with drainage and oral antibiotics.
- **Felon** – This is infection of the finger pulp. Treatment again is surgical drainage through a lateral approach, with appropriate antibiotics.
- **Bites** – Human bites are usually seen as part of a 'fight bite' – a punch to the mouth resulting in a 'bite' to the hand. If neglected these can result in serious infection. Surgical exploration should take care to identify any penetration to sheath or joint. Causative organisms are alpha-haemolytic streptococci and *S. aureus*. Early debridement and washout are essential. Animal bites present potentially serious infection sequelae. Pasteurella, alpha-haemolytic streptococcus and anaerobic microorganisms are the main isolates from the common bites of cats and dogs.
- **Flexor tendon sheath infection** (suppurative tenosynovitis) – Usually the result of an innocuous puncture wound. The presentation is usually with pain, fusiform swelling of the tendon sheath, with tenderness and erythema. The finger is held in a flexed position. Passive stretch of the tendon exacerbates the pain. Spread into the mid palmer space of the hand can occur. Treatment is timely surgical drainage of the pus, intravenous antibiotics and vigorous hand therapy to prevent stiffness.
- **Palmar space infections** – The mid palmar space lies between the flexor tendons above and the metacarpal bones below. The thenar space lies between the index finger and the thumb. Both are potential spaces that can develop abscess after penetrating injury. Symptoms are pain and swelling of the hand in the respective areas. Surgical drainage is required.
- **Septic arthritis** – Infection within the joints of the hand can occur as part of a penetrating joint injury or following blood-borne infection. Clinically the joint will be swollen and any movement of the joint will be restricted and painful. Treatment is drainage and washout with appropriate antibiotics, usually intravenous for an extended period (six weeks). These infections can produce joint stiffness and long-term problems from joint destruction and osteomyelitis.

Chronic regional pain syndrome (CRPS)

Also called reflex sympathetic dystrophy (RSD), Sudeck's atrophy, causalgia, this is a common complication to any hand injury or hand surgery. It is said to occur to a mild degree in up to 30% of wrist fractures and to a major extent in 2%. It is defined as an abnormal reaction to injury characterised by pain, swelling, stiffness, vasomotor changes and osteoporosis of the affected part. There are two types depending on whether there is an associated nerve injury.

- **CRPS type I (RSD)** – The clinical findings include regional pain, sensory changes, allodynia, abnormalities of temperature, abnormal sudomotor activity, oedema and an abnormal skin colour that occur after a noxious event.
- **CRPS type II (causalgia)** – Includes all type I symptoms, with a peripheral nerve lesion.

Treatment regimens involve treating the cause (adequately controlling pain with various modalities including sympathetic blockade, tricyclic antidepressants, vasodilators, steroids) in order to allow full functional rehabilitation. In a significant number of patients there is an associated altered cortical representation of the affected part, and therapy including mirror visual feedback and graded motor imagery may be required.

Summary

The hand is our most sophisticated versatile anatomical structure. From heavy lifting to fine accurate work, feeding to personal hygiene. We use our hands as an adjunct to language, using them to project emotions in a visual extension to our words. There are very few daily activities, which exclude their use. Even a minor hand injury can cause great anguish, and disability. Management of hand injuries requires a team approach and great attention to detail from all members of the team, especially the individual affected.

Further reading

Browner, B. D., Levine, A. M., Jupiter, J. B., & Trafton, P. G. (2008). *Skeletal Trauma: 2-Volume Set: Basic Science, Management, and Reconstruction (Browner, Skeletal Trauma)* (4th edition). Edinburgh: W. B. Saunders.

Bucholz, R. W., Heckman, J. D., Court-Brown, C. M., & Tornetta, P. (2005). *Rockwood and Green's Fractures in Adults* (6th edition). Philadelphia: Lippincott Williams & Wilkins.

Green, D. P., Hotchkiss, R. N., Pederson, W. C., & Wolfe, S. W. (2005). *Green's Operative Hand Surgery* (5th edition). Edinburgh: Churchill Livingstone.

Barton, N., & Mulligan, P. (1999). *Upper Limb and Hand (Modular Textbook of Orthopaedics Series)*. London: W. B. Saunders.

Chapter 13

Occupational therapy for hand injuries

Kerry Sorby

Introduction

This chapter will provide an overview of occupational therapy for the person who presents with a hand injury or condition affecting their ability to engage in their everyday occupations. The main focus of the chapter will be to present the principles of assessment and treatment that inform occupational therapy for this client group. Case studies 13.1–13.3 are used to illustrate these principles.

Case study 13.1

Diagnosis – Colles fracture

Joan – female, aged 66 years

Joan fell while out walking her dog. She sustained a Colles' fracture to her right dominant hand (fracture to the radius within 2.5 cm of the wrist). This was immobilised in a cast for six weeks and on removal she was referred to occupational therapy. She presented with pain, reduced range of movement in her right wrist (flexion/extension, abduction/adduction) and forearm (pronation/supination) and reduced grip strength.

Case study 13.2

Diagnosis – Closed humeral shaft fracture with radial nerve involvement

Michael – male, aged 28 years

Michael works as a plumber and was involved in a motorcycle incident. He sustained a closed fracture to his humeral shaft complicated by a high, radial nerve injury (the radial nerve is superficial in the midshaft region as it wraps around the spiral groove of the humerus).

Michael presented with a loss of wrist extension, loss of extension of all digits at the metacarpophalangeal joints and loss of thumb extension and abduction. This is also commonly known as a 'dropped wrist'. Michael was unable to position his wrist in extension; this significantly results in a weak grip and loss of hand dexterity. He was referred to occupational therapy for design and fabrication of a dynamic splint to be worn while the nerve regenerates, which may take three to four months (Cooper 2007).

> **Case study 13.3**
>
> **Diagnosis – Flexor tendon injury**
>
> **Peter – male, aged 23 years**
>
> Peter was stabbed in the palm (zone III) of his right dominant hand, resulting in tendon injury to both flexor tendons (flexor digitorum superficialis and profundus). He is a self-employed painter and decorator and lives with his girlfriend, who also works full-time. He was referred to occupational therapy one week post operatively.

Upper limb function provides the basis for fine motor skills of the hand to enable a person to participate in everyday tasks such as getting washed and dressed, toileting, preparing and eating a meal. For example, in order to pick up a chocolate bar to eat it, the muscles of the shoulder joint and girdle stabilise the arm in place. The movements of the elbow and forearm further position the hand to enable the fingers to flex around the chocolate bar wrapper. The co-ordination of 27 bones, 17 articulations, 33 muscles and three nerves within the hand allows timely and effective removal of the wrapper in order for the person to enjoy the pleasure of eating the chocolate bar.

Hand function requires the smooth fluid integration of sensory and motor components and therefore requires support of other body systems, in particular the central and peripheral nervous system. For example, muscles in the abdomen and trunk are required to maintain a stable base of support to allow the arm to move forward to reach a cup of coffee on a table. This very simple occupation requires normal functioning of visual components to locate the cup in order to then recognise its size, form and position. Synchronised movements of the arm and hand then enable the correct position of the hand: tactile and proprioceptive receptors provide the information to interpret the pressure and grip required to lift the cup of coffee to the mouth smoothly and safely.

It is important to remember that the hand is often also used to communicate thoughts and emotions (Goldin-Meadow 2006). A handshake may be used to greet a person or to close a business deal; one may gesticulate in anger when driving along a busy road, give a hug to comfort a loved one or to wave a goodbye. Therefore it is important for the therapist to recognise that any loss of hand function can become 'a significant source of stress and disruption in our daily lives' (Schier and Chan 2007). The occupational therapist needs to be aware of the impact the hand injury has on the person, their family/carers and their life roles. A loss of hand function may result in a loss of independence or dependency on others or a loss of activities within a role. Joan had to delegate shopping and meal preparation to her husband; Peter depended on his girlfriend to undertake all domestic chores as well as come to terms with her becoming the breadwinner, albeit on a temporary basis.

It is important to understand how the person's hand injury, and even the trauma that resulted in the injury, may impact on their psychosocial well-being. Issues related to self-efficacy and body image may hinder engagement in life roles and/or the therapy programme (Kimmerle et al. 2003).

Theories informing occupational therapy

It is important to emphasise that the occupational therapist should have a sound knowledge of hand anatomy, aetiology and pathology of the person's presenting clinical condition in order to understand how these may impact on their ability to undertake daily occupations. The occupational therapist can then choose relevant assessments to identify the person's unique needs. From this, the occupational therapist uses clinical reasoning skills to select the most appropriate interventions to maximise the person's functional potential.

As occupational therapy in this clinical area focuses on physiology, anatomy and biomechanics, the biomechanical frame of reference is the most likely to be used with a person who has experienced a loss of hand function. This frame of reference assumes that normal hand function can be resumed by the application of a graded treatment programme based on kinesiological principles (Hagedorn 2000) and/or the provision of equipment, assistive devices or splints to compensate for loss of hand function. A treatment programme is graded to encourage return of the person's normal range of movement, muscle strength and endurance. By focusing on performance components the biomechanical approach is considered to use a 'bottoms-up approach', this is viewed by some as reductionist and ignores the consequences of hand injury on occupations (Fitzpatrick and Presnell 2004). A person-centred approach, by comparison, would advocate a more 'top-down approach' the therapist would evaluate a person's roles and habits and then identify which components were inhibiting participation in these.

Stages of healing

Loss of function in the hand may result from involvement of one or more of the structures of bones, joints, nerves, tendons, skin and/or soft tissue. It is therefore essential that the occupational therapist has a sound knowledge of the normal healing process for the structures involved in the person's hand injury or condition. Tissues, as stated in the previous chapter, heal in three predictable stages, although the time scales of these stages will vary from person to person dependent on age, general health and mechanism of the injury/condition (Cooper 2007). These phases are inflammatory, regenerative and remodelling. These distinct phases will guide the therapist in choosing relevant assessment tools and interventions. In the inflammatory stage a static splint may be used to immobilise and/or protect tissue, for example a person with De Quervain's disease is provided with a thumb post splint to rest the extensor pollicis brevis and abductor pollicis longus tendons (Coldham 2006).

The stage where occupational therapy may be most active is during the fibroplasia stage whereby scar tissue is formed (one to six weeks post injury/surgery); interventions used should encourage a balance of promoting active range of movement and protection of the healing structures. In the final stage (remodelling), activities that promote gentle resistance are used to promote tensile strength and increase endurance in order to carry out a variety of occupations.

Arches of the hand

The hand comprises three arches, which provide a postural base to the hand to enable the fluid movement of the intrinsic muscles to manipulate a wide range of grips to facilitate hand function.

These arches are:

- **Longitudinal** – This is formed by the length of the hand from the wrist crease, along the second and third metacarpals to the tip of the distal phalanx of the index and middle finger (Figure 13.1).
- **Transverse** – The proximal transverse arch is formed by the carpal bones and is therefore considered to be a stable and rigid arch. The distal transverse arch is formed by the head of the metacarpal bones and is therefore more mobile (Figure 13.2).

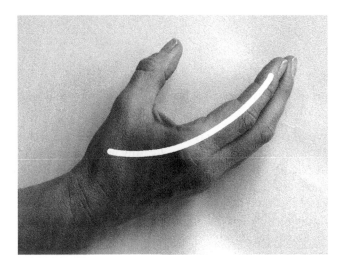

Figure 13.1 Longitudinal arch.

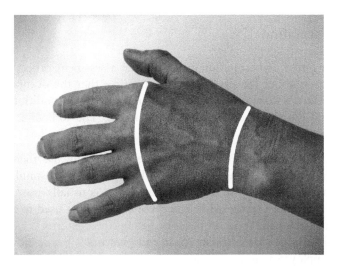

Figure 13.2 The transverse arches.

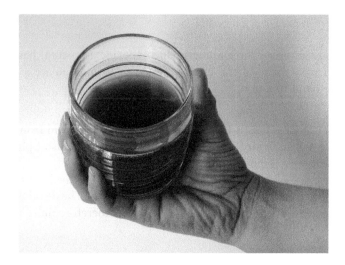

Figure 13.3 Oblique arch.

- **Oblique** – This is formed when the thumb moves in opposition to each finger (Figure 13.3).

The overall goal of therapy is therefore to maintain the arches of the hand in order to optimise participation in everyday tasks. Any injury to the hand which results in muscle imbalance, changes in tone and /or nerve innervations is likely to impact on the shape of the arches and thus loss of hand function (Sangole and Levin 2008). Maintaining the arches of the hand is the cornerstone of occupational therapy. For example, splints are often provided, when the arches of the hand have become 'flattened', to maintain the arches during the different stages of the healing process.

Choosing assessment tools

Gathering information

As in any area of occupational therapy the assessment process begins with gathering information about the person. It is imperative that the occupational therapist listens to the person's story regarding how their hand injury/condition has impacted on their individual lifestyle and choice of occupations. The following information should be considered:

- **Hand dominance** – How does the person usually use their affected hand? Many activities of daily living require both hands to be used simultaneously; for example, when eating a meal the non-dominant hand is usually used to position the fork to hold the food in place while the dominant hand is used to manipulate the knife to cut and place the food on the fork (using fine dexterity).
- **Occupation/leisure interests (past and present)** – Joan enjoys gardening; Peter is a self-employed painter and decorator and enjoys cycling and outdoor activities; and Michael works for the council as a plumber and enjoys socialising with his friends in

the pub. The occupational therapist needs to analyse how each hand injury impacts on each individual's engagement in valued occupations.

- **Injury** – What is the mechanism of the injury? How long ago did the injury occur? This information will be used to establish the stage of healing and inform the choice of interventions used.
- **Previous surgical intervention that may impact on hand function** – For Peter, the operation notes state that the surgical repair is technically considered to be strong and therefore an early active flexion protocol is recommended (see range of movement on p 241) (Cooper 2007; Rosenthal and Stoddard 2005).
- **Past medical history** – Some medical conditions can impact on the rate of normal bone/soft tissue healing (e.g. diabetes).
- **Pain** – This is difficult to quantify as it is a subjective experience and unique to each person. However, it is important to establish the person's perception of their pain levels, as it may influence their engagement in the treatment programme. Analgesia (painkillers) may need to be considered prior to therapy intervention. The person should be encouraged to define their pain in terms of character, intensity, duration and patterns. The use of pain diaries are useful to document a person's pattern of presenting pain symptoms over a period of time; the person is asked to record activities that they have undertaken and the pain they have experienced (perhaps from one appointment to the next). The therapist will be able to analyse the diaries and identify movements and/or grips that exacerbate or alleviate their presenting pain.
- **Present level of functioning** – The therapist needs to be aware of the impact of the hand injury on the person's life roles. For example: worker role for Michael and Peter; spouse, home-maintainer and dog-walker for Joan.
- **Person's aims of treatment** – Peter is self-employed and would like to return to work as soon as possible; Joan would like to be able to plant some bedding plants in her garden; and Michael would like to be able to drink a pint of beer with his dominant hand.
- **Person's level of motivation/compliance** – Lai (2004) identified a number of key factors that influence the person's ability to engage with hand therapy. These were: a positive attitude towards the hand injury and potential recovery, active involvement in the goal setting process and perceived support network from family, social and work environments.

The occupational therapist will use a combination of non-standardised and standardised assessment tools to establish a comprehensive assessment of the person's needs. Non-standardised assessments will include an initial interview, observation and palpation of the hand. This includes:

- **Condition of the wound/scar** – The colour, site and hypersensitivity of Peter's surgical scar will be monitored.
- **Temperature of skin** – Increased temperature may indicate the presence of inflammation or infection; decreased temperature may be indicative of poor circulation, which may result in delayed wound healing.
- **Oedema** – Peter presents with mild oedema following his surgery. On palpation, the oedema is soft and yielding: this is considered 'normal' at this early stage of wound healing. However, the oedema in Joan's hand feels woody and dense (Boscheinen-Morrin and Conolly 2001) *and* has persisted beyond the inflammatory stage, soft tissue has begun to become fibrosed. This has resulted in her hand becoming painful,

with increased joint stiffness and connective tissues adherence: this has impacted on her overall hand function.

- **Thickening/nodules** – This can be indicative of particular conditions. Thickening of the palmar aponeurosis is indicative of Dupuytren's disease; thickening of the A1 pulley is indicative of trigger finger.
- **Presence of deformities** – A rupture of the tendon of flexor digitorum profundus will lead to hyperextension of the proximal interphalangeal joint and flexion of the distal interphalangeal joint; this is known as a swan-neck deformity. An extensor tendon injury to the tip of a finger (zone I) may result in a 'mallet finger', characterised by loss of active extension at the distal interphalangeal joint.
- **Soft tissue tightness** – Movement at Joan's fingers maybe limited by soft tissue tightness due to inactivity while her cast was on.
- **Joint stiffness** – The therapist can passively move the joints through a range of movement to determine if there is a 'springy' end feel or 'hard' end feel. A *springy end feel* has a spongy quality at the end range of the person's movement. This indicates a potential for remodelling and hence is more likely to respond to therapy. A joint with a *hard end feel* is indicative of a stiffer joint (Cooper 2007) and is less likely to respond to therapy; surgical intervention may be required.
- **Positioning of the hand** – Does Michael 'hold' his hand in a protective/guarding manner? Is Peter willing for his hand to be touched or use his hand when removing his coat? Are the arches of Joan's hand maintained and is there evidence of muscle atrophy?

Further non-standardised assessments will be used to complement the above assessments. This will involve observation of the person carrying out activities of daily living skills. For example, Michael was observed to be having difficulty fastening his buttons; Joan was having difficulty pouring hot water from a kettle due to reduced grip strength in her wrist extensors; the wearing of his splint prevents Peter using his dominant hand to participate in occupations. Observation of a person informs the therapists about the coping strategies that the person uses to carry out the task independently – this may include adopting awkward or compensatory postures, imbalance of muscle groups, or even avoidance of using particular joints.

As previously stated, the hand is a very complex functional unit that can be involved in a diverse range of activities. The therapist therefore needs to have a range of assessments available to accurately assess how the person's clinical condition is impacting on their current level of functioning. A combination of non-standardised and standardised assessments will therefore be used.

Standardised assessment tools that have been included in this chapter have been selected because they are commonly used in clinical practice and have proven validity, reliability and sensitivity within the clinical area of hand therapy practice (Corr and Siddons 2005; Fess 1998). For a more comprehensive range of assessment tools the reader is referred to Simpson (2004). In order to ensure reliability and validity of the assessment tools used, the following points need to be adhered to:

- **The same therapist** should carry out the assessment on each occasion (intra-reliability).
- **Same time of day.** This may be very important when working with a person who has fatigue or whose level of functioning is likely to fluctuate (for example, a person with rheumatoid arthritis).

- **The same point in the treatment session.** Before the treatment session commences, midway through the treatment session or at the end of the treatment session.
- **Consistent** in the choice and use of equipment each time. The same goniometer/ tape measure should be used on each occasion.
- **Method** used is consistent within the same department. Within the department there may be guidelines/protocols for administering the assessments used: manuals for administering the tool may be available.
- All equipment is *calibrated and checked regularly*. A dynamometer should be calibrated annually.
- Consistent method of *documentation*. It is important that all staff record the assessment results in a consistent manner.

Measurement of pain

Pain is a fundamental aspect of hand injury; alleviation of pain is seen as an important clinical indicator for the person concerned (Chan and Spencer 2005). As previously stated pain is an individual, subjective experience and is therefore difficult to record objectively. Most measurements of the description pain are therefore self-reported. Examples of these are the visual analogue scale, the numerical rating scale and McGill Pain Questionnaire.

- **Visual analogue scale** – Joan is asked to indicate along a 10 cm line (ranging from no pain to worst pain) the amount of pain she is experiencing at the present time.
- **A numerical rating score:** Peter is asked to give a numerical figure to represent his level of pain (on a score from 0 = no pain to 10 = worst pain imaginable).

Both of these scales are popular within the acute clinical setting as they are quick and easy to administer, interpret and report. However, one needs to recognise that these measures only consider the person's perception of the intensity of their pain.

- **McGill Pain Questionnaire** (Melzack 1975) – This is also a self-reported measure, which includes a numerical intensity scale as well as a set of descriptor words and a pain drawing. It does take longer to administer (approximately 30 minutes) than the first two measures. However, it does include the site and the character of pain.

Measurements of range of movement

Goniometry is considered one of the most reliable methods of measuring joint range of movement (Bucher and Hulme 2002; Pratt and Burr 2001; Simpson 2004). A goniometer is the measurement tool that measures passive and/or active range of movement. The occupational therapist places the axis of the goniometer over the centre of the joint and the arms of the goniometer over adjacent joints. The therapist should be aware of the normal range of movement expected at the joint to be measured and results should be compared to the unaffected hand.

When measuring Joan's range of movement at her right wrist, one needs to consider that normal range of movement of the wrist is 70–80° of flexion and 70–75° of extension. Simpson (2004) and Boscheinen-Morrin and Conolly (2001) advocate placing the

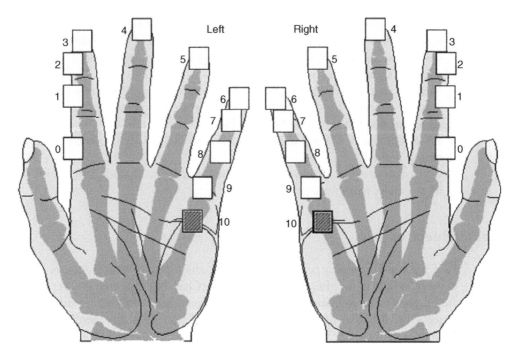

Figure 13.4 Kapandji range of motion chart.

proximal arm on the palmar surface of the forearm, placing the axis along the proximal end of the thenar crease and the distal arm on the palmar surface of the hand towards the middle of the third metacarpal. Composite finger flexion (the range of movement combined from the metacarpophalangeal joint and interphalangeal joints) was used with Peter. The distance between the pad of his fingertips and the distal palmar crease was measured with a ruler. Limited movement would be indicated if he could only flex his fingers to the mid-palm of his hand.

A quick, easy and practical method of measuring opposition of a person's thumb as movement returns is Kapandji's ten stages (Kapandji 1992; Figure 13.4). A person with full opposition will be able to oppose their thumb to the base of the little finger or the distal palmar crease (positions 9 and 10 on Figure 13.4).

Measurements of muscle strength

The hydraulic dynamometer is used to measure isometric grip strength and is considered to be a standardised and reliable assessment tool (Bucher and Hulme 2002; Fess 1998; Simpson 2004). Results can be interpreted by comparing with the person's unaffected hand and/or to American norms (Mathiowetz et al. 1985) or British normative data (Gilbertson and Barber-Lomax 1994).

This tool only measures an isometric grip so the assessment may need to be complemented by observation of occupations relevant to the individual (Tyler et al. 2005). Joan has a grip strength of 13.6 kg (30 lb), however the therapist would need to evaluate if Joan was able to sustain this grip strength to safely carry a supper tray from the kitchen through to the lounge area.

Measurements of sensation

In Bucher and Hulme's (2002) survey of 249 hand therapists and Jerosch-Herold's (2002) study of 225 hand therapists, the most commonly used assessment of sensibility of the hand was the Semmes Weinstein monofilament test, followed by static two-point discrimination (2PD). The monofilaments measure light touch and deep pressure and are useful when monitoring return of sensibility following a nerve injury such as Michael's. The monofilaments are gently applied to the skin until the monofilament bends; it is then lifted away from the skin. This procedure is repeated three times on each part of the hand along the sensory distribution of the affected nerve(s), any positive response is recorded from the patient. The Moberg pick up test may also be used; this involves a speed test, timing a person to pick up a series of standardised objects and placing them in a box. Comparison of results is made with the uninjured/unaffected hand.

Measurement of oedema

A volumeter is commonly used for measuring oedema of the whole hand (Pelleccia 2003). The hand is immersed in a water filled commercial measure and water is then displaced into a measuring cylinder. The more water that is displaced (compared to the unaffected hand) is indicative of oedema present. This method would not be appropriate for Peter due to his wound. It is also contraindicated for a person with an infection, in a cast or with an external fixator *in situ* due to the risk of cross-contamination between people using the equipment (Maihafer et al. 2003). However, this tool is not sensitive enough to accurately measure oedema at a single joint or digit (for example, for a person who has had fracture dislocation of the proximal interphalangeal joint of their little finger). In this case, circumferential measurements of the joint would be considered more effective for baseline and post-treatment comparison using a tape measure. Creases on the palmar aspect of the finger are used as an anatomical landmark from which to take the measurement (to ensure consistency between repeated measures).

The figure of eight method was used to measure oedema in Joan's hand. The tape measure was placed obliquely over the dorsum of the hand from the ulnar styloid to the midpoint of the second metacarpal, then anteriorly across the distal palmar crease to the fifth metacarpophalangeal joint and finally obliquely back over the dorsum of the hand to the radial styloid. This method was considered quick and easy to administer and cost-efficient with Joan (Pelleccia 2003).

Measurements of functional performance

As well as measuring impairment, it is also important to assess a person's current level of hand function. The tool most commonly used in Bucher and Hulme's survey (2002) was the Disabilities of the Arm, Shoulder and Hand (DASH) outcome measure (Hudak et al. 1996).

This 30-item self-reported measure was specifically designed for people with musculoskeletal conditions; it aims to enable the person to describe the impact that a person's clinical condition has on their current lifestyle and presenting symptoms. It was designed particularly for a person who has impairment at one or more joints in the upper extremity. It can therefore be used with Peter, Michael and Joan. One of the advantages of using this tool is that it allows the person to identify how their presenting symptoms affect participation in the occupations that are important to them and therefore provides the basis for collaborative goal setting with the therapist (Wong et al. 2007). It is available electronically, free of charge, from the Canadian Institute for Work and Health (www.iwh.ca.on.ca).

From the results of assessments, the patient's aims and objectives should be mutually agreed: a collaborative approach at the planning stage of the occupational therapy process facilitates compliance, adherence and concordance to the therapy programme (Steward 2004). Case-Smith's (2003) study of 33 people with upper extremity injuries found that the most common goal was driving and suggested that this was due to its importance in achieving other life goals. This would certainly be relevant for Peter and Michael who need to drive to meet the requirements of their worker role.

Occupational therapy intervention

The therapy programme devised will be individually tailored reflecting the person's unique presenting symptoms and goals of treatment identified as a result of the assessment process. Close liaison with the surgical/medical team is encouraged to consolidate the therapist's understanding of any clinical precautions that may impact on Peter's engagement in the therapy programme. Patient education is an integral part of any intervention. The challenge for the therapist is to 'translate' the surgeon's protocols into 'lay' terminology and advise the person how these can be applied to their everyday tasks and their therapy programme.

Below is a list of treatment interventions that may form the occupational therapists repertoire or 'toolbox'. An acronym to remember the scope of treatment is PROGRESS:

- **P**ain management
- **R**eturn to occupations
- **O**edema and wound management
- **G**rading and/or modifying activity
- **R**ange of movement
- **E**xercise as an adjunct to therapy
- **S**ensory retraining
- **S**plinting

The challenge for the therapist is to choose a range of relevant interventions to meet the individual's needs/goals.

- **Pain management** – Individuals' pain thresholds differ. The therapist needs to educate the person that pain 'should be respected as the natural response of tissue to excessive stress' (Rosenthal and Stoddard 2005). Peter is keen to return to work so has been a little zealous with his exercises: he needs to be advised of the importance of adhering to the treatment protocol to prevent rupture of the repaired tendon. However, pain has made Joan reluctant to participate in the therapy programme; she needs encouragement to move her painful and stiff wrist in order to prevent further adhesions.

- **Return to valued occupations** – It is important that the person with a hand injury/ condition optimises the gains made in the therapy room with active participation in occupations for self-care, work and productivity and leisure. Initially Joan was reluctant to participate in some occupations due to the pain and loss of hand function in her wrist. However, the challenge for the occupational therapist is to use their activity analysis skills to design a graded therapy programme for Joan at home. During her initial interview, Joan expressed that she was a keen gardener and is anxious about how her hand injury will impact on her ability to engage with the gardening activities she has planned for the summer. This would be a positive opportunity for the therapist and Joan to work collaboratively to design a graded programme to promote range of movement, strength and endurance of her wrist over the next six weeks period as her bone heals. Working with soil provides a natural medium for active resistive exercise for the wrist joint.
- **Oedema and scar management** – During the inflammatory stage, Peter's wound may be protected with dressings and this would need to be considered as splinting is also used at this stage. The therapist needs to liaise with the nursing and medical staff regarding local policies and procedures relating to wound care.

In the early phase, rest, ice, compression and elevation (RICE) are core components of oedema management. Active movements of unaffected joints should be encouraged. For example, while Joan was immobilised in a cast for six weeks she should have been encouraged to actively move the joints proximal to the injury (the shoulder and elbow joint) and distal to the injury (metacarpophalangeal and interphalangeal joints). Patient education is a central component of oedema management; teaching Joan techniques to engage in routine tasks, for example getting washing and dressed or preparing meals, may be sufficient to encourage normal active movement of the required joints.

The use of compression may continue into the next phase of regeneration. Active movement of the hand is the cornerstone of effective management at this time. Therefore, compression may only be used during periods of rest and at night (this may be in the form of taping or Lycra gloves) to complement activity during the day. Silicone gel may be used for scar management to promote a scar that is pale and supple.

During the final phase of healing (remodelling) most structures will be able to withstand active movement. Movement and compression remain the key components of management of oedema. A graded programme will be required to increase tensile strength of the wound and endurance.

- **Grading and/or modification of activities** – For each person in the case studies, they will need to use assistive devices, equipment, splints and/or modify activities to compensate for loss of hand function. Peter and Michael were unable to use their dominant hand while their splints are worn; therefore, they were advised to wear loose fitting clothes so that the sleeve can go over the splint. They will need to attend to most tasks unilaterally using their unaffected hand. Joan was advised how to modify her kitchen activities so that the weight or forces of objects could be graded as she regained strength in her wrist (for example, initially only filling the kettle with enough water for one person, preparing meals on the hob rather than the oven to avoid having to lift trays to put in or take out of the oven). Often remedial activities are used to promote strength and endurance. Although they are valued as an adjunctive to returning to occupations, a more person-centred approach would analyse activities that are purposeful and meaningful for the individual and grade/ modify these to promote range of movement, strength and then endurance. For example, Wilson et al. (2008) illustrate how origami is analysed and then graded to facilitate hand function.

- **Range of movement** – The therapist guided Peter through a graded programme of early active flexion exercises to gradually increase the stresses placed on the repaired tendon. Initially Peter was encouraged to passively flex his fingers; at three weeks active flexion was introduced. At six weeks, when his tendon was considered to be entering the remodelling phase, Peter was able to begin resistive exercises (Groth 2005; Rosenthal and Stoddard 2005). Similarly, Joan engaged in a range of baking and gardening activities that encouraged active and then resistive movement of her wrist joint.

- **Exercise** – This may include passive exercises to maintain range of movement, tendon/nerve gliding exercises, active assistive/active exercises to enhance range of movement and strengthening exercises to work on strength and endurance. Although exercises are considered to be a physiotherapy domain, they may be used by an occupational therapist as an adjunct to participating in a person's valued occupations. It is important that the person continues with their exercise regimen in their home/ work environments to optimise overall performance.

- **Sensibility retraining/desensitisation.** A person with sensory impairment following a peripheral nerve injury or a person with a hypersensitive scar can learn to adapt and use compensatory strategies to carry out everyday tasks. Sensibility retraining can commence once the person is able to feel moving touch; this involves the therapist applying different stimuli over the palm and fingertips so that the person can identify the stimulus visually when their eyes are open and then from sensory feedback with their eyes closed. Repetition of the stimuli promotes attention, feedback, memory and reinforcement (Boscheinen-Morrin and Conolly 2001).

- **Splinting.** This is a commonly provided intervention for a person with a hand injury/ condition. There are a number of excellent texts (for example, Cooper 2007 and Fess et al. 2005) dedicated to the topic of splinting the hand and therefore this section will only provide the reader with an overview of the principles informing the use of splinting.

In order to gain informed consent prior to the provision of a splint, the occupational therapist will need to inform Peter and Michael about the purpose of the splint, the potential benefits and risks involved with wearing a splint and the anticipated wearing regimen. Michael and Peter need to be aware of their commitment to the therapy programme that accompanies the wearing of the splint.

Purpose of a splint

There are four key reasons that an occupational therapist may provide a prefabricated splint or design and custom make a splint. These are:

- **To immobilise, stabilise or protect tissues in the acute phase of wound healing following an injury, surgery or exacerbation of disease** – A dorsal blocking splint was fabricated for Peter. The splinting material is moulded over the dorsum of the hand, blocking extension of the metacarpophalangeal joints, thus protecting the repaired tendon. The wrist is positioned in 20–30° of flexion, and the metacarpophalangeal joints in 50–70° flexion. Peter would be expected to wear the splint for six weeks post operatively.
- **To immobilise, stabilise or protect tissue when integrity has been compromised by a long-term condition** – Joan could have been provided with a functional wrist brace to decrease pain in her wrist and maintain structural and functional integrity of the joint (MacDonald and Sorby 2006).
- **To protect tissue that is at risk of deformity or contracture subsequent to paralysis or altered muscle tone** – Michael has been provided with a dynamic splint. The static base of the splint supports his wrist in extension and prevents overstretching of the wrist extensors (Fess et al. 2005). The dynamic component of the splint allows Michael's fingers to actively flex to grasp an object but then his fingers are pulled back into extension by springs/elastic to allow him to release the grasp.
- **To correct deformity** – For example, a static night resting finger(s) splint following surgical correction for Dupuytren's contracture, or a dynamic splint to correct a flexion deformity of a proximal interphalangeal joint.

Boscheinen-Morrin and Conolly (2001) advocate that to enhance compliance with the wearing regimen, 'the splint should be simple in design, be easy to don and doff, be free of pressure and be as cosmetically pleasing as possible.' Verbal and written instruction regarding the wear and care of the splint should always be provided to individuals (College of Occupational Therapists 2003).

There is inconsistency within the literature regarding wearing regimens for individual splints (Pratt 2004). Wearing regimens should reflect the purpose of the splint: the occupational therapist needs to use clinical reasoning skills to determine the **right splint for the right individual at the right time.** Clinical reasoning will be informed by the therapist's understanding of biomechanics, anatomy, kinesiology, the individual's clinical condition, splinting protocols and techniques and the person's motivation and identified needs (Lohman et al. 2007). The therapist is advised to liaise with the surgeon regarding protocols of care following specific surgical techniques. It is important to remember that the occupational therapist has a duty of care to follow up the splint for the length of time the person is to wear the splint.

Throughout the treatment programme, it is essential to utilise the therapist's use of self to support the person to manage their hand condition/injury.

'*When we touch our clients' hands, we touch their lives ... it is important not to lose sight of the whole person whose extremity we are treating*'.

Cooper (2007)

It is important to remember that while we as therapists may be familiar with surgical protocols or protocols of rehabilitation, this will be a new experience for the person concerned. As already discussed, loss of hand function may result in loss of several roles or engagement in valued occupations. Patient education is a core component of the whole occupational therapy process: to enable the person to understand not only about their hand injury/condition but the journey that they are likely to experience in order to maximise their hand function at the end of therapy.

Summary

This chapter has identified a range of assessment tools and treatment interventions that can be used for a person who presents with a hand injury or condition. As the hand is an intricate, multi-dimensional and dynamic unit, the impact of an injury on a person's hand function will vary according to individual lifestyle and occupational choice. Thus, every person presents as a unique, yet exciting challenge to the occupational therapist. The therapist will need to utilise his or her clinical reasoning skills to balance a treatment programme that not only is delivered at the right time to facilitate the healing and rehabilitation process but is also a programme that is individually tailored to meet the person's unique needs and lifestyle.

References

Boscheinen-Morrin, J., & Conolly, W. B. (2001). *The Hand. Fundamentals of Hand Therapy*. Oxford: Butterworth-Heinemann.

Bucher, C., & Hulme, K. (2002). Assessment following hand trauma: a review of some commonly employed methods. *British Journal of Hand Therapy*, 7(3), 79–85.

Case-Smith, J. (2003). Outcomes in hand rehabilitation using occupational therapy services. *American Journal of Occupational Therapy*, 57(5), 499–506.

Chan, J., & Spencer, J. (2005). Contrasting perspectives on pain following hand injury. *Journal of Hand Therapy*, 18, 429–436.

Coldham, F. (2006). The use of splinting in the non-surgical treatment of De Quervain's disease: a review of the literature. *The British Journal of Hand Therapy*, 11(2), 48–55.

College of Occupational Therapists. (2003). *Occupational Therapy Clinical Guidelines for Rheumatology*. London: College of Occupational Therapists.

Cooper, C. (2007). Fundamentals of clinical reasoning: hand therapy concepts and treatment techniques. In C. Cooper (Ed). *Fundamentals of Hand Therapy. Clinical Reasoning and Treatment Guidelines for Common Diagnoses of the Upper Extremity*. St Louis: Mosby.

Corr, S., & Siddons, L. (2005). An introduction to the selection of outcome measures. *British Journal of Occupational Therapy*, 68(5), 202–206.

Fess, E. (1998). Making a difference: The importance of good assessment tools. *British Journal of Hand Therapy*, 3(2), 3.

Fess, E., Gettle, K., Phillips, C., & Janson, J. (2005). *Hand and Upper Extremity Splinting. Principles and Methods*. St Louis: Mosby.

Fitzpatrick, N., & Presnell, S. (2004). Can occupational therapists be hand therapists? *British Journal of Occupational Therapy*, 67(11), 508–510.

Gilbertson, L., & Barber-Lomax, S. (1994). Power and pinch grip strength recorded using the hand-held Jamar dynometer and B + L pinch gauge: British normative data for adults. *British Journal of Occupational Therapy*, 57(12), 483–488.

Goldin-Meadow, S. (2006). Talking and thinking with our hands. *Current Directions in Psychological Science*, 15(1), 34–39.

Groth, G. (2005). Current practice patterns of flexor tendon rehabilitation. *Journal of Hand Therapy*, 18, 169–174.

Hagedorn, R. (2000). *Foundations for Practice in Occupational Therapy*. New York: Churchill Livingstone.

Hudak, P. L., Amadio, P. C., & Bombardier, C. (1996). Development of an upper extremity outcome measure: the DASH (Disabilities of the Arm, Shoulder and Hand). The Upper Extremity Collaborative Group (UECG). *American Journal of Industrial Medicine*, 29(6), 602–608.

Jerosch-Herold, J. (2002). A survey on the use of sensibility tests by hand therapists in the UK. *British Journal of Hand Therapy*, 7(2), 55–63.

Kapandji, A. (1992). Clinical evaluation of the thumb's opposition. *Journal of Hand Therapy*, 5, 102–105.

Kimmerle, M., Mainwaring, L., & Borenstein, M. (2003). The functional repertoire of the hand and its application to assessment. *American Journal of Occupational Therapy*, 57, 489–498.

Lai, C. (2004). Motivation in hand-injured patients with and without work – related injury. *Journal of Hand Therapy*, 17, 6–17.

Lohman, H., Poole, S. E., Scheirton, L. S., & Sullivan, J. C. (2007). Clinical reasoning applied to splint application. In B. Coppard, & H. Lohman (Eds). *Introduction to Splinting. A Clinical Reasoning and Problem Solving Approach* (3rd edition) Edinburgh: Mosby.

MacDonald, R., & Sorby, K. (2006). Protection and preservation: maintaining occupational independence in clients with rheumatoid arthritis. In L. Addy (Ed). *Occupational Therapy Evidence in Practice for Physical Rehabilitation*. Oxford: Blackwell Publishing.

Maihafer, G., Llewellyn, M., Pillar, P., Scott, K., Marino, D., & Bond, R. (2003). A comparison of the figure-of-eight method and water volumetry in measurement of hand and wrist size. *Journal of Hand Therapy*, 16, 305–310.

Mathiowetz, V., Kashman, N., Volland, G., Weber, K., & Dowe, M. (1985). Grip and pinch strength: normative data for adults. *Archives of Physical and Medical Rehabilitation*, 55, 69–74.

Melzack, R. (1975). The McGill pain questionnaire: major properties and scoring methods. *Pain*, 1, 277–299.

Pelleccia, G. (2003). Figure-of-eight method of measuring hand size: reliability and concurrent validity. *Journal of Hand Therapy*, 16, 300–304.

Pratt, A. (2004). Is eight weeks immobilisation of the distal interphalangeal joint adequate treatment for acute closed mallet finger injuries of the hand? A critical review of the literature. *British Journal of Hand Therapy*, 9(1), 4–10.

Pratt, A. L., & Burr, N. A. (2001). Review of goniometry use within current hand therapy practice. *British Journal of Hand Therapy*, 6(2), 45–49.

Rosenthal, E., & Stoddard, C. (2005). Questions hand therapists ask about treatment of tendon injuries. *Journal of Hand Therapy*, 18, 313–318.

Sangole, A., & Levin, M. (2008). Arches of the hand in reach to grasp. *Journal of Biomechanics*, 41, 829–837.

Schier, J. S., & Chan, J. (2007). Changes in life roles after hand injury. *Journal of Hand Therapy*, 20(1), 57–59.

Simpson, C. (2004). *Hand Assessment. A Clinical Guide for Therapists*. London: APS Publishing.

Steward, B. (2004). Compliance, adherence and concordance: a review of engaging patients in their treatment. *British Journal of Hand Therapy*, 9(3), 88–95.

Tyler, H., Adams, J., & Ellis, B. (2005). What can handgrip strength tell the therapist about hand function. *British Journal of Hand Therapy*, 10(1), 4–9.

Wilson, L., Roden, P., Taylor, Y., & Marston, L. (2008). The effectiveness of origami on overall hand function after injury: a pilot controlled trial. *British Journal of Hand Therapy*, 13(1), 12–20.

Wong, J., Fung, B., Chu, M., & Chan, R. (2007). The use of disabilities of the arm, shoulder and hand questionnaire in rehabilitation after acute traumatic hand injuries. *Journal of Hand Therapy*, 20, 49–56.

Chapter 14

Brachial plexus injury

Claire Ireson

Introduction

This short chapter will provide an overview of the anatomy of the brachial plexus and describes the management of people who have brachial plexus lesions resulting from trauma. Occupational therapists may encounter people with this injury at any stage of their treatment from the acute recovery phase to the later rehabilitation phases. It must be stressed that this is not a common injury and is unlikely to be seen regularly like other common upper limb and hand injuries in the general orthopaedic and trauma environment. Occupational therapists working with people with brachial plexus lesions in the latter stages of recovery usually work in specialist centres that have specific assessment and treatment protocols for this injury.

The brachial plexus

The brachial plexus is a network of nerves and is formed by the spinal nerves and roots of C5, 6 (upper trunk) C7 (middle trunk), C8 and T1 (lower trunk) and sometimes with a contribution from C4 and T2. Having divided into the upper, middle and lower trunks, these divisions divide further into the posterior, lateral and medial cords and then into supraclavicular and infraclavicular branches. These then become the nerves that occupational therapists will be most familiar with including the median, ulnar and radial nerves. The plexus is complex to understand and is often illustrated as a tree diagram to demonstrate the structures and how they divide (Moffat and Mottram 2000). All nerve supply to the upper limb passes through this plexus, therefore any injury can cause substantial functional impairment. The plexus begins at the scalenes, courses under the clavicle and ends at the axilla.

Brachial plexus lesions

The brachial plexus may be injured by a high-energy trauma to the upper limb and neck region particularly where the head and neck are moved violently away from the ipsilateral shoulder. Injury can result in partial or complete paralysis of the upper limb, depending on whether all five roots or just the upper or lower roots are affected. The extent of the lesion will determine whether the paralysis is temporary or permanent but in all cases it will be devastating for the individual.

Causes may be direct or by traction:

- Causes of direct injury:
  - Penetrating injury, e.g. stab wound, low to high velocity gun shot or animal bite
  - High pressure or direct blow
  - Falls from great height
  - Tumour
  - Post-mastectomy radiotherapy treatment
  - Iatrogenic.
- Causes of traction injury:
  - Road traffic accidents especially involving motorbikes
  - Sporting accidents including boating
  - Falls from great height
  - Obstetric procedures (Erb's palsy).

Traction injuries resulting from road traffic accidents involving motorbikes are the most common and are disproportionately prevalent in young males between the ages of 15 and 25 years (Narakas 1985). The position of the arm at the time of the injury will determine the nature of the injury. If the arm is held at the side then a C8–T1 injury is likely, however if the arm is abducted then C7 is often involved.

Traction injuries can be divided into pre-ganglionic lesions (proximal) and post-ganglionic lesions (distal). In pre-ganglionic lesions, there is avulsion of the nerve root from the spinal cord and there is less chance of recovery or surgical treatment. In post-ganglionic lesions, there may be continuity of the cell bodies with their axons leading to neuropraxia, axonotmesis (nerve sheath in tact) or neurotmesis (rupture of the complete nerve). In all post-ganglionic lesions the nerve roots are intact.

Symptoms and diagnosis

The following signs and symptoms may be present:

- Fractured clavicle
- Swelling around the shoulder region
- Neck and shoulder pain
- Paraesthesia, weakness in arm or paralysis
- Horner's syndrome (there is ptosis (drooping of the eyelid) and difference of pupil size indicating an incomplete lesion in the lower plexus, e.g. C5–7)
- Diminished or absent pulse (suggesting vascular injury).

Diagnosis of the exact level of injury is complex. Wynn Parry (1981) classifies and describes these in detail. Accurate and detailed sensory and motor testing should be undertaken alongside diagnostic imaging, e.g. magnetic resonance imaging (MRI) and electrophysiological testing. Motor and sensory testing can be challenging due to the variations occurring among the spinal nerves.

Treatment

Advanced trauma support will usually be required as a brachial plexus lesion is usually associated with multiple injuries resulting from the accident. Open wounds will need to be debrided and immediate vascular repair undertaken with nerves tagged for later repair.

Occupational therapists may encounter people who were treated long ago by the original management approach of fusing the shoulder, applying a bone block of the elbow and finger tenodesis, which led to one handedness. Today, improved microsurgical techniques mean there are far greater opportunities for functional restoration of the upper limb.

Early surgical exploration is recommended followed by surgical repair dependent on the type of lesion. This may include nerve transfers, nerve grafting, muscle and tendon transfers and neurolysis of scarring around the brachial plexus to optimise the individual's level of function. This treatment is almost always carried out by an expert surgeon within a tertiary specialist centre.

Non-operative management includes mobilisation, stretching and the use of splinting and bracing of the upper limb for support and to avoid contractures.

Complications

- Contractures
- Deafferentation pain (intractable pain caused by avulsion of the nerve roots)
- Bony deformities
- Scoliosis
- Posterior shoulder dislocation
- Agnosia of the affected limb
- Incomplete recovery even with surgical intervention.

Occupational therapy

Recovery from a brachial plexus lesion is a slow and long process for the individual who will undergo months of reassessment and rehabilitation of the upper limb. The sudden loss of function can be devastating, affecting all areas of occupational performance. The occupational therapist will be involved throughout the care of the person from the early post-lesion phase to recovery. Most occupational therapy departments will only see one or two cases per year (if any), and these are likely to be referred onwards to a tertiary centre. Many prosthetic centres are involved in the later stages of rehabilitation with the assessment and provision of specialist splintage known as flail arm splints and subsequent functional upper limb retraining.

Frampton (2000) recommends the use of comprehensive physical examination assessment checklists that include joint range of movement, pain, sensation and motor function assessment of the upper limb and hand along with assessment of activities of daily living.

Early stage intervention

In the early stage the individual will use a soft collar and sling (Figure 5.5, p 80) to support the glenohumeral joint and to prevent subluxation. This will hold the elbow at 90° and across the chest. The following interventions are then undertaken:

- Passive exercise to shoulder, elbow, wrist and hand to maintain range of movement and function where applicable
- Activities of daily living – use of adaptive and compensatory approaches for feeding, dressing, etc.
- Provision of appropriate splintage for elbow, wrist and hand to provide support and assist function. It will be apparent from the assessment which splint/splints are appropriate. The flail arm splint may not be appropriate at this stage if the person is awaiting surgery
- Pain control
- Postural advice (including sleeping)
- Social and work interventions.

Middle stage intervention

- Strengthening and re-education of re-innervated muscles using graded therapeutic upper limb activities
- Restoring and increasing joint range of movement using graded therapeutic upper limb activities
- Stretching soft tissues to prevent contractures and increasing range of motion (including use of serial splints)
- Sensory re-education and training
- Re-assessment of pain control
- Review of flail arm splinting or other joint splints as required
- Review of compensatory and adaptive approaches including reducing assistive equipment as required.

Late stage intervention

- Vocational rehabilitation and work resettlement
- Ongoing strengthening and mobilisation to meet goals and objectives of the individual
- Review of definitive splinting if required (see Chapters 5 and 13).

Flail arm splint

The flail arm splint is a specialised splint, often prescribed and fitted by the multi-professional team at a prosthetic centre. It is a light weight, modular splint which can offer varying degrees of support and movement. It provides shoulder support allowing some abduction, varying degrees of elbow flexion being locked according to the required angel of flexion and forearm and wrist support as required. Here, various terminal devices like those used at the end of a prosthesis can be fixed to act as tools to replace the function of the affected hand, or outriggers to support the digits can be manufactured, e.g. to support the digits in a functional static position to enable use of a keyboard or telephone keypad. A cable from the shoulder strap on the opposite shoulder operates the device.

If a full flail arm splint is not required then varying splinting can be offered to support the joints, e.g. the elbow and wrist. Wrist gauntlet splints can be used with the same terminal devices to increase bilateral activities. If there is some function of the wrist or hand then dynamic or static splinting using outriggers can be used. Retraining of the arm is similar to that of an amputee learning to use their prosthesis (see Chapter 15). The splint will require regular review as and when function returns to the partially damaged or repaired nerves. In some cases where there is no return of function the individual may continue to use the splint on a long-term basis.

Summary

Rehabilitation of the brachial plexus is a complex and lengthy process. After surgical repair, the occupational therapist will need to review the operation notes to understand what the nature and predicted outcome of the surgery will be. Once it is clear which nerves have been damaged and repaired and which tendons have been used for tendon transfers, specific treatment plans may be developed and evaluated.

The use of standardised upper limb assessment tools is recommended to ensure that there is accurate assessment, and baseline data from which to monitor change and progress.

References

Frampton, V. (2000). Brachial plexus lesions. In M. Salter & L. Cheshire. *Hand Therapy: Principles and Practice*. Oxford: Butterworth Heinemann.

Moffat, D. B., & Mottram, R. F. (2000). *Anatomy and Physiology for Physiotherapists* (2nd edition). Oxford: Blackwell Science.

Narakas, A. O. (1985). The treatment of brachial plexus lesions. *International Orthopaedics*, 9(1), 29–36.

Wynn Parry, C. B. W. (1981). *Rehabilitation of the Hand*. Oxford: Butterworth.

Further reading

Burke, S., Higgins, J., McClinton, M., Saunders, R., & Valdata, L. (2005). *Hand and Upper Extremity Rehabilitation: A Practical Guide* (3rd edition). Edinburgh: Churchill Livingstone.

Conolly, W. B., & Prosser, R. (2003). *Rehabilitation of the Hand and Upper Limb*. Oxford: Butterworth-Heinemann.

Lowe, C., & O'Toole, J. (2002). Therapists' management of brachial plexus injuries. In E. Mackin, A. Callahan, T. Skirven, L. Schneider, & L. Osterma. (Eds). *Rehabilitation of the Hand: Surgery and Therapy* (5th edition). Philadelphia: Mosby.

Chapter 15

Traumatic amputation: management and occupational therapy

Fiona Carnegie

Introduction

When working with amputees it is important for the occupational therapist to recognise that every person is an individual and the loss of a limb is devastating. This chapter will outline the causes of amputation, particularly focusing on the occupational therapy rehabilitation of the upper and lower limb amputees whose surgery resulted from a traumatic accident (either at the time of the trauma or as a result of failed reconstructive surgery) or other orthopaedic intervention, e.g. infected knee replacement. Over the past 20 years, this particular client group has changed. Older amputees, multiple amputees and those with complex conditions/trauma now frequently survive the acute phase of treatment as a result of surgical and technological advances and require specialist rehabilitation to return them back to functional independence.

Causes of amputation

In the UK, the National Amputee Statistical Database (NASDAB) provides demographic, diagnostic and activity information on an annual basis on all new patients who are referred to the prosthetic services. As can be seen from the figures in Table 15.1 the majority of referrals are for lower limb amputees. On comparing Tables 15.2 and 15.3 we can see that the majority of lower limb amputations result from dysvascularity, with only 9% being the result of trauma. Upper limb amputations, while much less common, occur mainly as the result of trauma.

In the UK, the majority of traumatic amputations that present result from road traffic accidents. In countries where there are armed conflicts, a lack of legislation around health and safety in the work place, or poor road safety records, the percentage of traumatic amputations is likely to be higher.

Table 15.1 Total referrals to prosthetic centres in the UK (2005/6) (NASDAB 2006)

Lower limb amputees	4567 (92%)
Upper limb amputees	242 (6%)
Congenital limb deficiency	163 (2%)

Table 15.2 Causes of lower limb amputation

Dysvascularity	70% (of whom 40% have diabetes mellitus)
Trauma	9%
Infection	5%
Neoplasm	3%
Neurological factors	1%
Other	11%

Table 15.3 Causes of upper limb amputation

Trauma	54%
Neoplasm	14%
Dysvascularity	12%
Infection	6%
Neurological factors	2%
Other	12%

Levels of amputation

Figure 15.1 shows the different levels of amputation.

The multi-disciplinary team

The amputee will be seen initially in the acute setting where the multi-disciplinary team central to their care will consist of the surgeon, nurse, physiotherapist, occupational therapist and social worker. The amputation will be carried out here and rehabilitation commenced.

Where the person and their multi-disciplinary team is considering whether an amputation might be the best course of action, e.g. in the case of a failed reconstruction or persistent infection, it is often beneficial for the individual to visit a rehabilitation unit to discuss the course of prosthetic rehabilitation. This will prepare them for the second stage of the rehabilitation process.

Once the acute phase is over the person may transfer as an inpatient to a rehabilitation unit or may return home and attend as an outpatient. During this phase of the amputee's care the team will usually be headed by a rehabilitation consultant and consist of the above team members but with the addition of a prosthetist, counsellor and/or a psychologist. Good communication and liaison is essential between each team

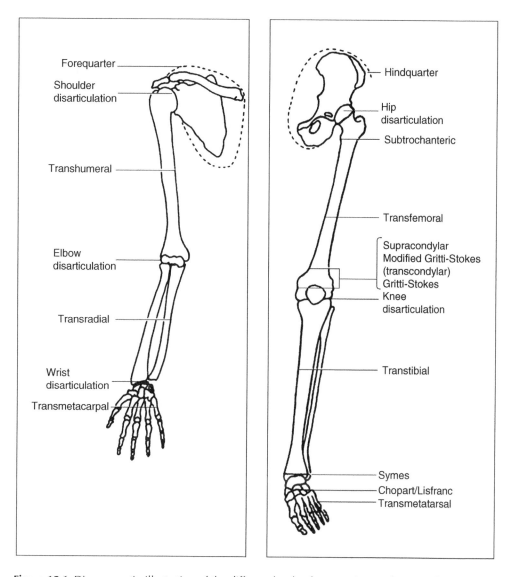

Figure 15.1 Diagrammatic illustration of the different levels of amputation. Redrawn with permission from Engstrom, B. & Van de Ven, C. *Therapy for Amputees*, 3rd edition, 1999. Edinburgh: Churchill Livingstone.

member and between the acute and rehabilitation teams in order to ensure a seamless and efficient service for the person and to avoid duplication of input. The individual and their family are central to the rehabilitation process.

Perioperative intervention

Where a pre-amputation assessment can be carried out, it is important to complete a holistic assessment of the individual and consider how other existing medical conditions or other injuries following the accident etc. may impact on their rehabilitation.

The condition of the limb requiring amputation (e.g. joint function, bone and skin condition) may determine the level of amputation and affect the amputee's long-term functional ability.

As a general rule retaining the proximal joint is an advantage but only when the joint is functional and the residual limb is long enough to form a useful lever to move a prosthetic limb. A skilled surgeon will create a residual limb, which will accommodate a prosthetic limb comfortably, carry the weight of the prosthesis, and, in the case of the lower limb amputee, carry the weight of the amputee. The bone ends will be smoothed and the muscles sutured together to form a covering over the bone ends. The nerves are cut under tension so that they retract up into the tissue; if the nerve is not cut short enough it may cause neuromas to form in the scar tissue, causing pain and restricting the amputee's functional ability.

An amputation can also be performed through the joint (joint disarticulation) and has the following advantages:

- A general anaesthetic may not be required. As the surgery is quick to perform, this may be necessary for those who are medically unwell, or at the scene of trauma.
- For lower limb amputees who are unlikely to be prosthetic users, an amputation through the knee joint (knee disarticulation) gives them a 'lap' when sitting, making functional tasks easier.
- It is the best level of amputation for a growing child as both growth plates are retained; when the child is fully grown they will have a good length of residual limb.

However, a disadvantage of an amputation through the joint is that it is difficult to obtain a cosmetically pleasing prosthesis. This is because a prosthetic joint is still required and this may alter the proportions of the prosthesis.

Psychological aspects of amputation

Amputees use varying strategies in the way they adjust to their new situation, for some this is very hard, especially those for whom it is a sudden and unprepared-for eventuality, e.g. a traumatic amputation (Livneh et al. 2000). However, some individuals have the opportunity to prepare for an amputation and be involved in the decision-making process, e.g. if it is required as a result of a complex injury where an amputation is the most advisable treatment option.

For some individuals there are many gains in having an amputation: the removal of an immobile, painful joint and provision of a prosthesis may lead to improved mobility and function, fewer hospital appointments, less formal or informal care, the possibility of returning to work and leisure pursuits. Therefore the gains in function and lifestyle outweigh the loss of their limb.

The way that the need for amputation is explained to a potential amputee is very important; when it is presented as the most beneficial option, it will be seen in a positive light. If, however, it is presented as a failure by the surgeon and the team, the amputee is likely to have a negative view of the surgery. The individual and their family require a realistic view of the future – this is important as the amputee must be aware of the time scales and the difficulties they may encounter during the rehabilitation process and beyond.

For some, previous losses have renewed significance in the light of the amputation. This is particularly the case for people who have had past bereavements, relationship breakdowns, unemployment or previous trauma. Counselling for the amputee may be needed at this stage or later in the rehabilitation process. Counselling may also help the amputee adjust to their new body image: accepting the appearance of their residual limb may be hard for some and they may require reassurance and encouragement. Family and friends may also find this situation difficult and will need help. Post-traumatic stress disorder can impact greatly on rehabilitation and these persons require patience and understanding, they and their family may need psychological support and therapists may benefit from advice from the psychologist. People with existing mental health problems require extra support especially when the amputation is as a direct result of their illness, e.g. attempted suicide or self-harm. It is important to liaise closely with the relevant mental health team.

Some amputees may experience short-term cognitive difficulties following surgery, as a result of the general anaesthetic; these usually resolve relatively quickly. Others may have difficulties due to systemic infections causing cognitive as well as physical complications. Others may have age related cognitive difficulties, e.g. dementia, or previous medical conditions e.g. stroke. These problems will have an impact on their ability to participate in rehabilitation.

Phantom limb sensation/pain

Many amputees experience a very real sensation of their missing limb immediately following surgery. They may find this very disconcerting and may be at risk of falling, especially when they first get up without supervision. For some the sensation is painful (Wright 2002). Treatment for phantom limb pain is still in the research phase and various methods can be trialled with individuals. All amputees should be encouraged to handle their residual limb to re-educate the nerve endings and desensitise the area. Other treatment methods include medication, acupuncture, transcutaneous electrical nerve stimulation (TENS) and mirror box (Chan et al. 2007).

Using a mirror box allows the person to look at a reflection of their remaining limb in the visual space, which would be occupied by their amputated limb. From this they can experience sensation and movement as though they were originating it from their phantom arm. In some patients, this has helped reduce the phantom pain (Murray et al. 2007). Some amputees experience chronic phantom limb pain and may require assessment by a specialist pain team.

Lower limb amputee rehabilitation

The older amputee

Over 50% of all amputees in the UK are over the age of 65 years (NASDAB, Information Services Division NHS (2007)). The major cause of amputation in this group is vascular disease (NASDAB). Traumatic amputations are less common in the older person but can happen and the rehabilitation process is very similar. They often have other coexisting medical conditions or disabilities, e.g. cardiovascular problems, stroke, diabetes, arthritis and cognitive problems. Smoking is a contributory factor of vascular disease and slows the healing process in trauma patients; therefore it is always recommended that amputees stop smoking. The rehabilitation process may take longer for older amputees due to limits in their physical fitness and the effects that any coexisting conditions may have on their functional ability. Their social situation and support networks are also critical to the outcome of rehabilitation.

The younger amputee

Traumatic amputees are in the main young adults (NASDAB, Information Services Division NHS (2007)). These people are usually otherwise fit and well. Some, however, may have other coexisting disabilities as a result of the trauma they experienced. Amputations may also be performed due to malignancy or infections and these individuals may experience fatigue and have anxieties about their future health.

Pre-prosthetic rehabilitation

The lower limb amputee should be encouraged to get out of bed as soon as possible, usually on the day following surgery, when the drains are removed. A joint assessment by an occupational therapist and a physiotherapist is beneficial at this stage to teach correct transfer techniques. Early mobility is encouraged in order to maintain muscle strength and exercise tolerance. Ideally this will be in a self-propelling wheelchair, encouraging independence.

Wheelchair

All lower limb amputees require a wheelchair in the early stages of rehabilitation in order to achieve independent mobility. Hopping using crutches or a walking frame is not recommended as an alternative at this stage, due to the risk of falling and the possibility of resultant injury and of increasing oedema in the dependent residual limb. These factors may delay prosthetic fitting.

Older or bilateral amputees are always likely to rely on using a wheelchair for part of each day. Younger, single limb amputees may also require a wheelchair for times when they are unable to use their prosthesis but this is dependent upon their medical state and physical fitness. Others will choose to hop with crutches at these times, which is acceptable once the residual limb is fully healed and all oedema is resolved. Use of crutches is contraindicated for older and/or overweight amputees due to the stress on their shoulders, wrists and remaining limb. Amputees require the same wheelchair assessment and training as any other person with mobility difficulties. However, their particular situation raises specific issues.

- Those with a transtibial amputation will require a stump board (Figure 15.2) to keep their residual limb elevated. This helps to reduce oedema, prevent knee flexion contractures and protect the residual limb from being knocked when mobilising.

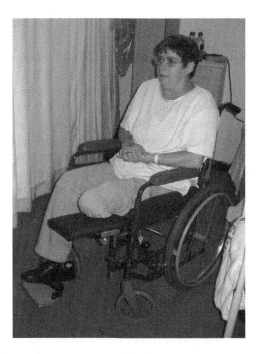

Figure 15.2 A transtibial amputee using a stump board.

- Those with a knee disarticulation may benefit from a stump board for comfort, to prevent pressure on the underside of the residual limb and protect the residual limb when mobilising.
- Bilateral amputees have an altered centre of gravity due to the loss of the weight of their legs. This results in their being more likely to tip backwards in the wheelchair. There are two possible solutions to make the wheelchair more stable:
  - To set the rear wheels back 76 mm (3 inches) making the wheelbase longer, thereby making the wheelchair less prone to tipping. The chair is then more difficult to propel, as more shoulder extension is required
  - To fit anti-tip bars at the back, which prevents the chair tipping but makes manoeuvring over small thresholds and outdoor mobility difficult.

An alternative to the above is to teach the amputee to use the instability of a wheelchair to their advantage by learning how to balance the wheelchair on its rear wheels and do a 'wheelie'. Younger amputees are usually able to learn this, allowing them to be more independent, particularly with outdoor wheelchair mobility as they are able to negotiate kerbs and obstacles without assistance.

A cushion is also required, especially if the amputee is going to be a more than occasional wheelchair user. Cushion prescription using standardised Tissue Viability Scoring System, e.g. Waterlow, is particularly important when an amputee has circulation problems and/or is going to spend long periods of time in the wheelchair. These amputees will require a pressure relieving cushion. For those with a hip disarticulation or a hemipelvectomy (who have lost one ischium) seating is a particular issue and they may require a ramped or specially designed cushion.

Transfers

- Hoisting – Some people are unable to transfer and require a hoist. There are special amputee slings available, which cater for the altered weight distribution of the bilateral or high single amputee and cover a greater surface area giving more security. Hoist companies are willing to assist with prescription advice.
- Sideways (single amputee) – A sideways transfer using a sliding board, e.g. from wheelchair to bed, involves the amputee positioning the wheelchair as close as possible to the bed. They remove the wheelchair armrest, put the sliding board under their bottom to bridge the gap and use their arms and remaining foot to push themselves over to the bed. Care is required: the brakes must be on and the front castors in line with the rear wheels so the wheelchair does not move. This type of transfer may also be carried out without the sliding board, provided the gap is small enough to negotiate safely. For this type of transfer the heights of the surfaces is critical, as the two surfaces need to be of the same height. It is also easier to transfer onto a firm surface, i.e. transferring on and off a pressure relief mattress is very difficult. If required the occupational therapist may need to supply appropriate furniture raising equipment.
- Standing pivot (single amputee) – With this method the amputee stands on their remaining foot and pivots round to the second surface (Figure 15.3). This method of transfer requires the amputee to have good balance and care must be taken if they have ulcers on their remaining foot or arthritis in their remaining knee. The remaining foot is placed in a position that will aid the transfer. It is usually easier for the amputee to transfer towards their remaining leg. An amputee who can do a

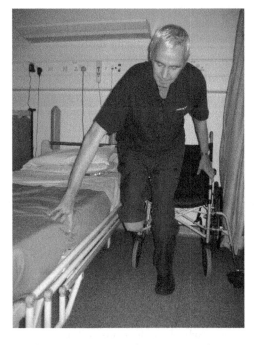

Figure 15.3 A single amputee demonstrating a standing pivot transfer.

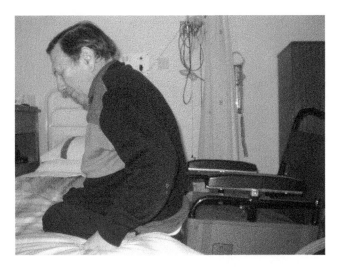

Figure 15.4 A bilateral amputee demonstrating a forwards/backwards transfer from wheelchair to bed.

standing pivot transfer may require a sliding board to manage a car transfer due to the gap between the wheelchair and the car seat.

Bilateral amputees

- Sideways – this transfer is similar to that described for the single amputee; the armrest is removed prior to the amputee moving across in front of the wheel onto the other surface. A sliding board may be used. The brakes must be securely on and the front castors in line with the rear wheels.
- Forwards/backwards – this transfer involves the wheelchair directly facing the second surface, both armrests stay in place and the amputee moves straight forward either lifting the body weight on their arms or 'walking' forward using their pelvis, onto the second surface (Figure 15.4).
- Using existing prosthesis – if the amputee was a single transtibial amputee and wore a prosthesis prior to becoming a bilateral amputee, they may choose to use their prosthesis to assist with transfers, using either a sideways or a standing pivot method of transfer.

Activities of daily living

The amputee should be encouraged and assisted to achieve independence with personal activities of daily living as soon as possible. Dressing and toileting can be commenced as soon as the amputee can transfer. Bathing and showering will depend on wound healing.

- Dressing – The single amputee can dress their lower half lying on the bed using the bridging technique, i.e. lifting their bottom off the bed by pushing down with their remaining foot (Figure 15.5). This is the safest method, as there is no risk of falling

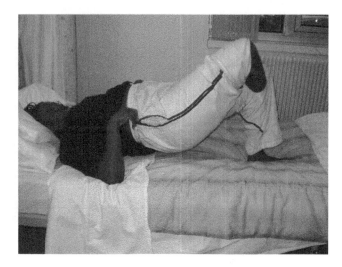

Figure 15.5 A transtibial amputee demonstrating the bridging technique for dressing their lower half.

but particular care is required if the remaining foot has injuries or compromised circulation. Alternatively, they can stand on their remaining leg to pull up their clothes. Good standing balance and muscle strength is needed to achieve this. A bilateral amputee will need to dress on the bed, rolling from side to side to pull up clothing. This expends a lot of energy and the task is more difficult if the amputee is lying on a pressure relieving mattress.

- Washing – A single amputee can have a strip wash, sitting for most of the task and standing on their remaining leg to wash their bottom and back of legs; this requires very good balance. Those with poor balance and bilateral amputees will require bed baths initially. For bathing they require the same assessment as any other person with a disability. A bilateral amputee who prefers a bath requires extremely strong upper limbs to lift themselves from the bath base up to a bath seat and then to the bath board. A safer and easier alternative to this is using a bath lift. If they are using a shower over the bath they need an extra wide shower board to give sufficient stability. If a bilateral amputee is using a shower they require a fixed seat which is wide enough to enable them to lean from side to side to wash thoroughly. If they have a level access shower a self-propelling shower wheelchair can also be used.
- Residual limb hygiene – It is very important that the residual limb is kept clean and dried thoroughly.
- Remaining foot hygiene – Single amputees need to be very careful to maintain good foot hygiene; this is particularly important for those who have diabetes, as they may have peripheral neuropathy and are prone to infection, and are at risk of further amputation.

Home assessment from acute care

Amputees are often discharged home from their acute hospital before commencing prosthetic rehabilitation. A home visit may be required to consider safe mobility and function within the home and the surrounding area including access (steps, door widths, wheelchair access), equipment (to aid transfers, bathing, toileting), and how the amputee will manage domestic tasks. Particular consideration should be given to toileting at night and first thing in the morning, as it is at these times that the phantom limb sensation can be most strong and cause accidents.

Sometimes the amputee may be confined to living in one room in the short term due to lack of environmental adaptation and time to make complex arrangements before hospital discharge. It may be necessary to arrange a homecare package to manage basic daily living activities. There is often a need to work collaboratively with social services occupational therapists and social workers, assessing for major adaptations, e.g. door widening, room layout or new bathroom facilities or the need for re-housing in the long term. It is important also to consider the home environment not only as a place where a wheelchair can be used but also as a place in which a prosthetic limb may be used in the future. Referrals to other services to address needs for ongoing rehabilitation in preparation for prosthetic rehabilitation, and for equipment or adaptations, may be needed following the initial visit and discharge home. The first visit home can be stressful for the amputee and their family and is often a time they are faced with the reality of the future.

Prostheses

A prosthesis attempts to replace what has been lost following an amputation. In the case of a lower limb prosthesis, it primarily replaces the mobility function.

Transtibial

Those with a transtibial amputation retain their knee joint so the prosthesis must replace the foot and ankle. The prosthesis (Figure 15.6) consists of a socket, shin piece and foot. The socket is held on to the residual limb by a variety of means. The main weightbearing area is the patella tendon. There are different types of feet available, giving various degrees of stability, and they are prescribed according to the functional requirements of the amputee.

Transfemoral

Those with a transfemoral amputation or knee disarticulation have also lost their knee joint. The prosthesis (Figure 15.6) consists of a socket, knee joint, shin piece and foot. There are many different types of socket, generally encompassing the whole of the thigh. Those with a knee disarticulation weightbear through their remaining femoral condyles, transfemoral amputees weightbear on their ischial tuberosity. There are various methods of suspension; in older people, a rigid pelvic band may be used and occasionally they will use a shoulder strap for added suspension. When the amputee has sufficient muscle strength around the residual limb and good proximal control, less suspension is used. There are many different types of prosthetic knee joints, giving different properties. Safety is always paramount, and individuals at higher risk of falling will be prescribed a knee that will remain locked when walking. Younger amputees often have better muscle

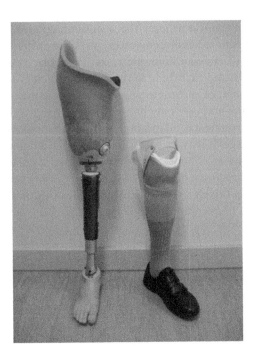

Figure 15.6 On the left is an example of an unfinished, transfemoral prosthesis with suction suspension at the fitting stage. On the right is a transtibial prosthesis, with cuff suspension and a cosmetic covering.

strength and balance, and are therefore expected to have a good gait pattern walking with a free knee. Their functional requirements will dictate the type of knee prescribed.

Hip disarticulation and hemipelvectomy amputations are rare; the prosthesis is large, replacing the hip, knee and foot. The socket surrounds the pelvis and is held on tightly with straps, and some amputees also use a shoulder harness.

Prosthetic rehabilitation

Often the prosthetic rehabilitation starts with use of an early walking aid, e.g. a PPAM aid (pneumatic post-amputation mobility aid) or a Femurette. These enable the therapist to fit a generic walking aid to the amputee for assessment and training, and gives psychological benefits to the amputee walking early. The PPAM aid also assists in reducing oedema due to the alternating pressure on the residual limb as the amputee walks.

Criteria for prosthetic prescription

Early walking aids can help the multi-disciplinary team assess whether prosthetic prescription is appropriate for the amputee. They should have reached independence in their daily living skills in full; being able to transfer independently, wash and dress themselves. Flexion contractures of the proximal joints may also preclude them from using a prosthesis.

The energy expenditure required for a single transtibial amputee is 25% greater than an able bodied walker, a transfemoral amputee uses 55% more energy (Schmalz et al.

2002). It is important that this is taken into account when considering prosthetic rehabilitation for an amputee, also that they have the cognitive skills to learn new concepts
and understand safety factors related to prosthetic rehabilitation.

Donning/doffing

Methods of donning and doffing prosthesis are many and varied. A transtibial amputee
will usually don the prosthesis in sitting. A transfemoral amputee using prosthesis with a
rigid pelvic band will don the prosthesis while sitting down. Most other types of socket
and suspension are put on while the amputee is standing up; this requires very good
standing balance. The residual limb may fluctuate in volume in the early stages after the
amputation so stump socks are used to ensure a good socket fit. The amputee therefore
needs to adjust the number of socks they use to compensate for the changes in volume.

Transfers

There are some amputees who are unlikely to walk with a prosthesis, e.g. frail older
people, for whom prosthesis may assist with transfers. This will only be appropriate
if they have had a transtibial amputation, the prosthesis enables them to have two feet
on the floor and they can use knee extension of both limbs to assist them to stand. For
transfemoral amputees a prosthesis is a hindrance with transfers, but those who can
use one are advised to lock their prosthetic knee before standing as this ensures that the
knee will not give way.

Standing balance

Standing is very important, as many tasks require a stationary posture. The amputee
must learn to weightbear through both their remaining limb and their prosthesis. Bilateral amputees have to weightbear continually through their prostheses and this can be
uncomfortable initially. They must practise static standing, doing simple tasks for short
periods of time until their balance is good enough for them to carry out more complex
tasks requiring dynamic standing balance (Figure 15.7), e.g. cooking, gardening.

Gait training

Initially the amputee learns to walk using the parallel bars for safety, support, and to
create a good gait pattern. At this stage they will usually be under the supervision of
a physiotherapist. They will then progress using appropriate walking aids; one stick
and one bar, then two sticks before coming out of the bars or a frame. Many younger
amputees want to progress very quickly to walking without sticks. If they do this too
soon they may develop a poor gait pattern resulting in possible long-term complications
of the hip and back. Younger amputees should achieve an excellent gait, whereas for an
older amputee, safety remains the prime concern.

Functional walking

Many amputees are able to transfer the skill of walking with a prosthesis into different
environments and when completing functional tasks, without any assistance. Others

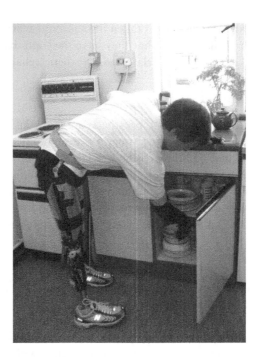

Figure 15.7 A transfemoral amputee bending down to reach a kitchen cupboard.

find this progression difficult, especially those who cannot maintain appropriate concentration, or those who use a frame and have to work out how to negotiate obstacles and carry items. It is important that the amputee is able to walk in confined spaces, such as at home, and on different surfaces (carpet, lino, etc.). For some amputees this is the extent of their ability, whereas others should be encouraged to manage steps, to walk on rough ground, travel on public transport or go shopping.

The bilateral amputee may have bulky walking aids (often two tripods), which can create difficulties walking at home, especially through doorways and in confined spaces. This may improve with practice or may require a change of equipment, e.g. use of a wheeled walking frame/quadrupod and stick.

Home assessment with prosthesis

A home visit is recommended, especially for the older, frail amputee and the multiple amputee, when they are walking independently and have achieved a level of mobility required in the home environment, e.g. managing steps/stairs/slopes/uneven ground. It is important to consider access and to assess how much the amputee will use a wheelchair and how often they will be walking. This is because it is easier for an amputee to climb steps than it is to walk up a ramp. Inside the property they will need two banisters on the stairs, sometimes rails at steps. Transfers when wearing their prosthesis also need to be reassessed and a suitable place to don the prosthesis needs to be determined. This is particularly important for bilateral amputees. Amputees who use walking aids may need assessment with a kitchen trolley for carrying items. Toileting at night must be considered, i.e. use of a commode near the bedside (Figure 15.8), use of a bottle, transfers into

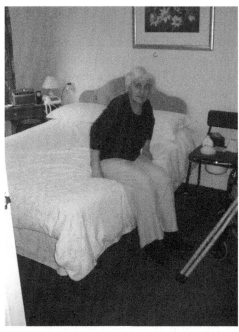

Figure 15.8 A transtibial amputee on a home visit.

a wheelchair, or donning prosthesis and walking to the toilet. Some amputees who live in a house will need a wheelchair upstairs as well as down.

Some amputees of working age require help to prepare to return to work, this may be in the form of discussion and advice regarding travel or their pattern of work. For example the occupational therapist may suggest a trial journey to work outside of the rush hour or perhaps staring back part time to build up stamina. In some instances the occupational therapist may need to visit the work place to advise about equipment or adaptations required to enable the amputee to fulfil their work role.

Case study 15.1

Diagnosis – Above knee amputation

Barbara – female, aged 73 years

Barbara had a total knee replacement to resolve osteoarthritis; this became infected and she had to walk with a fixed knee and in considerable pain. She visited a prosthetic centre and saw what would be available if she had an amputation. She chose to have an amputation and her rehabilitation included training in the use of wheelchair and a prosthesis. Her rehabilitation was slow. Six weeks after her first fitting she was able to walk with a prosthesis with a semi-automatic knee lock, using a walking frame. She was able to self-propel a standard wheelchair. She returned to living in her compact ground floor warden controlled flat. Her home visit included assessing her ability to walk and use the wheelchair within her home environment. She had her bath removed and a shower fitted with a wall mounted fixed shower seat. She is now able to manage in her home and walk 50 yards to her car and drive into town and to visit friends.

Rehabilitation of the upper limb amputee

The arm positions the hand so the hand can service its user. The hand is important as a precision tool, for power, gives considerable sensory feedback, and is significant in non-verbal communication. The loss of a hand involves loss of many functions; the amputee is the only one who can identify which loss is the most significant, not least of which may be the aspect of body image.

Early rehabilitation

Hand dominance

Those who have lost their dominant hand require exercises and activities to increase the dexterity of their remaining hand.

Oedema

As with the lower limb amputee it is important to try to keep the residual limb elevated in order to reduce oedema. This is very hard to achieve because the arm is usually dependent. When the patient is sitting they should be encouraged to keep the residual limb up as high as possible, on pillows or for a transradial amputee in a hand sling attached to a drip stand. Some surgeons may advocate stump bandaging; considerable care is required to maintain a consistent pressure. Muscle contraction and massage will help to reduce oedema; massage can also normalise sensation and will assist the amputee with adjustment to their altered body image.

Range of movement of remaining joints

It is important to maintain a full range of movement of the remaining joints, particularly the elbow for the transradial and the shoulder for the transhumeral amputee. The neck and spine also require excellent range of movement. When using an upper limb prosthesis, movement of the whole of the rest of the body is important for function and also the cosmetic appearance of the prosthesis; if the amputee walks with a natural arm swing the prosthesis is less obvious to the casual observer.

Activities of daily living

Eating

Some amputees will require equipment to assist them, e.g. a plate surround, or rocker knife; others prefer to learn new techniques, e.g. using the side of the fork to cut food or using food on the plate as a buffer.

Dressing

It is beneficial to advise amputees to wear clothes with minimal fastening to start with, to reduce their frustrations. Some amputees prefer to learn how to manage buttons and laces, etc. with one hand, while others benefit from special adaptations, e.g. use of hook and loop fastenings, or elastic shoelaces.

Washing

Washing the remaining hand is difficult and frustrating. Some will just rub the fingers together, while others use their residual limb to wash against. When bathing the hand can be washed between the knees. Washing the remaining arm's axilla can also prove a problem; some can reach their hand into the armpit, others can use their knee when sitting in the bath. Some may need a long-handled sponge.

Writing

When the non-dominant hand is amputated, the primary problem, particularly for the transhumeral amputee, is holding the paper still; placing a weight on the paper can stabilise it. Those who lose their dominant hand need to learn to write with their remaining hand; they are advised to use a felt tip pen, draw rather than write initially (writing too early may lead to frustration), to hold the pen in a relaxed grip and not to press too hard on the paper. Typing is often an important skill and can be an alternative to writing; care is required so that the amputee does not over use the remaining hand. Special keyboards adapted for one handed use are available. Positioning and posture are also important when using the keyboard to reduce the possibility of back and arm strain.

Prostheses

There are three types of prostheses: replacing cosmesis, or function, or trying to replace both. The hand is so complex that it is not possible to satisfactorily replace all of its functions in one prosthesis.

- The cosmetic prosthesis (Figure 15.9) primarily replaces the cosmetic function of the arm; for the transradial amputee this has a foam hand, which has wires in the fingers so that they can be positioned as the amputee chooses, and the socket is secured onto the person by body contours, over the olecranon and condyles. The transhumeral amputee will have an elbow joint also to position the forearm, and for them the socket goes over the shoulder and is usually held on by straps to the other axilla.
- The body-powered prosthesis replaces the function of the hand, having a socket, elbow (for a transhumeral amputee), forearm section and wrist rotary and terminal device, which may be a split hook or a cosmetic hand or any of the 20 or so working devices: pliers, potato peeler, tool holder, typing peg, spade grip, etc.
- A harness is fitted so that body movement results in opening or closing of the terminal device or operation of the elbow joint.
- The externally powered prosthesis has a motorised hand or hook, which is operated by myoelectric or switch control; the power may operate the terminal device (hand or hook) and/or the wrist and/or the elbow, as follows:

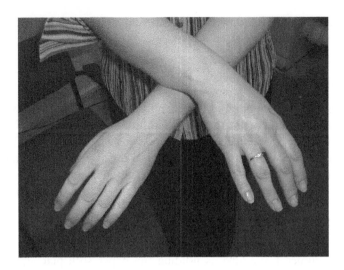

Figure 15.9 An example of a cosmetic upper limb prosthesis.

- Myoelectric control – electrodes are sited in the socket close to the skin which pick up the muscle contractions, amplify them and these send a signal to the motor in the terminal device to open or close/ the wrist to rotate/ the elbow to raise or lower
- Switch control – there is a switch in the socket or in the harness which when activated drives the motor in the terminal device, wrist or elbow.

Prosthetic assessment

For upper limb amputees it is helpful if they are shown all types of prostheses, and informed of the advantages and disadvantages of the different systems. This information can be given before amputation when possible, and can enable them to make informed choices. The external-powered prosthesis is not suitable as a first prescription, as it is heavier than the others, and the socket, in the case of myoelectric control, must be close fitting; oedema will continue to have a small effect for many months.

Prosthetic training

Cosmetic training

It is important to check that the amputee can don and doff the prosthesis independently and that the socket is comfortable. There are a few functional activities that can be practised, e.g. holding a knife, which can be used to stop food falling off the plate (the cosmetic hand cannot hold a knife securely enough to cut food). The prosthe-

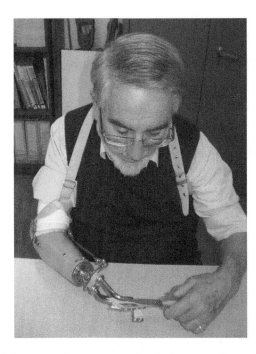

Figure 15.10 A transradial amputee learning to work a body-powered prosthesis by practising using scissors to cut up stamps.

sis can be used to steady objects, paper, etc., and to carry things over it, e.g. a bag or coat.

Body-powered training

The amputee must learn how to operate the terminal device, and the appendages may require altering to harness the body movement exactly. Initially the amputee will practise using the prosthesis alone, usually with the split hook with one or two bands, e.g. picking up solitaire pieces, progressing to playing the game; it is easier to operate the terminal device in standing at first. They will then progress to simple two-handed tasks, e.g. cutting paper (Figure 15.10), using the scissors in the remaining hand and holding the paper in the split hook, taking care to have the hook at the correct angle.

The last stage of the training is to carry out tasks that the amputee may need to do in everyday life, and this will vary with each individual, e.g. holding a knife or fork in the split hook, opening containers. It is helpful for them to see and try out some of the other terminal devices, e.g. the spade grip, camera holder, pliers, etc.

The transhumeral amputee will need to learn to operate the terminal device and the elbow lock. This maybe a hand-operated device, or there may be the option of an automatic action to lock and unlock it; this requires determination to master, involving depression, internal rotation and abduction of the shoulder joint (it is like nudging someone in the ribs).

Case study 15.2

Diagnosis – Traumatic transhumeral amputation

Gary – male, aged 23 years

Gary was involved in a car accident and sustained a traumatic transhumeral amputation. He was in hospital for three weeks and discharged to his parents' home. His mother was very anxious and had sessions with the psychologist. After two months, Gary was fitted with his first prosthesis: a body-powered prosthesis with split hook and automatic elbow joint; he learnt to use it effectively within three sessions of training and returned to his work in printing. Six months after the injury he had training with a myo-electric prosthesis but has chosen to use the body-powered limb, as it is lighter and more functional. He wears the prosthesis all day every day, using the split hook for most tasks. He has special terminal devices for technical drawing and a camera holder and fishing rod holder for his hobbies. During his rehabilitation these activities were simulated within the treatment environment and information passed on to his employers who were only too happy to assist in facilitating Gary's return to work.

Externally powered training

The amputee must learn how to operate the terminal device, which may be a hand or a hook. When operated by switch control the movement required is similar to the body-powered prosthesis. When using the myo-electric method of control the amputee must gain control of the hand/hook, this is done by carrying out simple tasks with the one hand, similar to the activities used for the body-powered training. Once the amputee has control of the terminal device practical tasks can be carried out, e.g. use of knife and fork, opening jars (Figure 15.11), carrying things. Then a transradial amputee will learn to use the hand in different positions, above the head, behind the back, this being the main advantage that the hand has over the body-powered prosthesis. It should be possible to operate the myo-electric controlled hand in any position.

The socket of the transhumeral prosthesis restricts the positions it is possible to move this arm into approximately 45° flexion and abduction. The transradial amputee has use of the elbow and shoulder; they can operate the prosthesis easily in the mid position and lift the prosthesis away from their body. The transhumeral amputee has an artificial elbow joint and the socket usually extends over the shoulder resulting in reduced shoulder movement. The transradial prosthesis is more functional than the transhumeral but also the residual limb is more useful as it can be used to stabilise objects, to carry, etc. Therefore it is difficult to predict if an amputee will benefit from prosthesis or not. Some amputees will wear their prosthesis all their waking hours, others will wear it for specific tasks and some, after learning to use it, decide to manage without.

Bilateral amputees

The bilateral upper limb amputee has considerable difficulty achieving functional independence. If there is a difference in residual limb length, the longer side is likely to become the dominant one. Bilateral transradial amputees will be able to feed themselves, manage clothing without fastenings and manage urination; but will have dif-

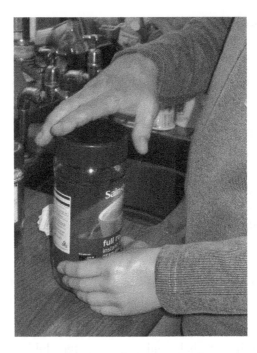

Figure 15.11 An amputee using an electric prosthesis to open a jar.

ficulty cleaning themselves after a bowel movement. They will require considerable motivation, as to achieve these tasks will need determination and excellent problem-solving skills. Body-powered prostheses and myo-electric prostheses may assist function. Some amputees use a mixture of different types of prostheses, e.g. one cosmetic and one body-powered.

For those who have bilateral transhumeral amputations, the level of independence they can achieve is highly dependent on their character, motivation and physical fitness. They will have to use other parts of their body to increase the possibility of independence. Some amputees learn to use their feet for fine function and if they are agile enough may feed themselves with fork in their toes; this is generally only possible when the amputations occur in young people under the age of 20.

Children

Children who have single or multiple amputations are often very resilient, however, when discussing amputation and treatment following it with young children, it is particularly important how language is used (see Case study 15.3, p 276). Young children usually learn to walk with great ease; they are in an active learning phase of life and have less fear. A single transtibial amputee will be able to run like their peers.

Activities which could be used to encourage children with lower limb prosthesis include:

- Standing to play at a table/sand box
- Walking with a push-along-toy or trolley

- Kicking a football
- Sitting down and getting up from the floor
- Sitting and standing from appropriate height chairs

Children who have an upper limb amputation will benefit from learning how to use a prosthesis. Training is similar to that used with adults but using age related activities. Activities suitable for use with a pre-school or primary school aged child might include:

- Games involving grasp and release
- Threading activities
- Cutting and sticking
- Simple construction games
- Writing and computer work
- Eating
- Dressing.

In the long term some of these children will opt not to use prostheses and learn how to manage tasks one handed. The occupational therapist's role is to enable them to achieve independence as far as they are able and to help them to see themselves as competent, confident individuals. Often the child's parents will benefit from support and advice on how to help and encourage the child in the quiet moments at home when questions and concerns are voiced. Amputations occurring in young people may be more complicated physically and emotionally. It is important to be aware of the child's friends and siblings, their schoolteachers and classmates. It can sometimes be helpful to visit the school to assess and address the child's needs there.

Case study 15.3

Diagnosis – Symes amputation

Charlie – male, aged 3 years through to 7 years

When Charlie was 3 years old he slipped under a mowing machine. He was rushed to hospital and underwent an amputation through the ankle joint (Symes amputation). After four weeks he was discharged home with a wheelchair and was referred for prosthetic prescription. This was very straightforward and he learnt to walk (and run) with ease and returned to nursery as if nothing had happened. His family had a great deal of adjusting to do, resolving of guilt and blame, requiring support from therapists and a counsellor.

When Charlie was aged 7 he required further surgery. He became very agitated and distressed about this. When asked about his concerns he explained that he had been lied to four years earlier, he had been told he was going to the theatre (to him that was a fun outing to see a show) and this had not been the case. Was he being lied to again? It was then possible to understand his concerns and explain to him what was going to occur in language appropriate to a 7 year old.

The surgery forced the family also to revisit the traumatic events of four years previously, which was distressing for them. Following this surgery, Charlie had to return to using a wheelchair and was unwilling to return to school until he was walking again. He is now back walking, running, jumping the same as his friends. He will have prosthetic hardware to enable him to do all the tasks he wishes but he will always remain an amputee.

Amputees with additional problems

When amputees have additional disabilities careful assessment is required regarding functional ability and whether prosthesis will be helpful. In the case of a head injury, where hemiparesis is evident, the side of the amputation and hemiparesis is significant in how they manage walking aids and the cerebral deficit caused by the head injury. If they have arthritis the strength in remaining joints will need to be assessed, toleration of the weight of the prosthesis, and how they will manage to don and doff the limb. The main difficulty will be: for those who have sensory loss, communication during prosthetic training; in the case of blindness the use of a walking aid and a white cane when walking; and for an upper limb amputee the lack of sensory feedback when using an upper limb prosthesis.

As early gait training involves partial weightbearing, both with the early walking aid and initially with the prosthesis, if injuries to the remaining leg involve partial weightbearing, prosthetic rehabilitation may have to be delayed as it is not possible to partially weightbear on both limbs.

Driving

In the UK the amputee must inform the Driver and Vehicle Licensing Agency and their insurance company of the amputation. A single left lower limb amputee can drive an automatic car that is unadapted. If the right leg has been amputated they will need to have the accelerator pedal moved to the left side. A bilateral amputee will need to use hand controls. A left upper limb amputee will find it easier to drive an automatic car; a right limb amputee will need to be able to steer while changing gear and may need adaptations for secondary controls. Those with multiple amputations or additional disabilities should be encouraged to attend a mobility centre for a driving assessment.

Support networks

For many amputees their previous support networks will be sufficient. Others may find it helpful to be in touch with other amputees, this could be through amputee-specific groups, e.g.: the Limbless Association, which has a regular magazine, a befriending service and advice line regarding sports, disability awareness, etc; Reach, a similar group for those with the upper limb affected; or Steps, a group for children with abnormalities of the lower limb. Others choose to find support from activity-specific groups, e.g. the Disabled Biker's Association and the One-armed Golfer's Association. Many amputees find that the amputation causes them to re-evaluate their lives and sometimes they make active choices to change direction: going to college to study, retraining for alternative employment, starting a new sport or hobby.

Summary

The rehabilitation of the amputee starts before the amputation and continues long after discharge. The initial stage is acute rehabilitation, then the prosthetic phase, and then adjustment to using the prosthesis at home, at work and during leisure pursuits.

They will have to make changes to their homes, habits and lifestyle, and the prosthetic service will support them with changes in prescriptions as the needs arise. It will be at least two years before the amputee reaches their full potential.

References

Chan, B., Witt, R., Charrow, A. P., Magee, A., Howard, R., Pasquina, P. F., Heilman, K. M., & Tsao, J. W. (2007). Mirror therapy for phantom limb pain. *New England Journal of Medicine*, *357*(21), 2206–2207.

Information Services Division NHS. (2007). *The Amputee Statistical Database for the UK Annual Report 2005/2006*. Online. Available at: www.nasdab.co.uk (accessed 7 April 2009). Edinburgh: Information Services Division NHS Scotland on behalf of NASDAB.

Livneh, H., Antonak, R., & Gerhardt, J. (2000). Multidimensional investigation of the structure of coping among people with amputations. *Psychosomatics*, *41*(3), 235–244.

Murray, C. D., Pettifer, S., Howard, T., Patchick, E. L., Cailletter, F., Kulkarnie, J., & Bamford, C. (2007). The treatment of phantom limb pain using immersive virtual reality: three case studies. *Disability and Rehabilitation*, *29*, 1465–1469.

Schmalz, T., Blumentritt, S., Jarasch, R. (2002). Energy expenditure and biomechanical characterics of lower limb amputee gait: The influence of prosthetic alignment and different prosthetic components. *Gait Posture*, *16*, 255–263.

Wright, A. (2002). Neuropathic pain. In J. Strong, A. M. Unruh, A. Wright, & G. David Baxter (Eds). *Pain: A Textbook for Therapists*. Edinburgh: Churchill Livingstone, pp. 365–368.

Further reading

Atkins, D., & Meier, R. (Eds). (1989). *Comprehensive Management of the Upper-Limb Amputee*. New York: Springer-Verlag.

Barsby, P., Ham, R., Lumley, C., & Roberts, C. (1995). *Amputee Management – a Handbook*. London: King's College School of Medicine and Dentistry.

Carnegie, F. (2002). Children with limb deficiency. In C. Swee Hong & L. Howard (Eds). *Occupational Therapy in Childhood*. London: Whurr Publishers.

Engstrom, B., & Van de Ven, C. (Eds). (1999). *Therapy for Amputees*. Edinburgh: Churchill Livingstone.

Appendix

Useful organisations and contacts

Action for Sick Children (www.actionforsickchildren.org.uk)
Children's health care charity formed to ensure that sick children always receive the highest standard of care possible.

American College of Rheumatology (www.rheumatology.org)
The American College of Rheumatology is an organisation of and for physicians, health professionals, and scientists that advances rheumatology through programmes of education, research, advocacy and practice support that foster excellence in the care of people with arthritis and rheumatic and musculoskeletal diseases.

Arthritis and Musculoskeletal Alliance (ARMA) (www.arma.uk.net)
ARMA is the umbrella body providing a collective voice for the arthritis and musculoskeletal community in the UK. It works to improve the quality of life for more than 8.5 millions people with these conditions in the UK. There are 34 member organisations representing service user, professional and research groups.

Arthritis Care (www.arthritiscare.org.uk)
Arthritis Care exists to support people with arthritis. It is the UK's largest user led organisation working with and for all people who have arthritis.

Arthritis Foundation (USA) (www.arthritis.org)
The foundation helps people take control of arthritis by providing public health education, pursuing public policy and legislation, and conducting evidence-based programmes to improve the quality of life for people with arthritis in the USA.

Arthritis Research Campaign (ARC) (www.arc.org.uk)
The Arthritis Research Campaign raises funds to: promote medical research into the cause, treatment and cure of arthritic conditions; educate medical students, doctors and allied health care professionals about arthritis; and provide information to the general public.

Arthritis Society (Canada) (www.arthritis.ca)
The mission of the Arthritis Society is to search for the underlying causes and subsequent cures for arthritis, and to promote the best possible care and treatment for people with arthritis.

Baby Hips (Ireland) (www.babyhips.ie)
This website is a resource for parents of babies undergoing treatment in a hip spica cast for developmental dysplasia of the hip (DDH).

Back Care (www.backcare.org.uk)
Back Care is a registered charity that aims to reduce the burden of back pain by providing information and support, promoting good practice and funding research. It acts as a hub between patients, health care professionals, employers, policy makers, researchers and all others with an interest in back pain.

Bone and Joint Decade (2000–2010) (www.boneandjointdecade.org)
The Bone and Joint Decade encompasses diseases associated with musculoskeletal diseases such as joint diseases, osteoporosis, rheumatoid arthritis, osteoarthritis, low back pain, spinal disorders, severe trauma to the extremities, crippling diseases and deformities in children. The Decade is a multi-disciplinary, global campaign that will implement and promote initiatives in all parts of the world.

British Association of Hand Therapists (BAHT) (www.hand-therapy.co.uk)
BAHT is a registered charity whose aim is to advance and promote the study and general knowledge of the treatment of the hand.

British Elbow and Shoulder Society (BESS) (www.bess.org.uk)
BESS promotes the study of the shoulder and elbow and promotes interdisciplinary practice, education and research regarding the management of these two joints.

British Limb Reconstruction Society (BLRS) (www.boa.ac.uk)
The society brings together surgeons involved in the techniques of limb lengthening and correction of both congenital and acquired deformities of the upper and lower limbs as well as the reconstruction of post-traumatic limb defects. It aims to advance education in this field of practice.

British Orthopaedic Association (BOA) (www.boa.ac.uk)
The BOA is the professional association for trauma and orthopaedic surgeons in the UK. Objectives include advancement in the science, art and practice of orthopaedic surgery with the aim of bringing relief to people of all ages experiencing the effects of injury or disorders of the musculoskeletal system. It provides education and practice management services for orthopaedic surgeons and health professionals.

British Orthopaedic Research Society (BORS) (www.borsoc.org.uk)
The British Orthopaedic Research Society (BORS) is a multi-disciplinary association devoted to pursuing research relevant to orthopaedic and musculoskeletal surgery.

British Pain Society (www.britishpainsociety.org/)
The British Pain Society is a representative body for all professionals involved in the management of pain in the UK. The society aims to achieve the highest possible standards in the management of pain through education, training and research in all fields of pain and by facilitating the exchange of information and experience.

British Society for Paediatric and Adolescent Rheumatology (BSPAR) (www.bspar.org.uk)
BSPAR is a multi health care professional organisation that aims to advance paediatric rheumatology care in the UK and Ireland, by raising the standards of clinical care, enhancing the quality of training and promoting research.

British Society for Rheumatology (BSR) (www.rheumatology.org.uk)
BSR is a medical society committed to advancing knowledge and practice in the field of rheumatology. It works at national and local level to promote high quality standards of care for people with these conditions.

British Society for Surgery of the Hand (BSSH) (www.bssh.ac.uk)
BSSH is an information and education body for Hand Surgery in the UK for all health care professionals. It strives to improve the care of people with hand injuries and hand disorders through education and research, and by promoting and directing the development of hand surgery.

British Trauma Society (www.trauma.org/bts/)
The British Trauma Society considers trauma care as a multi-disciplinary concern and brings together committed clinicians with an interest in trauma care.

College of Occupational Therapists Specialist Section: Trauma and Orthopaedics (COTSSTO) (www.cot.co.uk/specialist/trauma/intro/intro.php)
COTSSTO aims to promote best occupational therapy practice and improve the skills and knowledge of occupational therapists working with people with orthopaedic conditions, amputation or limb deficiency.

Contact a Family (www.cafamily.org.uk)
Provides support and advice to parents, whatever the medical condition of their child. They have information on over 1000 rare syndromes and rare disorders and can put families in touch with each other

Disabled Living Foundation (DLF) (www.dlf.org.uk)
The Disabled Living Foundation provides free, impartial advice about all types of equipment for disabled adults, disabled children, older people, and their carers and families.

Douglas Bader Foundation (www.douglasbaderfoundation.co.uk)
The mission of the foundation at its inception and today is to continue Douglas' work in conjunction with and on behalf of individuals with a disability.

European League against Rheumatism (EULAR) (www.eular.org)
An organisation which represents the patient, health professional and scientific societies of rheumatology of all the European nations. EULAR endeavours to stimulate, promote, and support the research, prevention, treatment and rehabilitation of rheumatic diseases.

In Car Safety Centre (www.incarsafetycentre.co.uk)
A specialist company providing advice and guidance, purchase or hire of car seats, and harnesses for children including those children with special needs including hip spicas.

International Society for Fracture Repair (ISFR) (www.fractures.com)
ISFR is embodied in an organisation of individuals from around the world who are dedicated to the advancement and interchange of science of fracture repair and its application to improvement of patient care.

Muscular Dystrophy Campaign (www.muscular-dystrophy.org)
A charity that focuses on all muscular dystrophies and related muscle diseases. It is dedicated to improving lives of all those people affected by providing information, advice and support.

National Amputee Statistical Database (NASDAB) (www.nasdab.co.uk)
Demographic and clinical information is presented regarding the cause and level of amputation referrals made to prosthetic centres within the UK.

National Institute for Health and Clinical Excellence (NICE) (www.nice.org.uk)
NICE is an independent organisation responsible for providing national guidance on promoting good health and preventing and treating ill health. It has guidance on public health, health technologies and clinical practice.

National Library for Health: Musculoskeletal Specialist Library (www.library.nhs.uk/musculoskeletal)
This electronic library exists primarily to support the work of NHS health professionals in the field of musculoskeletal disorders in the UK. By providing easy access to NHS Core Content and a variety of other hand picked resources it aims to provide the latest and best available evidence and information to support practice.

National Library for Health: Specialist Child Health Library (www.library.nhs.uk/ChildHealth)
The specialist electronic library addresses a wide range of topics related to the health and well-being of children.

National Library for Health: Trauma and Orthopaedic Specialist Library (www.library.nhs.uk/trauma_orthopaedics)
The Trauma and Orthopaedics Specialist Library forms part of the wider National Library for Health (NLH). to enable clinicians and allied health professionals to have seamless access to the best current know-how and knowledge to support health care related decisions.

National Osteoporosis Society (www.nos.org.uk)
The National Osteoporosis Society is a national charity dedicated to improving the prevention, diagnosis, and treatment of this fragile bone disease.

Online Mendelian Inheritance in Man (OMIM) (www.ncbi.nih.gov)
The OMIM database is a catalogue of human genes and genetic disorders for use primarily by physicians and other professionals concerned with genetic disorders, by genetics researchers, and by advanced students in science and medicine.

Orthoseek (www.orthoseek.com)
Orthoseek is a source of authoritative information on paediatric orthopaedics and paediatric sports medicine.

Orthoteers (www.orthoteers.org)
Orthoteers is one of the biggest online repositories of orthopaedic information on the web. It includes sections on rehabilitation, regional anatomy and conditions, trauma, biomechanics and an image gallery.

Patient UK (www.patient.co.uk)
The aim of this website is to provide non-medical people and health care professionals in the UK with good quality information about health and disease. Evidence based information leaflets, reviews of health and illness related websites and links are available.

Perthes' Association (www.perthes.org.uk)
The Perthes Association aims to help and advise families of children with Perthes' disease and associated conditions.

Prevention of Falls Network Europe (ProFaNE) (www.profane.eu.org)
ProFaNE is a thematic network with 25 partners focusing on the issue of prevention of falls and improvement of postural stability among older people. The aim is to bring together workers from around Europe to focus on a series of tasks required to develop multi-factorial prevention programmes aimed at reducing the incidence of falls and fractures among older people.

RADAR: The Disability Network (www.radar.org.uk)
RADAR is a disability charity working to represent the need and expectations of disabled people in the UK.

REACH: The Association for Children with Hand or Arm Deficiency (www.reach.org.uk)
REACH pools knowledge of its membership to offer a level of support to all children with hand or arm deficiency by providing information, experiences and guidance.

Scoliosis Association (www.sauk.org.uk)
SAUK aims to provide information about scoliosis, eliminate fear and stigma, and offer contacts for shared experiences.

SCOPE (www.scope.org.uk)
SCOPE is a disability organisation whose focus is on people with cerebral palsy. It aims to help disabled people achieve equality in society in which they are valued and have the same civil rights as everyone else. It provides information, campaigns and research.

Scottish Intercollegiate Guidelines Network (SIGN) (www.sign.ac.uk)
SIGN aims to improve the quality of health care for patients in Scotland by reducing variation in practice and outcome, through the development and dissemination of national clinical guidelines containing recommendations for effective practice, based on current evidence.

Shoulderdoc (www.shoulderdoc.co.uk)
An educational website for patients and health care professionals covering common shoulder conditions and some elbow problems.

Society for Back Pain Research (www.sbpr.info)
The Society for Back Pain Research promotes the study of all clinical and scientific aspects of spinal pain, including the neck, and to encourage research into its causes, treatment and prevention.

Spinal Injuries Association (www.spinal.co.uk)
The Spinal Injuries Association (SIA) is the leading national charity for spinal cord injured people. It aims are to offer support, services, information for people with spinal injury throughout their lives and campaigns actively on their behalf

Steps (www.steps-charity.org.uk)
Steps is a charity that aims to drive forwards the provision of quality support and information to empower everyone affected by lower limb conditions.

Trauma Audit and Research Network (TARN) (www.tarn.ac.uk)
A network for providing accurate and relevant information for health care professionals to facilitate effective care for injured patients.

Trauma.org (Care of the injured) (www.trauma.org/)
Trauma.org is an independent, non-profit organisation providing global education, information and communication resources for professionals in trauma and critical care.

United Brachial Plexus Lesion Network (www.ubpn.org)
The United Brachial Plexus Network (UBPN) is an organisation devoted to providing information, support and leadership for families and those concerned with brachial plexus injuries worldwide.

United Kingdom Limb Loss Information Centre (www.limblossinformationcentre.com)
The UK Limb Loss Information Centre is an offshoot of the Douglas Bader Foundation created to guide individuals with congenital or acquired limb loss and their friends, family and carers through the emotional, physical and psychological process of coming to terms with limb loss.

World Orthopaedic Concern UK (www.wocuk.org/)
World Orthopaedic Concern aims to improve the standard of orthopaedic, trauma and reconstructive surgery in developing countries through education and training of surgeons, medical students, paramedical personnel and technicians.

WorldOrtho (www.worldortho.com)
WorldOrtho is an interactive website, created and maintained by the Department of Orthopaedic Surgery at Nepean Hospital, Sydney, Australia. Regularly updated, it provides a comprehensive database of educational, research and patient care information on orthopaedics, trauma and sports medicine.

Index

Printed and bound in the UK by
CPI Antony Rowe, Eastbourne